CLINICAL EPIDEMIOLOGY
HOW TO DO CLINICAL
PRACTICE RESEARCH

CLINICAL EPIDEMIOLOGY
HOW TO DO CLINICAL
PRACTICE RESEARCH

Third Edition

R. Brian Haynes, MD, PhD, FRCPC, FACP, FACMI
Professor of Clinical Epidemiology and Medicine
Michael G. DeGroote School of Medicine
Faculty of Health Sciences
McMaster University
Hamilton, Ontario, Canada

David L. Sackett, OC, MD, FRSC, FRCP (Canada, London, Edinburgh)
Director, Kilgore S. Trout Research & Education Centre
   at Irish Lake, Canada

Gordon H. Guyatt, MD, MSc, FRCPC, FACP, FACCP
Professor of Clinical Epidemiology and Medicine
Michael G. DeGroote School of Medicine
Faculty of Health Sciences
McMaster University
Hamilton, Ontario, Canada

Peter Tugwell, MD, MSc, FRCPC
Professor of Medicine, and Epidemiology and Community Medicine
University of Ottawa
Ottawa, Ontario, Canada

LIPPINCOTT WILLIAMS & WILKINS
A **Wolters Kluwer** Company

Philadelphia • Baltimore • New York • London
Buenos Aires • Hong Kong • Sydney • Tokyo

Acquisitions Editor: Sonya Seigafuse
Managing Editor: Kerry Barrett
Project Manager: Nicole Walz
Senior Manufacturing Manager: Ben Rivera
Senior Marketing Manager: Kathy Neely
Creative Director: Doug Smock
Cover Designer: Louis Fuiano
Production Services: Laserwords Private Limited
Printer: Edwards Brothers

3rd Edition

Clinical epidemiology: how to do clinical practice research / R. Brian Haynes ... [et al.].– 3rd ed.
   p. ; cm.
   Includes bibliographical references.
   ISBN-13: 978-0-7817-4524-6
   ISBN-10: 0-7817-4524-1
   1. Clinical epidemiology. 2. Medicine–Research–Epidemiology. I. Haynes, R. Brian.
[DNLM: 1. Biomedical Research–methods. 2. Epidemiologic Methods. 3. Research Design.
WA 950 C6413 2005]
RA652.C45 2005
614.4–dc22
                                                    2005008293

Care has been taken to confirm the accuracy of the information presented and to describe generally accepted practices. However, the authors, editors, and publisher are not responsible for errors or omissions or for any consequences from application of the information in this book and make no warranty, expressed or implied, with respect to the currency, completeness, or accuracy of the contents of the publication. Application of this information in a particular situation remains the professional responsibility of the practitioner.

The authors, editors, and publisher have exerted every effort to ensure that drug selection and dosage set forth in this text are in accordance with current recommendations and practice at the time of publication. However, in view of ongoing research, changes in government regulations, and the constant flow of information relating to drug therapy and drug reactions, the reader is urged to check the package insert for each drug for any change in indications and dosage and for added warnings and precautions. This is particularly important when the recommended agent is a new or infrequently employed drug.

Some drugs and medical devices presented in this publication have Food and Drug Administration (FDA) clearance for limited use in restricted research settings. It is the responsibility of health care providers to ascertain the FDA status of each drug or device planned for use in their clinical practice.

The publishers have made every effort to trace copyright holders for borrowed material. If they have inadvertently overlooked any, they will be pleased to make the necessary arrangements at the first opportunity.

To purchase additional copies of this book, call our customer service department at (800) 638-3030 or fax orders to (301) 824-7390. International customers should call (301) 714-2324. Lippincott Williams & Wilkins customer service representatives are available from 8:30 am to 6:30 pm, EST, Monday through Friday, for telephone access. Visit Lippincott Williams & Wilkins on the Internet: *http://www.lww.com*.

10 9 8 7 6 5 4 3

To JoAnne, Graeme, and Lindsay for love
and astonishing forbearance
—Brian Haynes

Go raibh míle maith agat, Barbara
—Dave Sackett

To the wonderful women who sustain all my
efforts, Maureen, Robyn, Paige, and Claire
—Gordon Guyatt

To Jane, David, and Laura for their love and
support throughout my work and personal
travails
—Peter Tugwell

CONTENTS

PREFACE

This book is about the methods for health care research. We've written *Clinical Epidemiology: How to Do Clinical Practice Research* for investigators at any stage of their careers, from beginning students to seasoned investigators. It is about how to do clinical-practice research, including some aspects of interventional health services research. In other words, it is about how to find answers to questions about such matters as the prevention and treatment, diagnosis, prognosis, and cause of health care problems; the measurement of health status and quality of life; and the effect of innovations in health services.

This book isn't about biostatistics. We've pitched the mathematical–statistical level at that of a smart person who has passed high school algebra. We've done this for two reasons. First, we think that the major methodological challenges in clinical-practice research have to do with preventing bias, not with performing statistical analyses. Second, we think it's vital to work with a statistician co-investigator rather than try to master and apply modern statistical techniques yourself (unless you are already a statistician!). For biostatisticians who might otherwise find this book useful, we apologize in advance for any oversimplified statistical bits.

WHY THIS BOOK?

This question has several answers. The simple one is that we enjoy what we do as clinical researchers and take pleasure in teaching what we do to anyone who is interested.

A more complex answer is that we are trying to fill the gap between superficial cookbooks and the "counsels of perfection" that tell readers what they must do to achieve methodological purity. The former neglect key issues at the clinical–methodological interface, and the latter fail to elucidate the rough-and-tumble practicalities of doing clinical-practice research. We propose to take you behind the pretty protocols and fastidious final reports to convey the often wrenching, sometimes comical, and usually manageable challenges that you will confront as you design, conduct, analyze, and interpret clinical-practice research. Along the way, we'll expose some of the politics of doing research, several ridiculous situations we got into and learned how to get out of, regrets we've had, and research projects that turned out better than we had any right to expect. It is the lessons we learned in getting into and out of these methodological pickles that distinguishes this book from the research methods book that was to have accompanied the first edition of this one.

Finally, the four of us delight in the fun and learning of joint-authorship. Our publisher's plea for a third edition spanned the period in which the practice of clinical epidemiology evolved into evidence-based medicine (EBM), and different combinations of us authored different texts in that new discipline.[1,2] The need for a practical book on how to generate the "E" for "EBM" gave us a chance to get back together, and we gleefully seized that opportunity.

An underlying theme in this book is that doing clinical-practice research is like shooting the rapids in a canoe. If you want to stay afloat without damaging your canoe, you need to learn how to anticipate trouble, to change your course in an instant when necessary, and to keep your sights on your ultimate goal, without worrying too much about pure paddle strokes or staying dry. To do this you'll need a deeper and more practical understanding of research methods than you can get by memorizing a printed page. You'll need to learn how to preserve the original intent of your investigation when confronted by barriers that preclude conducting your investigation precisely as you planned it. Better still, by working alongside us as we learned our lessons, you can design studies that will be less likely to stray into troubled waters in the first place, and less likely to capsize when they do.

To help you learn this blending of the science and art of research, we invite you to accompany us through the planning and execution of our own studies. Some of them happened when we were just beginning to learn how to paddle our own canoes; others are currently being planned (and teaching us some new strokes!). We'll provide scenarios describing the clinical stimulus and circumstances that led us to generate the questions we asked, show you what we planned to do, describe what happened, tell you how we coped with problems that arose, and admit what we would have done differently if we had a chance to do it all over again. We are the first to acknowledge that this won't substitute for you getting your own paddle in the water on your own projects. Nonetheless, we're convinced that joining us will provide you with a practical approach to designing and carrying out your own projects that you can't get from studying research methods in isolation, or from reading the fancified (and often fanciful) accounts of other people's research.

WHO ARE WE?

We are clinical epidemiologists, those odd folks with one foot in clinical care and the other in clinical-practice research. As clinical epidemiologists, we apply a wide array of scientific principles, strategies, and tactics to answer questions about health and health care, especially the latter. The principles we use are drawn most often from the discipline of epidemiology—but we purloin research principles from, and collaborate with, colleagues from

---

[1]Sackett DL, Straus S, Richardson SR, Rosenberg W, Haynes RB. *Evidence-based medicine: How to practice and teach EBM*, 2nd edition. London: Churchill Livingstone, 2000.

[2]Guyatt GH, Rennie D (eds). *Users' guides to the medical literature: A manual for evidence-based clinical practice*. Chicago: AMA Press. 2002.

any methodologically oriented, scientifically based, discipline—statistics, psychology, the social sciences, economics, health policy, health informatics, and beyond.

We'll introduce ourselves:

Brian Haynes
(http://www.fhs.mcmaster.ca/ceb/who/faculty/haynes.htm)

I am an internist, mainly interested in diabetes care, and a clinical epidemiologist. My main research interests at present are in "knowledge translation research" (KT research). This term is quite new, covering a spectrum of investigations aimed at enhancing the application of research knowledge, reducing the gap between what we (now) know about how to prevent and manage illness and the care that people with potential and real health problems receive. Before KT research became a popular term, my research was in finding ways to help patients follow prescribed treatments (patient adherence); developing and testing ways to help health practitioners do the right thing at the right time (clinical quality improvement); developing methods for improving the retrieval, grading, organization, dissemination, and uptake of current best evidence (health informatics); and testing health care interventions (clinical trials). I've enjoyed and enormously benefited from engaging in research in a highly collegial environment and highly endorse seeking or creating such a setting for anyone interested in a happy and productive academic career.

Dave Sackett

Twice a resident in internal medicine (1961–66 and 1983–85), I practiced for 38 years as a "hospitalist" in the United States, Canada, and England. Asked to found the clinical epidemiology department at McMaster, I had the meager sense and massive luck to surround myself with brilliant methodologists and students (including the co-authors of this book), all of who continue to try their damndest to teach me how to be a better clinical-practice researcher, teacher, writer, and mentor. In the twilight of my career, I confine my academic attention to clinical trials of anything that moves (and some stuff that doesn't), and to helping young investigators (including especially nearly a hundred "Trout Fellows") design and do the clinical-practice research that patients want done.

Gordon Guyatt
(http://www.fhs.mcmaster.ca/ceb/who/faculty/guyatt.htm)

I function clinically as a hospitalist, academically as an applied health care researcher, and politically as an activist and health journalist. My research has little focus; I follow the questions that happen to grab my interest and the opportunities that an extremely kind fortune has laid in my path—particularly the brilliant ideas and luminous energy of the young investigators with whom I work. I have contributed to clinical trials methodology, quality-of-life measurement, and guidelines methodology. This has come together in my most important academic role, that of an evangelist for evidence-based medical practice. That is still perhaps less important than my work in advocating for a society guided by social solidarity, and reflected in equitable access to high-quality health care.

Peter Tugwell
(http://www.ohri.ca/profiles/tugwell_summ.asp)

I am an internist with a special interest in rheumatology, and a clinical epidemiologist. My research has been split between a focus on musculoskeletal disorders and methods development. Initially my focus was on clinical trials and outcomes but that spread to causation through the opportunity to participate in the first science panel commissioned by the US Federal Justice System to establish an evidentiary base that can be used for class action suits—in this case for the putative causative association between silicone breast implants and connective tissue diseases. I have had the pleasure of being actively involved in the formal training and subsequent mentoring of many clinical epidemiologists both in Canada and from many other countries. This has led to my most recent career shift into the application of clinical epidemiology methods to reducing health disparities through better dissemination and use of evidence by patients, policymakers, practitioners, the press, the private sector, and the general public. In addition, my initial two years of experience as Americas Editor of the Journal of Clinical Epidemiology has impressed me with the pace of innovation in clinical epidemiology methods.

WHAT TYPES OF QUESTIONS DO WE ADDRESS?

We believe that bridging research and clinical practice, by being qualified and maintaining competence in both, has important advantages for the inspiration, relevance, and feasibility of the projects we undertake. Many of the best questions we have pursued come from our interactions (and failures!) with patients at the bedside and in the clinic, coupled with our understanding of what constitutes a researchable question. But we make no claim that trying to be competent in both research and clinical practice is either necessary or sufficient for conducting applied clinical research. Indeed, "big league" clinical research these days is very much a team sport, requiring people with many types of skills, including experts in research design, measurement, statistics, the clinical problem of interest, and, increasingly, the social sciences.

We are intent on using sound research principles, tempered with practicality, to find the best answers to "real world" questions about clinical practice and health care. These key questions have to do with

- how to screen for and diagnose disease and risk factors for disease;
- how to prevent, treat, ameliorate, or rehabilitate health problems;

- how to predict the course of disease;
- how to determine the cause of health problems;
- how to measure "burden of illness," "quality of life," and the effects of health services innovations;
- how to systematically summarize evidence from research;
- how to increase the quality of health care and improve its outcomes.

Each of these broad questions contains an array of finer questions. For example, questions about a health care intervention include examining whether such intervention does more good than harm under relatively ideal circumstances (*efficacy*: can it work?); whether it works under "real world" conditions (*effectiveness*: does it work?); whether it is good value for money and other resources (*cost-effectiveness*: is it worth it?); and how to transfer sound research findings about an intervention into effective care for individuals and communities (*translation*: is it translatable?). Similarly, additional questions about diagnostic tests include how many people a test labels correctly (*accuracy*), what proportion of people are labeled correctly as having a disorder when they do (*sensitivity*), what proportion of people are labeled correctly as not having a disorder when they don't (*specificity*), and what are the consequences of diagnostic errors of both types. And so on.

DON'T READ THIS BOOK LIKE A NOVEL!

Although there is some cross-linking, individual Chapters 1 to 11 at the beginning of the book both target specific types of research questions and provide stand-alone answers. Thus, if you've done some clinical trials and are motivated to do your first diagnostic test study, Chapter 8, Evaluating Diagnostic Tests, is the place to start (unless your trials haven't gone so well, in which case you might want to back up to the beginning!).

Chapters at the end of the book go into some universal issues you'll need to consider in surviving and thriving as a clinical-practice researcher, including organizing your time, getting grants, putting ethical principles into action, writing papers, analyzing data, and so on.

A WORD ABOUT PERSONAL PRONOUNS AND "PRIVATE" STORIES

When we began writing this book, we discussed how we would address you, the reader, when describing our work and views. We decided that we would use "we" and "us" and "our" when we mean the lot of us or when we mean you and us together; "I" and "me" and "mine" when one of us is describing work and thoughts that belong more or less uniquely to one of us (thus, the lead author of each chapter is identified); "you" when we would like you to try something yourself (and sometimes when we're just being preachy...); and "they" when talking about other people's research or principles. Our intention in using "I" is to be clear when we express our personal opinions. (Surprise! There isn't universal agreement on research tactics.) We'll switch to "we" when we want to change the perspective to tactics we all agree on or when describing activities we have done together or with others.

Play (with) Our CD

We've provided a searchable CD of the book for those of you who enjoy electronic access, or prefer lugging portable computers rather than books.

Visit Our Web Site

We invite you to visit our book's Web site at *http://hiru.mcmaster.ca/ CLEP3*. There, you will be able to let us know what you think of the book, ask questions, suggest corrections or improvements, find chapter updates, and learn how we and others are using the book in teaching clinical practice research. All welcome!

Brian Haynes
Dave Sackett
Gordon Guyatt
Peter Tugwell

ACKNOWLEDGMENTS

Many people offered comments and suggestions for improving the book as it moved through its various stages of evolution, and a few people helped a lot. We are grateful for all their contributions and acknowledge them according to the roles they played or chapters they commented on:

Editing, artwork (including the book's cover), organizing, and seeking permissions: Lindsay Haynes

Chapter 2: Sohail Bajammal, Debika Burman, Jeff Eng, Michelle Kho, Mark Morreale, Xiaomei Yao

Chapter 3: Karin Kallender, Jessie McGowan, Joan Peterson, George Wells,

Chapters 4–6: Neill Adhikari, Doug Altman, Warren Cantor, Iain Chalmers, Mike Clarke, Charlie Dunnett, Donald Eby, Mike Gent, David Grimes, Manoj Kumar, Michel Lievre, Joy MacDermid, Victor Montori, Heather Murray, Graham Nichol, Moacyr Nobre, Andrew Oxman, Stefan Sauerland, Ken Schulz, William Tarnow-Mordi, Ross Upshur, Andrew Vickers, and Danny Whelan

Chapter 7: Sohail Bajammal, Charlie Goldsmith

Chapter 8: Sohail Bajammal

Chapter 9: Heiner Bucher, Scott Richardson, Andreas Laupacis, Stephen Walter, Roman Jaeschke, Deborah Cook, George Wells, and, most notably, Adrienne Randolph and Tom McGinn.

Chapter 10: Jessie McGowan, Joan Peterson, George Wells

Chapter 11: Maarten Boers, Joan Peterson, George Wells

Chapter 17: Nancy Wilczynski

Performing Clinical Research

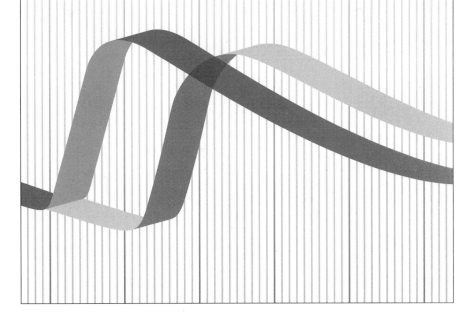

1

FORMING RESEARCH QUESTIONS

Brian Haynes

Just in case you didn't read the Preface, we'll quickly review the *modus operandi* of the approach that we'll take through the first 11 chapters of *Clinical Epidemiology*. Each of these initial chapters begins with a clinical research scenario that provides a behind-the-scenes look at our own research. We've taken this approach in part to elucidate, illustrate, and titillate, but mostly to keep this as an unvarnished account of real research rather than a theoretically pristine but unattainable counsel of perfection.

Each of the longer chapters also begins with a chapter outline to help you to jump in wherever you like. Here's the one for this chapter.

Chapter Outline

1.1   Where do researchable questions come from?
1.2   Key considerations in developing a study question
1.3   Composing the final prestudy question
1.4   Composing secondary questions
1.5   Dealing with contingencies

CLINICAL RESEARCH SCENARIO[1]

Observational studies of various sorts during the first half of the 20th century had established a relation between cerebrovascular strokes in the anterior part of the brain and narrowing of the carotid arteries in the neck and within the skull. This led to the invention of two surgical procedures. The first, carotid endarterectomy (CE), was introduced in 1954 to remove obstructions in the carotid artery as it passes from the aorta through the neck to the anterior brain. The second, extracranial–intracranial arterial bypass (EC/IC bypass), was developed in the late 1960s for individuals who had partial obstruction in the part of the

---

[1]As in other chapters, the text in shaded areas is about investigations we have conducted. The descriptions of these studies are interwoven with the appropriate sections on research methods.

carotid artery protected by the skull. Because CE cannot be performed in this part of the artery, the EC/IC bypass procedure "bypasses" the obstruction by freeing a branch of the superficial temporal artery (STA) on the outside of the skull then creating a hole in the skull over a branch of the middle cerebral artery (MCA), and then joining the STA to the MCA using microsurgical techniques that include an operating microscope and sutures that are invisible to the human eye. By the late 1970s, neither of these procedures had been tested in a well-conducted randomized controlled trial (RCT), although there had been an inconclusive trial of CE (in which surgical calamities were excluded from the analysis—a study in how *not* to analyze a clinical trial!) (1), and a second study was abandoned because of a 35% perioperative stroke and death rate among the first 43 patients admitted to the study (2).

In the late 1970s, a group led by Henry Barnett, a neurologist at the University of Western Ontario (UWO); David Sackett, a clinical epidemiologist at McMaster University; and Skip Peerless, a neurosurgeon at UWO, set about the task of evaluating surgical interventions intended to prevent strokes in the areas of the brain fed by the carotid artery. The key target at first was the surgical procedure that was by then relatively entrenched, CE. Testing the waters with surgeons who performed this procedure, and whose cooperation would be essential, it proved difficult to arouse enthusiasm for evaluating the procedure.

The target then shifted to the newer surgical approach, EC/IC bypass. This elegant procedure had been developed in Switzerland by Yasargil (3), brought to Canada by Peerless, and spread during the next 10 years to many countries. It was technically feasible, with high rates of bypass patency, but was very expensive, requiring both high surgical expertise and sophisticated equipment. Most surgical teams able to perform EC/IC bypass were in university centers, whereas CE had disseminated widely into the community hospitals as well. Although there were many case reports and case series attesting to the merits of EC/IC bypass, none of these compared it with medical treatment alone. This time it proved possible to recruit enough interested neurosurgeons and neurologists to form a study team. I was just completing my clinical training in internal medicine at the time, having previously completed my research training under Dave Sackett. My role in this process was to help develop the background literature review and the justification, including sample size considerations, a proposal for the study question, and a preliminary outline for the study design. Heady stuff for a young squirt anticipating an academic appointment the following year!

An RCT of EC/IC bypass was conducted, beginning in 1978 and reported in 1985 (4). The study showed no benefit for surgery; in fact, evaluation of the functional status of patients showed that the surgery delayed natural recovery from stroke for up to 1 year (5). With this result, skepticism began to grow about whether CE was any more respectable than its downstream cousin, EC/IC bypass. The conditions had now become more favorable for testing CE–under certain conditions. Many surgeons remained opposed to testing CE, and those who were potentially willing to participate in such a trial wanted to ensure that the procedure was given a fair chance to succeed. To them, this meant that only surgeons with a "good track record" for CE would be included in the study, that the obstruction in the carotid artery would be severe enough that patients would be likely to benefit from its removal (although many surgeons were offering the procedure for lesser degrees of narrowing), and that the patients themselves would be healthy enough to undergo surgery and live long enough thereafter for a benefit from surgery to be observed.

1.1 WHERE DO RESEARCHABLE QUESTIONS COME FROM?

Eugene Ionesco, the father of the "theater of the absurd," once said, "It is not the answer which enlightens, but the question." This certainly applies to health care research–new knowledge originates from having asked answerable questions. To find new and useful answers to important problems that have not already been resolved, you need to know a lot about the problem and precisely where the boundary between current knowledge and ignorance lies. Without knowing a lot about the problem, it is difficult to imagine that plausible diagnostic tests and interventions will be developed. Without knowing the current state of knowledge, it is difficult to know whether one is headed in the right "next-step" direction. Thus, the first answer to the question introducing this section is that researchable questions come from finding the "cutting edge" of knowledge for a health problem with which you are familiar. This is not as demanding a condition for applied health research as it can be for basic science because good applied research usually builds on basic research. Indeed, it has been said that in applied research, the questions are easy but getting the answers is hard. This may be true–but composing important questions that can be answered validly by current applied research methods is still a considerable challenge.

1.2 KEY CONSIDERATIONS IN DEVELOPING A STUDY QUESTION

As the clinical research scenario at the beginning of this chapter illustrates, many factors contribute to the formulation of a study question. Further, particularly in applied research, developing a question is an iterative process, not a "light bulb" phenomenon. To be sure, the light bulb must come on, but there is much work to be done both before the light will shine and afterwards. The iterative components include, to name a few, the basic dimensions of the clinical problem, the plausibility and feasibility of the design, the colleagues you will work with, the other resources you can muster to address the question, and the contingencies that emerge as you conduct the trial. The main interplay will be between what you would really like to do and what is really possible to do. This is anything but a linear process, but we'll have to present it as such, given the nature of the printed word—forewarned is forearmed—don't stick to the sequence discussed in subsequent text if your question could benefit from a different sequence. But the principles illustrated in the following sections will usually apply during the course of developing a study question, even if the sequence differs.

Basic Dimensions

The basic dimensions of a problem that lead to the formulation of important research questions include understanding the biology and physiology of the problem, its epidemiology (i.e., determinants and distribution, prevalence, incidence, and prognosis), and frustrations in its clinical management that lead to unsatisfactory results for patients. For example, for strokes, the association of anterior brain infarcts with atherothrombotic narrowing of the carotid arteries fits with the biology of the small clots often found at these narrowings, which can break off and impact in the smaller arteries of the brain, causing a stroke. The occurrence of strokes also fits with the physiology of impairment of blood flow that occurs when the narrowing exceeds 75% of the normal luminal diameter of the carotid artery in the neck. The fact that biology and physiology do not provide an adequate basis for how to deal with the problem is evident from the results of the EC/IC bypass study. Indeed, in this trial, patients with the best surgical results, in terms of increased blood flow to the brain, fared worst for prevention of stroke.

As for the epidemiology, we know that stroke is one of the leading causes of death and major disability and that the risk of recurrence after a minor stroke is considerable, at about 10% in the first year and then about 5% per annum thereafter (6). No one who deals with stroke victims can escape the conclusion that strokes would be better prevented than treated, if a safe and affordable preventive intervention is available, because the damage caused by a completed stroke is irreversible in the brain and the loss of function strokes incur is often unrecoverable. Case series and hospital surveys have documented that both EC/IC bypass and CE procedures can be performed with a lower perioperative morbidity and mortality than the observed rates of events mentioned earlier, although some studies of the quality of care for CE showed that perioperative rates of morbidity and mortality were higher than the risk of stroke recurrence in some hospitals, especially in community hospitals with low volumes of cases. Further, in the time frames of the EC/IC bypass and CE trials, these interventions were based on biology, physiology, and anecdotal experience, and they had not been tested in large randomized trials. Thus, the basic elements were in place for an initial study question for this trial along the lines of "Does CE do more good than harm in preventing stroke recurrence in patients with carotid circulation strokes?"

Advanced Considerations

Once these basic issues have been addressed, and an initial direction for a question seems promising, some additional key questions must be addressed.

Key questions checklist:

✓ What is the appropriate stage for evaluation?
✓ Can internal validity be achieved?
✓ To what extent is external validity (generalizability) achievable?
✓ What will your circumstances permit?
✓ What can you afford?
✓ What is the best balance between "idea" and "feasibility"?

✓ *What is the appropriate stage for evaluation?*

The suitable stage of evaluation depends mainly on what previous assessments have been made for the question you are most interested in. Most research is incremental, and deliberately so. The less assessment that has been done, the more one can and should consider a less definitive and much less expensive research design (right—it's about the bottom line).

Most diagnostic tests and treatments, particularly those in current use but incompletely assessed, are evaluated along a spectrum stretching from the explanatory end (can it work under ideal circumstances?) to the management end (does it work under usual clinical circumstances?). We'll return to these concepts in subsequent chapters. Studies for which scientific measures are taken to minimize bias will be somewhere in the middle of this spectrum, but will most often be toward the explanatory end because of the high cost of management studies. No study could be on the extreme of the explanatory end because circumstances of testing are never ideal. Indeed, even if they could be "ideal," this would differ from the "real world" so much that it would render the results of the study practically meaningless. On the management end, it is not possible or ethical to scientifically and unobtrusively evaluate treatments and tests without introducing so much risk of bias that the results are undependable. This is, admittedly, a matter of debate, with advocates of outcomes research and observational studies claiming that the results of RCTs can be reproducibly achieved in careful observational studies that are based, for example, on medical records. In our view, the degree of reproducibility in observational studies is unacceptable, and a careful RCT will be substantively better than an observational study at finding the truth. We'll take this up again in Chapters 4 to 6, on clinical trials.

Studies of causation, prognosis, and clinical prediction should also be staged according to the quality of preceding evidence, using the best study design that you can afford that goes beyond what has been done to date.

✓ Can internal validity be achieved?

Internal validity depends on both study design features ("methods") and on feasibility. Most of the study designs in this book are relatively straightforward, and we will deal with issues of validity from a methodological perspective throughout the book. Problems with feasibility, however, often stand in the way of success in implementing them. One such problem may be measurement. The basic principle of measurement was espoused by Lord Kelvin long ago (1883 to be exact): "... when you cannot measure it, when you cannot express it in numbers, your knowledge is of a meager and unsatisfactory kind." Crudely put, if you can't measure it, you can't study it. For example, researchers interested in studying emerging diseases such as severe acute respiratory syndrome or West Nile virus infection first needed to come up with a test or at least a "case definition" before their research could proceed.

A second problem can be follow-up. It is difficult (but not impossible) to do follow-up studies of individuals with addictions or of those who are homeless. One can restrict entry to those individuals who are willing and able to be followed, but this may fundamentally alter the question that is posed because those who will enter may act differently from those who refuse.

Studies based on medical problems that are rare also pose a special challenge: it may require a national or international effort to assemble enough patients. Especially when you are starting out as a researcher, this type of question might be left to someone else or to later years.

✓ To what extent is external validity (generalizability) achievable?

External validity refers to the ability to generalize the results of a study to other settings and patients, whereas internal validity refers to the soundness of the study to answer the exact question that it posed among the participants who began the investigation. A study that is internally invalid should not be undertaken (Period! Full stop!). In contrast, a study with limited external validity may be well justified if it represents a step forward in testing an idea at a reasonable price. Nevertheless, a question that includes a broad spectrum of patients that is similar to the range of presentations one sees in clinical practice has more appeal from a practical perspective than one that doesn't. The extent to which external validity can be achieved usually comes down to, you guessed it, money: explanatory studies ("ideal circumstances") generally cost less than management studies ("usual circumstances"). The choices and their trade-offs will be described in several chapters, as we go along. The general rule is don't sacrifice internal validity for generalizability— but pose a question that is as generalizable as you can afford.

✓ What will your circumstances permit?

Allowing for the desirability of having our reach exceed our grasp, the natural tendency of us all to "ask the big question" should be tempered by who we are and what circumstances we find ourselves in. The big question of whether CE does more good than harm is too challenging for anyone to tackle, let alone for someone who is just starting out. For example, CE can be and is offered to patients with asymptomatic narrowing of the carotid artery and for all degrees of stenosis. Attempting to answer the question for all indications would be exceedingly difficult. For our CE study, the prevailing clinical conditions meant limiting the question to symptomatic patients for whom surgeons and neurologists felt the procedure was likely to be beneficial, with surgery being done by operators with a record of low perioperative complication rate. As for who would be allowed to conduct the trial, it was very interesting as the junior on the team to see the "politics" of science play out, with the credentials of the senior neurologist, neurosurgeon, and methodologist being on the line before surgeons who were of mixed mind about whether CE "worked" but of a single mind that it was essential to sorting this out that these senior investigators be completely credible and trustworthy.

For CE, the matter of "uncertainty" evolved in a particularly interesting way. The EC/IC study cast enough uncertainty on the biologic-physiologic hypothesis for CE that it became possible to discuss the testing of CE with many surgeons. At one such meeting, Henry Barnett asked exactly the right questions: "Based on the evidence to date, how many of you believe that carotid endarterectomy does more good than harm for patients with stroke and carotid stenosis? And how many of you believe that it doesn't?" To the amazement of many (including me), the number of hands that went up was about equal for each question, providing sufficient basis for most believers of both persuasions to join forces to settle the matter once and for all. The circumstances were ripe.

✓ What can you afford?

If you decide to pursue an investigation, the next consideration is what you can afford. Key aspects of cost include the time to complete the study, the amount of effort required in relation to the expected benefit, the enthusiasm for this effort, and the availability of funds. For time, the longer the study will take, the more important the question needs to be, and the less likely it needs to be that someone else is going to "scoop" you by being in the field ahead of you. Investigations involving large numbers (i.e., of years, investigators, patients, research and support staff) generally cost lots of money. Funding agencies and their peer reviewers are generally averse to awarding lots of money—but if a good match exists between their interests and the importance and timeliness of the question you wish to pursue, and if you have a sound plan to answer the question and the resources (i.e., investigators, patients, and commitment) and reputation to do so, then large budgets are at least conceivable. Having said that, if you will need a lot of funds for the question you are posing, it is best for first projects either to be part of a team that is already successful (as was the case for me in the EC/IC study) or to start small, in the form of either a preliminary study to address issues of feasibility for a larger trial or a study that addresses an interesting question (that is not necessarily of earth-shattering importance). In other words, take a small step forward rather than a leap.

Some of the studies that we will display for you in this book, including the CE trial in this chapter, address relatively big questions, but some are quite small. An example of the latter is in Chapter 2 on conducting systematic reviews. Systematic reviews are research studies in themselves and are best done with a protocol that begins with a clear, answerable question and with methods for finding and reviewing articles, minimizing bias, and summarizing and analyzing results. One of the most rigorous ways of conducting such reviews is to prepare such a protocol and to submit it to a funding agency for peer review and funding. Although many systematic reviews are done by voluntary labor, the range of external funding for reviews is as much as $500,000. No small change! And the real reward from this activity is that it helps define exactly what questions have not yet been answered, setting the stage for next-step original investigations. This is worth considering before doing "first original studies" and, in fact, all major investigations.

✓ What is the best balance between "idea" and "feasibility"?

For the CE study, it was believed (but not known at the time) that the degree of carotid stenosis would affect both the risk for stroke and the benefit from surgery. To capture this potentially high-risk, high-response group, the study was set up as two separate trials, one for patients with high-grade stenosis (70%–99%) and one for patients with moderate-grade stenosis (30%–69%). Sample sizes were estimated on the basis of a 7% annual event rate for patients with high-grade stenosis and a 4% rate for those with lower-grade stenosis. This estimation assured those who felt strongly that stenosis was correlated with event rates that an early result could be achieved for patients with higher degrees of stenosis and that their results would not be "diluted" by the anticipated larger numbers of patients with lower degrees of stenosis. Further, statistical rules were developed for monitoring the accumulating results so that either of these trials could be stopped early if the results—either better or worse than estimated—warranted. This approach proved not only "politic" but also propitious. Indeed, the risk and the responsiveness for the high-grade group were both underestimated, leading to stopping the trial with a positive result when patients had been in the trial for an average of just 18 months of a planned 60-month trial. These results were quickly conveyed to participating investigators and their patients so that they could be taken into account for subsequent care decisions. For patients in the moderate-grade stenosis group, the trial was continued for its planned duration, and a positive, but less beneficial result was observed.

Formulating a question that strikes a justifiable balance between the idea(s) for your study and the feasibility of answering them is important for success. Early on in the course of testing, this can mean focusing on just those patients who have high risk for adverse outcomes of their condition and who are likely to be highly responsive to the intervention. This restriction clearly limits the number of individuals to whom the results may apply, but if it is relatively easy to find patients who have both of these characteristics, it greatly reduces the cost of initial testing. Chapter 6 will provide more details about this strategy and the trade-offs it involves.

1.3 COMPOSING THE FINAL PRESTUDY QUESTION

The CE trial study question, as stated by the steering committee (7), was: "The study will determine if carotid endarterectomy is beneficial to patients with carotid stenosis and transient cerebral ischemia or partial stroke by comparing patients randomly assigned to receive carotid endarterectomy in addition to best medical care with those assigned to receive best medical care alone. The study is addressing the following specific questions: (a) Does carotid endarterectomy reduce the risk of subsequent stroke and stroke-related death? (b) Does the degree of carotid stenosis identify patients who will benefit most from carotid endarterectomy? and (c) Will carotid endarterectomy maintain or improve the functional status of patients over time?"

This statement of the study question (or related questions) contains four elements that we recommend that are captured in the acronym, *PICO*: *P*atients, *I*ntervention (for intervention studies only), *C*omparison group, and *O*utcomes. For good measure, and to avoid embarrassment in Chile,[2] one could add *T*ime (*PICOT*).

If you have been following the steps above in preparation for a study question of your own, you will have noticed that your question has changed several times. It's now time to compose the question in a way that will "take charge" and direct the investigation that ensues. This should be a touchstone that you can refer to at times when the study boat hits a log and starts to sink, so that you can plug the hole in a way that suits the purpose of the expedition.

How inclusive should you be in describing the study question? The CE question posed earlier in the text is quite general about all aspects of the study, and one could more completely describe just one of the two simultaneous CE studies as: "Among competent, consenting patients with recent transient ischemic attacks or partial strokes in the circulation of the carotid artery, and ipsilateral stenosis of 70% to 99%, as judged by expert central review of selective angiograms, who are receiving optimal medical care and do not have elevated surgical risk, does the addition of CE, by surgeons who have an established 30-day perioperative complication rate of less than 6% for persistent stroke or death, reduce the subsequent risk of major stroke and stroke death over a period of 5 years, compared with patients who receive optimal medical care but do not receive CE?" This question could then be iterated for the second study—less than 70% stenosis.

---

[2]As one of us discovered after emphasizing the importance of PICO to future researchers in a Catholic university in Chile, "pico" is a slang term for an expansible part of the male anatomy...

Ninety-nine–word questions are difficult to comprehend, so we don't recommend this much detail in the question itself, but it is important to bear these details in mind when conducting the study and reporting its results, so that the results will not be overgeneralized.

1.4 COMPOSING SECONDARY QUESTIONS

It will be obvious from the preceding section that the CE study had several questions. Several basic principles guide the development of additional primary and secondary questions for studies. First, all primary questions must be asked "up front," at the beginning of the investigation. The same is true, as far as possible, for all secondary questions. This approach ensures that the questions are "hypothesis-driven" (i.e., based on your predictions of what will happen) rather than "data-driven" [i.e., made up after the study results are (partly) in, especially to "explain" findings that may well be simply the play of chance]. This approach also allows for proper planning and data collection for these additional questions, including estimates of sample size to determine whether the study is large enough to support reliable answers. These efforts can pay off; it will be less costly to run a study where some of the questions can be answered by data collection from only a subset of patients and where questions for which there can be no chance of a clear result are discarded along with their burden of data collection.

Second, these "add-on" questions should never compromise the primary question. For example, obtrusively measuring the adherence of the patients to their prescribed medications in a management study would undermine the validity of such a study if this measurement is not an intended part of the intervention. As another example, adding greatly to the data collection for a study can compromise the willingness of investigators and patients to participate.

Third, additional questions should not be a large part of the budget because this risks not receiving funding for the major study question. If they do add significantly to the budget (as even some simple measures can), then the secondary questions should be clearly separated in the budget so that reviewers and funding agencies can lop them off if they are not convinced that they are worth the cost, even if the main study question is.

1.5 DEALING WITH CONTINGENCIES

The CE study was originally designed for four separate study groups delineated by the stenosis levels defined in the preceding text and by the presence or absence of ulcerated plaque in the area of the stenosis for each of these two grades of stenosis. It was estimated that 3,000 patients, distributed among the four study groups, would be needed to provide separate answers concerning the benefit of surgery for each level of stenosis and presence or absence of plaque. Early on in the course of the trial it was determined through central review of the reports from surgeons at the various study sites that the presence or absence of plaque could not be reliably determined. Thus, the question concerning plaque versus no plaque could not be answered (remember Lord Kelvin!). The sample size estimates were altered to fit the two remaining study cohorts, 600 for the high-grade stenosis group and 1,300 for the moderate-grade stenosis group.

During any trial, you can expect that contingencies will arise that require modification of the protocol and changes in the question that is addressed. Sometimes, as in the example from the CE trial, the contingency will be profound enough that a study question will have to be dropped—if this is the main study question, then the trial may have to be abandoned entirely. Fortunately for the CE trial, there was more than one question, and the early detection of problems in reporting plaque led to a timely reduction in the sample size required. One could easily point fingers and say that the trial should not have proceeded in the first place if this measurement issue had not been addressed, but that is a different matter!

Most of the contingencies that arise will not sink the study if you keep a close eye on the process of the study (e.g., are patients being recruited at the anticipated rate) and if adjustments are made that counter the problem without compromising the basic intent of the study. For example, in the CE trial, because of slow recruitment, the upper limit of 80 years for patient age was relaxed if the surgeon judged that the perioperative risk was acceptable. In any event, only patients who were mentally competent and gave their informed consent were included.

The leaks in the protocol that become apparent as the study enters the water, and those that occur once underway, need to be plugged. You can plug the low recruitment leak (a very common one!) by recruiting more investigators or by relaxing entry criteria, but these changes need to be recorded and their effect, if any, on the study question needs to be described in reports of the investigation. For example, during the CE trial, standards for care for hypertension, for cholesterol lowering, and for antiplatelet treatment changed because of new evidence. The latter, in particular, had the potential for lowering the risk of stroke, the major study outcome measure. In each instance when major new findings and recommendations came out, they had to be considered by the study's steering committee and a decision had to be made about incorporating them into the protocol in a way that preserved the integrity of the study, if possible—or not, if need be. Although none of these factors changed the course of the trial for CE, the CE study results led to one other major trial being aborted.

REFERENCES

1. Fields WS, Maslenikov V, Meyer JS, et al. Joint study of extracranial arterial occlusion. V. Progress report of prognosis following surgery or nonsurgical treatment for transient cerebral ischemic attacks and cervical carotid artery lesions. *JAMA* 1970;211:1993–2003.

2. Shaw DA, Venables GS, Cartlidge NE, et al. Carotid endarterectomy in patients with transient cerebral ischaemia. *J Neurol Sci* 1984;64:45–53.

3. Yasargil MG, ed. *Microsurgery applied to neurosurgery.* Stuttgart: Georg Thieme, 1969:105–115.

4. The EC/IC Bypass Study Group. Failure of extracranial-intracranial arterial bypass to reduce the risk of ischemic stroke: results of an international randomized trial. *N Engl J Med* 1985;313:1191–2000.

5. Haynes RB, Mukherjee J, Sackett DL, et al. Functional status changes following medical or surgical treatment for cerebral ischemia: results in the EC/IC Bypass Study. *JAMA* 1987;257:2043–2046.

6. Dennis MS, Burn JP, Sandercock PA, et al. Long-term survival after first-ever stroke: the Oxfordshire Community Stroke Project. *Stroke* 1993;24:796–800.

7. North American Symptomatic Carotid Endarterectomy Trial (NASCET) Steering Committee. North American Symptomatic Carotid Endarterectomy Trial: methods, patient characteristics, and progress. *Stroke* 1991;22:711–720.

2

CONDUCTING SYSTEMATIC REVIEWS

Brian Haynes

Chapter Outline

2.1 Why to do systematic reviews and how to get academic credit for doing them
2.2 Types of questions that can be addressed by systematic reviews
2.3 Basic principles of conducting a systematic review
2.4 How many systematic reviews should you do?

Appendices

2.1 Search strategies
2.2 Instructions for reviewing citations (e-mail note for our CDSS review)
2.3 Sample CDSS review data abstraction form

CLINICAL RESEARCH SCENARIO

The developers and manufacturers of computerized decision support systems (CDSSs) make many optimistic claims indicating that they support more rational, efficient, and effective decisions. The last term, "effective," is the same that we use to describe many medical interventions and asserts that the CDSS will do more good than harm or, at least, will help those who use it to improve patient care. Such claims are music to the ears of those involved in the delivery of health services, including investigators who are looking for ways to improve research dissemination and uptake: it would be terrific if CDSSs could capture, package, and promote the use of new knowledge in a way that is much more effective than the usual means of dissemination, such as journal articles, training, word of mouth, and industry representatives.

Unlike licensed medicines, however, there is no legislated requirement for evidence of efficacy in randomized controlled trials (RCTs) before CDSSs can be marketed. Therefore, trials of CDSSs are voluntary and are bound to be limited in number and scope. In addition, because they are most often done by CDSS developers themselves, lack blinding (because of the obvious nature of the intervention), and encounter many other methodological challenges, CDSS trials are often viewed with even greater skepticism than are trials of new drugs or operations.

Dereck Hunt, a graduate student at the time, and I developed a CDSS to help with the care of patients with diabetes (1) (a story we'll return to in Chapter 7). We decided that we needed to test the CDSS in a proper RCT. To prepare for such a trial, we wanted to learn how often and how well other systems had been studied, what steps had been taken to deal with the obvious methodological issues that arise in such studies, and what their results could tell us about the effects of such systems. To realize these ambitions, we set about doing a systematic review (SR) of clinical trials of CDSSs, adding Amit Garg, Neill Adhikari, Heather McDonald, also graduate students, and others to the team. The key question we wanted to answer in the review was this: "In acute inpatient care, emergency rooms, and ambulatory care clinics, can CDSSs, when compared with care unassisted by CDSSs, improve the process and outcomes of patient care?"

2.1 WHY TO DO SYSTEMATIC REVIEWS AND HOW TO GET ACADEMIC CREDIT FOR DOING THEM

SRs are research projects in their own right—plain and simple. A research question for the review is posed up front, the "participants" are original published research reports (or sometimes SRs of them), rigorous search procedures are used to find all eligible reports, the reports are selected according to explicit criteria and are rated for quality, the findings of eligible reports are summarized and are often statistically combined, and anyone reading the review ought to be able to reach the same summary of findings, if not the same conclusions about their interpretation.

SRs are also the best way to begin any new primary-data research project because they establish what we already know and, more importantly, don't know. In recognition of this, the Medical Research Council in the United Kingdom requires a current SR as the foundation for requests for funds to conduct clinical trials. An SR defines the "cutting edge," helps you to define methods and justify the sample size for the new investigation, and shows grant review committees that you have done your "homework" in identifying the "frontier" for new research. *En passant*, you can use an SR at the beginning of a project to feed the Beast of Publish or Perish, providing the grist for the first publication to come from the project.

An SR paper in a peer review journal or in the Cochrane Library should also count academically as a research publication. Although some academic institutions and funding agencies discount SRs when they are considering a person's publications for purposes of promotion and tenure, most don't these days, especially when they see the luscious citation counts that a good review will generate. If your institution discounts SRs, we suggest three approaches. First, make sure you mix them with lots of original data publications: most promotion committees count publications rather than trying to rate their quality, but you must have some original data studies to win your spurs, so don't pin your career on SRs alone. Second, lobby your institution: SRs are scientific investigations that are essential to the efficient advancement of science and to clarification and communication of its important findings. Third, if all else fails and if your institution really does discriminate against SRs as worthy publications, don't include the term "review" or "meta-analysis" in your title: few appointment, promotion, and tenure committees have the time, resources, or inclination to look at the actual articles.

2.2 TYPES OF QUESTIONS THAT CAN BE ADDRESSED BY SYSTEMATIC REVIEWS

The typical SR is very narrow in scope—for example, addressing the effectiveness of a single health care intervention (e.g., aspirin) compared with a placebo or no treatment, for a single disease condition (e.g., prevention of stroke in a person with atrial fibrillation). These narrow reviews can make an important contribution in summarizing current knowledge, especially about whether aspirin can be "better than nothing," but clinical users want more—at the least a comparison with other treatments (e.g., anticoagulants) for the same condition. With more work (often substantially more), SRs can be broadened to include more treatments for the same condition [e.g., Taylor et al. (2)], or for related conditions, as for the massive Antithrombotic Trialists reviews that deal with antiplatelet and anticoagulant treatments for ischemic vascular conditions (3).

The CDSS review presented here is different in that it assesses the effects of a technology that can be applied across a broad range of related and unrelated medical problems. This limits the ways that results can be compared across studies because the patients, diseases, and outcomes will be diverse: apples and oranges, perhaps, but the resulting fruit salad can be satisfying, too.

Whereas an SR looking at the benefits of a treatment will need to stick to one condition at a time (even if multiple conditions are included in the same review), an SR questioning the adverse effects of a treatment can include all conditions that the treatment is used for. Therefore, reviews attempting to quantify the adverse effects of an antibiotic need not restrict their purview to a single type of infection if the drug is used for many types, although it might not make any sense to combine these studies to assess the efficacy of the drug.

Although most reviews to date have focused on questions about the effects of treatments, SRs may also summarize evidence concerning diagnostic and screening tests (4), disease prognosis (5), etiology (6), cost-effectiveness, and even other reviews (7). SRs of diagnostic tests are on the rise, with the Cochrane Collaboration presently gearing up for such reviews. Meanwhile, there are good articles on how to do them well (8,9).

2.3 BASIC PRINCIPLES OF CONDUCTING A SYSTEMATIC REVIEW

SRs are retrospective, observational studies. Biases are rampant in such studies, and careful protocols and procedures are needed to eliminate the biases that can be eliminated and to minimize the ones that can't.

The key steps for conducting a SR appear in this checklist:

✓ Pose your research question(s).
✓ Conduct your literature search.
✓ Specify your selection and assessment methods.
✓ Detail your data extraction procedure.
✓ Indicate your analysis approach.
✓ Choose your sample size.
✓ Plan your budget.

We will now take up each of these steps in turn, describe how we grappled with them in our SR, and discuss the scientific principles that determined our choices of methodological strategies at each step.

✓ *Pose your research question(s).*

We posed this question: "When provided for health professionals in acute inpatient care, emergency rooms, and ambulatory care clinics, can computerized decision support systems (CDSSs), when compared with care unassisted by CDSSs, improve the process and outcomes of patient care?" We defined a CDSS as "any software designed to directly aid in clinical decision making in which characteristics of individual patients are matched to a computerized knowledge base for the purpose of generating patient-specific assessments or recommendations that are then presented to physicians or other health care professionals."

Computers are now ubiquitous in health care settings, and it was important in our review to specify the exact application we were interested in and the effects that we wished to document. This required us to first develop a definition of "computerized decision support," and then circulate this to colleagues and members of the American Medical Informatics Association (many of whom have been involved in the development of CDSSs) for comment. On the basis of their suggestions, we generated the definition that appears above, which guided our efforts to sharpen the focus of our review. For example, we used this definition to exclude "neural nets" from consideration because these computer programs lack a "knowledge base" that one can examine first hand.

Compared with CDSSs, you might think that it is easier to define interventions such as medications, but even for these, it is important to describe the exact conditions and clinical indications that the review will focus on. To provide clinical relevance, credibility, and a clear focus, it is essential that members of the review team (even if it has only one member, you!) have or acquire the expertise to understand both the intervention being studied and its clinical application. For example, a review of antiplatelet agents for stroke that failed to distinguish between primary prevention (among people at risk for having a stroke but who have not had one to date) and secondary prevention (among people who have had at least one stroke) would not be useful to anyone attempting to make clinical decisions. Therefore, the review team for antiplatelet agents should have a clinician experienced in dealing with stroke risk, at least as a consultant. Better still, an antiplatelet agent review team should also include someone familiar with adverse effects of the agent (e.g., a clinical pharmacologist) so that the review procedures can be developed to extract data on not only the benefits of the intervention but also the adverse effects.

The question in our earlier reviews of CDSSs was phrased more loosely, seeking information from "controlled trials," including nonrandomized trials and before–after studies. When we found in the update for our first review that a fairly robust number of randomized trials (i.e., >20) had been conducted, we eliminated before–after studies from consideration. Some people disagree with this approach and feel that all types of studies should be included in an SR regardless of the rigor of the study design. To our way of thinking, however, there is a hierarchy of research designs, with randomized trials on top. If there are enough RCTs to address your review question, it makes no more sense to combine RCTs with studies of lesser design (e.g., natural "experiments" and before–after studies) than it makes sense to try to extend a bottle of wine by adding its chemical cousin, vinegar.

On the other hand, if there is little or no wine, vinegar can be useful. If you are using an SR to define the current state of knowledge, then including the "best studies available" makes sense even if the best studies are not RCTs. First, this allows you to characterize the "state of the art," justifying your proposal to do a better study than has been done so far. Second, observational studies and nonrandomized trials that are otherwise well executed (e.g., inclusion and careful description of appropriate patients, sound measurements of clinical effects, complete follow-up) can provide estimates of the prognosis of a medical condition and potential effects of an intervention that can help in estimating the sample size needed for a proper trial. It is important to note here that observational studies and nonrandomized trials generally overestimate the effects of interventions because they lack equivalent control groups. Therefore, these effects should be partially discounted when used to estimate the sample size for subsequent, stronger studies. Finally, observational studies are often the only feasible way of looking for rare or delayed adverse effects of interventions or exposures.

✓ *Conduct your literature search.*

Three steps are needed in the literature search for an SR: search for prior reviews, search for original published articles, and search for unpublished papers.

Search for Prior Reviews

The literature review for an SR begins with a search for other reviews that match the study question, using search strategies that are highly sensitive for retrieving reviews from electronic bibliographic databases.

> We retrieved and reviewed previous review articles on the subject of CDSSs. We searched for SRs in the Cochrane Library (including the Cochrane Database of Systematic Reviews and the Database of Abstracts of Reviews of Effects), the National Library of Medicine's MEDLINE, Excerpta Medica EMBASE, the American Psychological Association's PsycINFO, International Information Service for the Physics and Engineering Communities (INSPEC), and tracked citations of key articles through Science Citation Index (SCISEARCH). Systematic and narrative reviews were also retrieved in searches for original articles (i.e., articles that publish original data; see the section "Search for Original Articles" below).

It's pointless to do an SR that has just been done and done well. It is fruitful, however, to start from scratch if you believe that the best available SR is biased or to start where a good but dated and inconclusive SR left off. To find other review articles, Shojania and Bero (10) have developed and tested a lengthy general search strategy for reviews that has become the basis for a PubMed Clinical Queries search for retrieving SRs (*http://web.ncbi.nlm.nih.gov/entrez/query/static/clinical.html*). More recently, we have developed and validated a fairly simple search strategy, search:.tw. or meta-analysis.mp,pt. or review.pt. or di.xs. or associated.tw., with a sensitivity of more than 99% for retrieving SRs in MEDLINE through Ovid's MEDLINE search engine, and translations for PUBMED (11). There's not much point in worrying about the logic of this strategy, memorizing its terms, or understanding the Ovid syntax. If you have access to Ovid, the strategy is stored in the "limits" screen after you have entered the content terms for your review. Alternatively, these strategies appear in MEDLINE format on our Web site: (*http://hiru.mcmaster.ca/hedges/*). Just copy and paste the "sensitive" search strategy into PubMed.

This strategy will retrieve virtually all the SRs in MEDLINE. To narrow the search to SRs on the topic of interest to you, you will need to combine this strategy with "content terms." The content terms for CDSSs appear in Table 2–1, and the process is illustrated in Figure 2–1. The terms

TABLE 2–1   Search Terms for Finding Systematic Reviews about Computerized Decision Support Systems for Ovid's MEDLINE[a]

"Sensitive" search strategy to retrieve reviews (connected by logical "OR")	*Review.pt* OR *meta analysis.mp,pt* OR *tu.xs*
Logical (Boolean) connector	AND
Content terms (connected by logical "OR")	*Decision making, computer-assisted (sh)* OR *artificial intelligence (sh)* OR *diagnosis, computer-assisted (sh) OR therapy, computer-assisted (sh) OR hospital information systems (sh)* OR *CDSS*

[a]It's not necessary to understand library jargon to use these search terms, but for what it's worth, "pt" means "publication type;" ".mp" collects citations that have *any* of these terms in the title, abstract, or indexing terms in the database; "tu.xs" means "therapeutic use as an exploded subheading;" "sh" means subheading. This collection is then "ANDed" with the exhaustive search strategy for retrieving all review articles, as shown in Figure 2–1.

for content are derived by looking for the appropriate "Medical Subject Headings" (MeSH) in MEDLINE (*http://www.ncbi.nlm.nih.gov/entrez/meshbrowser.cgi*), and by adding any additional "text words," terms that you feel might appear in the text of articles about CDSSs but might not be represented in MeSH. MeSH is rather course-grained and indexing is somewhat inconsistent, so it pays to combine words and abbreviations that you feel authors of articles will use in their titles and abstracts ("free-text" words), including abbreviations. For example, the abbreviation CDSS is not a MEDLINE indexing term, but searching on "CDSS" alone in MED-LINE retrieves more than 100 references, many of them relevant.

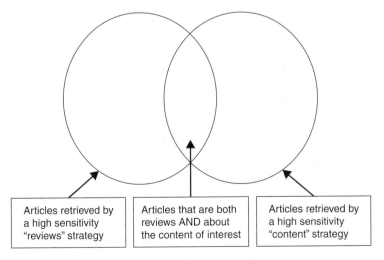

FIGURE 2–1   Combining two search strategies using Boolean logic.

It is inevitable with any highly sensitive search strategy that you will retrieve many more irrelevant than relevant articles. In this stage of looking for SRs, you will also retrieve many relevant RCTs of CDSSs. You'll want to set these aside for future consideration as you look carefully for SRs that, you hope, are on target for content, well done, and up-to-date. If you find one, then you're done, if not, you will need to press on with the steps below.

The search approach just described refers to MEDLINE. All other databases have their own approach, although the basic logic is the same. Once you've derived the MEDLINE strategy you wish to use, get help from an expert librarian searcher to help translate it. Alternatively, find a good SR on the topic similar to the one you are interested in and adopt its search strategy to your purpose. The Cochrane Library is an excellent source for such search strategies, as described in subsequent sections.

Search for Original Articles

The next step in doing an SR is to search for original published articles that report studies that match the study question, using search strategies that are highly sensitive for these types of studies. For the CDSS review that follows, we had been doing updates from time to time, so we built on our own previous reviews (12). Incestuous, perhaps, but also profitable; if your interest in an area continues, then updating your SR on the topic is usually good for a publication every few years, depending on the rate of publication of new studies. When you do update, however, it will be important to be open to new sources of original articles and ways of retrieving them. For example, the SR search strategy above is likely to be better than any one previously used and should be used for updating, with clear indication in your methods section of the period it was used for.

Study identification for our previous review involved searching MEDLINE, EMBASE, INSPEC, and SCISEARCH, from January 1974 to February 1992, for studies in any language. Conference proceedings and reference lists of relevant articles were also reviewed, and authors were contacted. We used a similar strategy for the update, searching for any additional original articles on CDSSs from February 1992 to January 1997. The Cochrane Library was added as a database for this and subsequent searches. This search was then updated again to January 2004. The MEDLINE search strategy included the MeSH terms "computer-assisted decision making," "artificial intelligence," "computer-assisted diagnosis," "computer-assisted therapy," and "hospital information systems." The complete MEDLINE, EMBASE, and INSPEC search strategies appear in Appendix 2.1 of this chapter. We also searched SCISEARCH (*http://library.dialog.com/ bluesheets/html/bl0034.html*) for articles that cited the primary studies from the previous reviews, as well as new relevant articles. Reference lists from all relevant articles were examined, and authors of relevant studies were contacted and asked if they were aware of any additional published or unpublished studies that we had not identified.

Most review articles, and especially those of the Cochrane Collaborative Review Groups [which are detailed in the Cochrane Library (*http:// www3.interscience.wiley.com/cgi-bin/mrwhome/106568753/HOME*)], provide detailed search strategies for original articles. You can use or modify these "industrial-grade" searches and you will usually require a librarian's assistance to do so. If you try to develop a "gold standard" search strategy yourself, you will usually be left wondering if you have retrieved all relevant studies. It is important to report the exact steps of the final search strategy you use so that you and others can replicate (and perhaps improve on) your search.

Here are some additional tips for searching the literature:

- Looking at the bibliographies of other review articles on the topic helps plug holes in your collection.
- Librarians can help a lot with searches, especially in "negotiating" the idiosyncrasies of the various bibliographic databases and your local library's access to them. However, it is important that they build on the search techniques developed for other SRs rather than try to develop their own search strategy from scratch.
- To find all the original articles on a topic; you will want to use the most sensitive search strategy you can find. Here is the most sensitive search strategy we have developed for retrieving RCTs from MEDLINE: "clinical trial.pt. OR random:.mp. OR tu.xs." This strategy is designed for use in Ovid's version of the MEDLINE database, available through most medical school libraries, and has a sensitivity of 99.3% and a specificity of 70.5%. Ovid has also implemented these terms as one of its "limit" options, so you don't need to remember the terms. The equivalent strategy for PubMed is available from the Clinical Queries search screen (*http://web.ncbi.nlm.nih.gov/entrez/ query/static/clinical.html*). Sensitive searches for studies about treatments, diagnostic tests, prognosis, etiology, and reviews appear in Table 2–2. In all cases, you will need to "AND" a collection of content terms to the appropriate strategy in the table.
- Unlike the situation for types of studies shown in Table 2–1, no "gold standard" exists for the terms that have to do with content (e.g., "computerized decision support systems") for comprehensive searches, so the best approach is likely to begin with the search strategies used in the best available review articles on the topic, especially those in the Cochrane Library if your topic is an intervention, and to see if you can do better, for example, by "ORing" in additional content terms if you feel any potentially useful terms have been omitted. The sensitivity of a search strategy is increased by "ORing" together all the terms that you can imagine might be used by authors and indexers to describe the types of studies you are interested in. For example, our sensitive search strategy for articles on CDSS was "computer-assisted decision making OR artificial intelligence OR computer-assisted diagnosis OR computer-assisted therapy OR hospital information systems." The "dark side" of sensitivity is

TABLE 2–2 **Sensitive Search Strategies for Retrieval From MEDLINE in Ovid[a]**

Purpose of Studies	Strategy	Sensitivity (%)	Specificity (%)
Treatment	Clinical trial.mp. OR clinical trial.pt. OR random:.mp. OR tu.xs	99	70
Diagnosis	Sensitive:.mp. OR diagnos:.mp. OR di.fs.	98	74
Prognosis	incidence.sh. OR exp mortality OR follow-up studies.sh. OR mortality.sh. OR prognos:.tw. OR predict:.tw. OR course:.tw.	90	80
Causation	Risk:.mp. OR exp cohort studies OR group:.tw.	93	63
Other reviews	review.pt. OR meta analysis.mp,pt. OR tu.xs.	98	69

[a]To use these strategies in Ovid, include the clinical topic terms for your search as one line, then click "limit" at the top of the search screen, go to the "Clinical Queries" box, and select the appropriate strategy. You can also "do it yourself" by typing the appropriate strategy from this table on a second line, then put "1 AND 2" on the third line.

false-positive retrievals—the more sensitive the strategy, the more good (true positive) and bad (false positive) articles it will retrieve.

• It is useful to combine the citations from different bibliographic databases into reference management software[1], for example, Reference Manager, ISI ResearchSoft: Thomson Corporation, *http://www.refman.com*, so that citations that are retrieved from more than one source are downloaded, merged, and formatted in the style that you need for subsequent referencing.

• For a topic with only smaller studies reported, the published studies can be expected to overestimate the effect of an intervention because positive studies are more likely to be published than ones with indeterminate results, a phenomenon known as *publication bias* (13,14). Publication bias measures the association between whether or not studies are published and the magnitude and direction of effect. Funnel plots can be used to depict the possibility of publication bias (15). Funnel plots graph a measure of study precision, such as the 95% confidence interval or standard deviation around a point estimate, against a measure of study effect, such as the absolute risk difference or odds ratio. If there is no publication bias, this plot should appear as an inverted funnel. Smaller studies statistically give a wide range of effect sizes and are less precise. Therefore, the widest spread will be at the base of the inverted funnel if all small studies are reported. If this does not occur, then it follows that some smaller studies have not been reported, typically those that give smaller effect sizes, leaving a hole in the lower-left sector of the inverted funnel when study precision is on the y axis and measure of study effect is on the x axis. Statistically, the existence of a dearth of data from small negative studies can be verified by several methods including the adjusted rank correlation test (16), the regression asymmetry test (17), and the trim-and-fill method (18).

- Heterogeneity of results from one study to the next causes problems for the interpretation of trials. "Homogeneous results" is a methodological condition for combining the results of trials in a meta-analysis in which each trial's result is treated as if it contributes to the testing of the same intervention, under similar circumstances, as for all other trials included in the analysis. If the results of different trials aren't similar or "homogeneous," then it may be that the trials aren't really testing the same intervention under similar circumstances of providers, patients, care settings, and so on. Unfortunately, formal statistical tests are typically low in power to detect heterogeneous results, so lack of a statistically significant degree of heterogeneity often constitutes no more than a whitewash, or at least isn't very informative. Recently, Higgins et al. (19) have developed a much more informative statistic, I^2, which calculates the percentage of total variation across studies that is due to heterogeneity, an approach that has recently been endorsed by the Cochrane Collaboration. Even when heterogeneity is found, it is often ignored by reviewers! From a practical perspective, for any meta-analysis the degree of heterogeneity should be assessed, and any evidence of heterogeneity should lead to examination of the primary studies to assess sources of heterogeneity (differences in patients, settings, interventions, co-interventions, outcome measures, etc.) and should prompt consideration of whether meta-analysis is warranted at all.

- Studies published in all languages should be included in the review if possible. Trials published in languages other than English appear to be of similar quality (20), can improve the precision of findings (21), and may also provide a way to reduce publication bias (22). Some controversy exists, however, about just how far one needs to go. The best way to answer this question is to examine the results of language-restricted and language-unrestricted reviews on the same topic. When David Moher et al. did so, they found no difference *on average* in the results that were reported from meta-analyses (23).

Search for Unpublished Studies that Match the Study Question

Looking for studies that have not been reported in the regular journal literature can be important, especially if the number of large studies (i.e., >1,000 participants, >100 endpoints) on a topic is small. Unpublished studies are typically found by reviewing abstracts of studies presented at scientific meetings and by contacting the authors of potentially relevant studies, by contacting authors of published studies and reviews, and by notifying people who are interested in the topic. For example, for our review of CDSSs, we circulated a request for published and unpublished studies to some members of the American Medical Informatics Association who we knew to be interested in CDSSs. For interventions that are produced by corporations (e.g., pharmaceuticals), it is also important to contact the relevant companies. As a courtesy and an inducement to reply, it is customary to offer respondents a bibliography of the published studies that you have retrieved.

Although looking for studies not reported in the regular journal literature is done for some reviews, it isn't done for most, and there are some reasons for this. First, it is a painstaking process to look through abstracts of scientific meetings to try to determine the fate of incompletely described studies that might or might not be relevant, especially if these meetings are not narrowly dedicated to the topic of interest. Second, trials that are not published may not be written up in a fashion that is satisfactory for accuracy and completeness. Third, unpublished trials may not have been completed for reasons such as low feasibility, poorly conceived interventions, and fatal design flaws, particularly when the interventions are as diverse as those within the definition of CDSSs. The situation may be different for, say, drug regimens once dose-ranging studies have been completed, where one can expect the regimen to be quite standardized. Finally, it may also be unnecessary to seek unpublished studies if large studies have been published on the topic of interest: additional small studies are unlikely to change the conclusion or increase the precision of estimates of effects.

✓ *Specify your selection and assessment methods.*

Four key steps are needed for study selection and assessment, beginning with scanning citations and their abstracts from database and hand searches, developing and applying eligibility criteria, assessing articles for eligibility, and assessing the scientific merit of each eligible study.

Scan Citations and Abstracts for Relevance

All citations we retrieved were reviewed and rated as "relevant," "possibly relevant," or "not relevant." The current review builds on two previous reviews, with similar but not identical procedures. To assess interrater reliability up to 1997, a random subset of 120 citations from the entire citation list was reviewed by two reviewers working independently. The raw agreement between independent observations was 83% and the level of agreement beyond chance was 58% [weighted kappa (24) was 58% (95% confidence interval was 42%–75%)]. For 1997 to 2004, all citations and their abstracts and indexing terms were reviewed by at least two reviewers working independently, and all full-text articles were retrieved if one or more reviewers indicated that they were relevant or possibly relevant. (Instructions for this phase of the review appear in Appendix 2.2)

The precision of a search is the proportion of retrieved articles that are relevant to the topic. The precision of "sensitive" database searches, intended to catch all trials and reviews on the topic, is typically small. For example, the precision for the sensitive search strategy for trials using the Ovid search engine, "clinical trial.pt. OR random:.mp. OR tu.xs," without any content terms included is about 1%. That is, only about 1 in 100 of the citations retrieved will "pan out" as a "true gold," relevant article. If you had to retrieve all the full-text articles to find the 1 in 100 that is relevant, it could become overwhelming. Fortunately, bibliographic databases provide full journal titles and indexing terms for all articles and abstracts for most. This permits screening of the retrieved items to identify articles that are likely to be relevant. Unfortunately, this is a tedious task that could potentially miss relevant articles, especially if you are searching by titles of articles alone and if your attention wanes. For this reason, screening of citations should be done with a download that includes all elements in the database for each item (i.e., full citation, abstract, and indexing terms), not just the titles, and the review should be done in duplicate, by at least two reviewers, with provision for identifying articles that are clearly or probably relevant, those that are possibly relevant, and those that are clearly not relevant. The screening should be done by at least two readers, especially if it cannot be documented that duplicate reading gives identical results (i.e., 100% agreement beyond chance). When you are screening, it is important to give citations "the benefit of the doubt" so that no relevant study is missed.

You can save a lot of time and effort in the initial assessment of relevance of citations by having the reviewers assess 100 or so citations and then compare difficulties and disagreements so that everyone is in agreement about what's potentially relevant and calibrated on how to look for it. This calibration step often identifies areas of uncertainty or confusion among the reviewers, as well as problems in the clarity of the review question, the definition of the intervention, and types of studies that should be considered. Reviewers should also be given clear instructions to avoid spending more than an hour at a time in screening, so that "reviewer fatigue" (a semidelirious state) is avoided.

If you are the only person doing the review (bad idea!), it is even more important to do at least a part of the screening in duplicate (separating the two assessments by, say, a week or two) to document the reproducibility of your assessments.

We also include another category for screening—"I" for "special interest"—to allow us to indicate articles that we would like to see in full text that aren't necessarily directly relevant to the review question but may add some dimension for discussion (e.g., ethical issues), or those articles that are of special interest for some other reason.

Develop and Apply Criteria for the Studies That Will Be Included

The full-text publications of all of the potentially relevant articles, in all languages, were reviewed, and studies were included in the review if: (a) the study participants were health professionals in independent clinical practice or postgraduate training; (b) the intervention was a computer-based CDSS evaluated in a clinical setting; (c) the outcomes that were assessed included effects on clinician performance (a measure of the process of care) or were effects on patients (including any aspect of patient well-being); and (d) the study prospectively collected data with a contemporaneous control group so that patient care with a CDSS was compared with care without one.

Although some reviewers would insist that all studies on the topic be included, in my view the criteria that you use to select articles for detailed review should represent a balance of rigor and feasibility. As stated earlier in this chapter, including poor with good studies in a review debases the quality of the final product—unless there are few or almost no good studies, in which case, sticking with only the good studies will make for a rather thin assessment of the state of knowledge. The more good studies there are, the higher should be the bar for eligibility criteria. The criteria can include both methods and content. For example, you could set the research criteria for diagnostic test studies as:

- inclusion of a consecutive series of participants suspected, but not known, to have the disorder or derangement of interest
- objective diagnostic ("gold") standard (e.g., laboratory test not requiring interpretation) OR current clinical standard for diagnosis (e.g., a venogram for deep venous thrombosis), with documentation of reproducible criteria for subjectively interpreted diagnostic standard (i.e., report of statistically significant measure of agreement beyond chance among observers)
- each participant must receive both the new test and some form of the diagnostic standard
- interpretation of diagnostic standard without knowledge of test result
- interpretation of test without knowledge of diagnostic standard result.

If you apply these criteria to a number of articles that describe the performance of tests for the disorder you are interested in, and if you find that none of them meets all the criteria, then you will need to relax the criteria, for example, by replacing the first one with "inclusion of a spectrum of participants, some, but not all, of whom have the disorder or derangement of interest." This criterion permits the inclusion of a broader range of studies, including ones that have selected patients already known to have or to be free of the disease of interest. This approach is definitely not as relevant from a clinical perspective and will overestimate the sensitivity and specificity of the test when applied in usual circumstances where you don't know if a person does or doesn't have the disease of interest. However, if this is the best evidence available on a test that is currently in clinical use, then it will still be of use to summarize the available evidence, if only to indicate that the test has limitations and that it needs to be tested more definitively.

Another take on the issue of how inclusive to be in selecting studies is to incorporate all studies, assess their merit for both clinical relevance and scientific merit, then determine the relation between merit and results.

Indeed, this is the "party line" of the inner circle of SR methodologists. Following this line, if no relation is shown, then include all studies in the final analysis. If there is a relation, do an overall analysis and a preplanned subgroup analysis of the best studies. It takes a lot of studies on a topic to be able to pull this off well; if you have only a few studies to work with, the analysis will lack the power to detect a relation between methods and results, creating the illusion of security. On the other hand, if you have many studies to work with, you will need many resources to do the review. If you have the resources available or can get them, fine. Otherwise, you might want to heed a favorite saying of one of the previous chairs of my university department, George Browman: "Don't let the excellent be the enemy of the good."

The data extraction form for our CDSS review, beginning with the criteria for inclusion, is in Appendix 2.3 of this chapter. Here are some tips on data extraction forms:

- If a form already exists for rating potentially relevant studies of the sort you will be reviewing, and if it has been assessed for reliability (e.g., by comparing duplicate independent assessments of a series of articles), use it if it serves your purpose. If not, you will need to modify an existing form or develop your own. Developing data extraction forms for individual studies in SRs (as in other studies) is an iterative process. One investigator usually takes the lead in drafting the form, members of the study team try it out independently on a few articles, and then everyone meets to discuss their success in figuring out what's needed, how the instructions could be improved, how the form could flow better, and so on, until everyone is as happy with the form as can be. Going through this process at the beginning of the review of articles can be boring and tedious. But it is a lot less boring and tedious than waiting until all the articles have been rated, only to discover that different reviewers have interpreted criteria differently or with varying degrees of rigor.
- Having only one reviewer is most dangerous because the errors of that reviewer will not be discovered through examination of disagreements. If there can be only one reviewer, then a duplicate assessment of the articles by the same rater at a later time is better than nothing at all.

Assess Articles for Eligibility and Document the Reproducibility of this Assessment

Each potentially relevant article was assessed independently and in duplicate.

The agreement between reviewers on the eligibility of studies for the SR was assessed. The raw agreement was 98% and the level of agreement beyond chance was 86% [kappa statistic 86% (76%–97%)]. All disagreements were resolved by consensus—we went through disagreements one by one to determine if the article contained the information we needed to settle the disagreement (whether for or against including the article); if not, we decided whether additional information should be sought from the author. If so, the article was discussed again after attempting to contact the authors.

A good approach to extracting information from an article is to mark the article for the information that corresponds to the criteria (e.g., using a highlighter). If the information is difficult to find, indicate in the extraction sheet exactly where in the article the information is located. If the information in the article is unclear or ambiguous, indicate the problem and your reasoning in making a decision about eligibility. This makes discussion of disagreements much simpler and more efficient.

The kappa statistic is commonly used to compare duplicate ratings. As noted in the introduction to this book, we've excluded detailed descriptions of statistical methods but have promised to point you to appropriate resources. Statistical texts that include analysis of rates and proportions—that is, most basic stats texts (24,25)—will provide one or more methods of assessing agreement between observers.

For Eligible Articles, Assess the Scientific Merit of Each Study and Document the Reproducibility of this Assessment

At least two authors assessed all selected studies independently for methodological quality. A 10-point rating scale (see Appendix 2.3) was used, and disagreements were resolved by consensus. The scale assessed five potential sources of bias including the method of allocation to study groups (i.e., random versus nonrandom allocation), the unit of allocation (i.e., clinic versus physician versus patient), baseline differences between groups, the type of outcome measure (i.e., objective versus subjective), and the completeness of follow-up. The unit of allocation was included because of the likelihood of contamination in trials in which interventions are applied to clinicians and end points are measured for patients. For example, the lowest score for unit of allocation was given when individual patients were allocated to intervention and control groups because a clinician may treat some patients with, and others without, the aid of the CDSS; knowledge gained by the clinician from the CDSS may then be applied to control patients, leading to an underestimate of the system's effect. A similar situation can occur when individual clinicians within a team or group are the units of allocation; the presence of a CDSS, or of colleagues who are using a CDSS, in the clinical setting may influence the treatment given by clinicians allocated to the comparison group.

All studies were initially graded for adequacy of follow-up of patients. In some trials, however, only a subset of the randomized patients were assessed for outcomes, for example, only those attending an appointment during the study period as a subset of all those randomized from a patient roster. This was especially common in trials assessing the role of CDSSs in preventive care. For these studies, the completeness of follow-up criterion was inapplicable, and the remaining score was pro-rated so that the maximum possible score remained as 10 points.

The agreement between reviewers for the scientific merit of the new studies was high. A total of 30 new studies were assessed, and eight discrepancies occurred for baseline similarities, four for group formulation, three for outcome measure scores, two for the unit of allocation, and one for the follow-up. All disagreements were resolved by discussion.

The merit assessment for our CDSS review was tailored to include key methodological features that are important to the validity and interpretation of trials of CDSSs. For example, given that it is impossible to blind users of such systems, cluster randomization becomes an important method to reduce bias from "contamination," as detailed in the project noted in preceding text. For testing less complex interventions, such as medications for which blinding of patients and providers is possible, a simpler approach will do. The Jadad scale, which assesses randomization, blinding, and drop-outs, is the most popular approach for assessing the quality of a clinical trial study and has the advantages of being validated and simple to apply (26). Since the development of the Jadad scale, Ken Schulz has demonstrated the importance of concealment of randomization (27), and this is a justifiable addition to any validity assessment (more details on this in the section on Allocation below). David Moher et al. have provided much more detailed assessments of the options for assessing study quality and their performance (28,29,30). Juni et al. (31) demonstrate some of the problems with ratings scales and make the case for limiting assessments to individual items that have been shown to have an impact on effect sizes.

✓ *Detail your data extraction procedure.*

For each article that met eligibility criteria, we used a word processor to cut and paste the original abstract from MEDLINE onto the abstraction form. We then went through the entire article to create our own detailed extract with each feature needed for our review.

The payoff from all the hard work you've done to this point begins to emerge with data extraction from the eligible studies that you've identified. The basic notion here is that you should extract and organize all the information from each article that you will need so that you will not need to return to the original article. This takes careful planning! Details will include identifying the exact questions addressed by each study; describing the participants; indicating the method and unit of allocation; and extracting measurements of the clinical processes and events that are pertinent to your review. The details appear in subsequent text, and a sample from the review featured in this chapter is in Appendix 2.3.

Identify Question(s) Addressed by Each Study

We reviewed the author's statement concerning the question(s) addressed by each study (typically in the last paragraph of the Introduction of the article, just before Methods), and compared this with the description of what was done in the execution of the study.

In extracting information about the question(s) addressed by the study, it is important not to rely too much on what the authors claim as their purpose. The study design may not match the question exactly. For example, the authors may have set out to test a CDSS to increase the uptake of preventive care in general practice settings but may have ended up being able to recruit only a handful of practices that were already doing a good job of preventive care, limiting the likelihood of showing an effect and the generalizability of the result. The study, as executed, dictates what purpose was addressed, not the good intentions of the investigators, and not the stated design of the study. Therefore, the purpose of the study can be best interpreted by reviewing the details of what was done rather than by taking the author's statements at face value.

Specify Study Participants

The text of the article was perused as far as needed for details of who was invited, and how many entered and completed the study, for practices, practitioners, and patients.

It is important to extract details about who was approached to participate, what proportion of those who were approached agreed, and what proportion of them actually contributed data for the course of the trial (i.e., percentage follow-up). Authors often do not report or keep track of how many people were approached, so it may not be possible to provide information on this aspect of recruitment in your review. However, authors definitely should know, and report, how many people entered the study and how many completed it. If this isn't clear from the report, then the author should be approached to provide the details.

In health services research intervention studies (including evaluations of CDSSs), there are usually two levels of participants to account for: practitioners, who are usually the intermediaries of CDSS "advice," and the patients these practitioners serve. Features and numbers of both these groups should be extracted from the study reports.

Specify Method and Unit of Allocation

Information was extracted from each report concerning the method of allocation to comparison groups (including how random allocation was conducted and whether allocation was "concealed") and the unit of allocation (i.e., individual patients, care providers, or practice groups).

The validity of testing interventions in health care (and no doubt in other domains) is related to how comparable the study groups are to begin with. Two key features of allocation of participants to intervention and control groups are important to extract. First, determine whether the allocation was (really) random (32). Random allocation is the preferred method for forming comparable groups in controlled trials because it distributes both known and unknown factors that might influence the outcome randomly among the groups being compared. Determining the likelihood of various outcomes (more about this in Chapters 5 and 6 on therapeutic trials), and whether they should be attributed to the play of chance or to the effects of the intervention, forms the basis for statistical analysis of the findings. In assessing whether a study used random allocation, it is important to pay attention to the details of what was done. Random allocation means that a participant's placement into a group is determined by a chance process (e.g., flipping an unbiased coin, looking at a randomization table in a statistics text or, more often these days, using a computer-generated random sequence from a statistics program), not on an arbitrary method (such as the day of the week when they arrived for care) or an intentional method (such as the investigator deciding who is in which group). In determining what the investigators did, it is important to watch for "weasel words" that imply randomization but that mean something less, such as "based on date of birth" or "hospital identification numbers." For example, Lazar et al. indicated in one report of a trial (33) that, "Patients who met the eligibility criteria for inclusion into the study were prospectively randomly assigned to a GIK or no-GIK group, based on the last digit of their hospital identification number." In their next report for the same trial (34), they simply indicated that, "Patients were randomly assigned to a GIK or no-GIK group."

Second, it is important to determine, if possible, whether the allocation was "concealed" so that investigators and participants did not know what the next allocation would be when the participant was entering into the study (27). Here are some working definitions:

Allocation concealed. The authors were deemed to have taken adequate measures to conceal allocation to study groups from those responsible for assessing patients for entry in the trial (e.g., central randomization; sequentially numbered, opaque, sealed envelopes; sealed envelopes from a closed bag; numbered or coded bottles or containers; drugs prepared by the pharmacy; or other descriptions that contain elements convincing of concealment).

Allocation not concealed. The authors were deemed not to have taken adequate measures to conceal allocation to study groups from those responsible for assessing patients for entry in the trial (e.g., no concealment procedure; sealed envelopes that were not opaque; or other descriptions that contain elements not convincing of concealment).

Unclear allocation concealment. The authors did not report or provide us with a description of an allocation concealment approach that allowed for classification as concealed or not concealed.

In our experience, many investigators don't know the meaning of concealed allocation and have difficulty fielding questions about how this was handled in their studies; hence, we include "unclear allocation concealment" as one of the possibilities in data extraction.

Additional tips on extracting information from articles and studies:

- It is important to do your own extract, based on a template of the details you want to report in your review, by going through the complete text of the article (and beyond, to the author or prior articles on the same study, if necessary). The original abstracts of articles are almost always incomplete for the details you will need. The details that you need from the article will often be scattered in different sections, not "where they should be." Further, you will often find discrepancies from place to place in an article and will need to make a judgment, often with the help of the authors, on what actually transpired.

- Extracting all these details serves several purposes. First, it provides the information that will later form the summary tables for the review. Second, it facilitates checking by a second reviewer. Third, it means seldom needing to go back to the original article when the extraction is complete. This is important for the preparation of the draft of the review and becomes progressively more important when updates of the review are prepared. Finally, if there are disagreements among the studies and no obvious source for the disagreements (such as poorly conducted versus well conducted studies), the details that you extract systematically from each study can be incorporated into a "meta-regression analysis" comparing results against study characteristics.

Measure Clinical Processes and Events That Were Considered in Testing the Intervention

One of the reviewers extracted information concerning patients, setting, intervention, and outcomes, checked by a second reviewer. We included information concerning effects on patient care processes (e.g., whether a service was provided) and clinical outcomes (i.e., whether patients' clinical problems were affected).

Ideally, it is best to focus attention only on studies that provide information on the effects of CDSSs on *both* clinical processes and outcomes. We were able to do this in a review of interventions to improve patient adherence (35). For the adherence review, it became obvious that changes in patient adherence often did not result in any appreciable benefit to patients, and risked increasing adverse effects. From a health care perspective, an intervention that doesn't improve clinical outcomes for the better isn't worth paying much attention to; indeed, it should be condemned as a waste of time and other resources. With the current state of CDSS research, however, there are too few studies that measure both processes and outcomes to do justice to the current state of evolution of CDSSs by insisting on both process and outcome measures in each study. From a strictly clinical perspective, this choice means that the review is much less interesting and important, except for raising warning bells about the promises of CDSS developers and purveyors. This general lack of relevance for clinical practice will need to be emphasized in the write-up of the review.

The studies were grouped naturally into four major topic areas: drug dosing, diagnosis, preventive care, and studies of active medical care.

Observational research, such as reviewing the research to date on a topic, often involves looking for patterns that may not appear in looking at individual studies. In the case of studies of CDSSs, the studies seemed to fall into the four groups just mentioned. It is important to look for these patterns, to increase the opportunity for comparing "like with like" and finding conclusive results within these similar groups. For example, studies of preventive care reminders are homogeneous enough in their objectives, interventions, and results to confidently conclude that reminder systems have a positive influence on completion of most preventive tasks (with the possible exception of things most doctors don't like to do, such as digital rectal examinations!). Studies on the use of computers to assist with diagnosis are much less conclusive about benefits. But it's also important to avoid getting trapped by the "natural categories" you perceive. For example, if you were to insist on treating CDSSs for disease X (say, hypertension) as "naturally" different from CDSSs for disease Y (say, hyperlipidemia), so that findings are summarized only within these disease-specific categories, you might conclude that CDSSs "work" in hypertension, but not in hyperlipidemia, when in fact they may have about the same effect in just about any chronic disease with self-administered oral medications (and only seem to be different for hyperlipidemia because there were too few studies or studies of too small size to detect the effect).

There's obviously room for judgment—and controversy—in how you "lump or split" studies, and our advice is to look for the patterns but keep an open mind about whether the ones you choose to emphasize represent the best interpretation of the evidence. This is a topic worth raising in the Discussion section of your paper, along with other confessions about the weaknesses and alternative explanations of your findings and conclusions. (Alas, paragraphs on weaknesses are often most prominent in the Discussion sections of the strongest studies and missing from the weakest studies...)

✓ *Indicate your analysis approach.*

Studies were grouped within the four categories and their findings for each process and outcome effect were summarized for comparison. Subsequently, all studies that evaluated the effects of using a CDSS on patient outcomes and that reported no statistically significant improvement were analyzed to determine the power of each to detect a medium and clinically important difference in outcomes between the groups (12). An example of a moderate and clinically significant change would be a 25% absolute increase in the proportion of patients at a general medicine clinic who had adequate blood pressure control. The approach described by Cohen was used, and, in each case, an α probability of 5% along with a medium effect size were used for the calculations (36).

"Power," the ability of a study to detect an effect when it is present, is a key problem in the research in any field. Many preliminary studies are simply too small to dependably detect even a sizable benefit. This is certainly true for studies of CDSSs, with sample sizes as low as 20 patients. For example, for a study of a CDSS for preventive care that increased the rate of diabetes screening from 50% to 75%, the investigators would need to recruit about 77 participants per group to be 90% sure of detecting the effect at a level of statistical significance of 5%. With only 20 participants in the trial, a negative result is almost certain—by default. A way to deal with this is meta-analysis, or combining the results of different studies, if there are several studies on the topic and if their conduct and findings are homogenous enough to be combined. Unfortunately, this degree of similarity among studies is seriously lacking for CDSSs. These studies vary for the settings, patients and clinical problems, providers, interventions, duration of follow-up, and outcome measures, so no meta-analysis is warranted. The fallback here is to determine the "power" of the negative studies for finding a clinically important effect, so that you can report how many of the "negative" trials were large enough for this to be a convincing result. The officially disparaged approach, "vote counting," would be to simply treat all studies as equals and "count the votes" for and against the intervention having an effect, based on the number of studies finding, and failing to find, statistically significant results.

Meta-analysis is a statistical technique for summarizing and combining the results of two or more investigations. Meta-analysis is often inappropriate, although it is commonly done. For a meta-analysis to be justified, the clinical condition being studied must be the same in each investigation included in the analysis, the study methods should be of comparable quality, the interventions should be the same, and the outcome measures must be the same. It is generally easy to justify a meta-analysis for medications (such as warfarin versus placebo or aspirin) prescribed for a condition (such as atrial fibrillation) and for outcomes (such as stroke and bleeding). It is impossible to justify a meta-analysis of, say, interventions to promote adherence to medications when the clinical problems, settings, interventions, measurements of adherence, and outcome events differ from study to study (35).

If the results of investigations are to be summarized by meta-analysis, how the results are compared across studies is important. Simply counting successes and failures, with each study counting as one "test" won't work because of the reasons given in the earlier paragraphs. Adding up results across studies is even worse, as the following example shows.

TABLE 2-3   2002 World Series of Baseball Game Scores

Game	Anaheim Angels	San Francisco Giants
1	3	4
2	11	10
3	10	4
4	3	4
5	4	16
6	6	5
7	4	1
Total	41	44

Table 2-3 reports the results of the 2002 World Series of baseball. The San Francisco Giants scored the most runs. Did they become world champs? No way!–the Anaheim Angels were champs that year because they won four of the seven games. To the victors go the spoils: this one game difference means bragging rights, a place in history, a lot of bread for the Angels, and chopped liver for the Giants. For the game five blow out, the Angels' embarrassing loss wouldn't have mattered a whit more if the score had been 1 to 100, except for the transient humiliation. The same is true for tallying studies for a meta-analysis; it's what happens within studies ("games") that matters most.

To make matters more complicated than baseball scores, it is also important to "weight" the studies according to the number of participants they included. Therefore, a study of 100 participants ought to count much less than a study of 1,000. In fact, this is the basis for the statistics for meta-analysis: it is the summary of results within studies, added across comparable studies, according to the relative size of the studies. The statistical details of meta-analysis are beyond the scope of this book but are well covered in many books and papers. A quick summary of some of the options from the Cochrane Reviewers' Handbook (37) appears in Table 2-4. The most recent version of the handbook is at *http://www.cochrane.org/admin/manual.htm.*

The terms in Table 2-4 are defined in the Cochrane Reviewers' Handbook Glossary (38), which is included with the Cochrane Library. An example of a meta-analysis appears in Figure 2-2. This simple and elegant display includes all the relevant data concerning study endpoints for each included trial, the graphical representation of the individual study results, and their meta-analytic "bottom line" in the form of a diamond below the individual study results. Following along the top row of Table 2-4, the analysis in Figure 2-2 is based on dichotomous data and uses odds ratios for the occurrence of any disabling stroke or death among patients who had a recent transient ischemic attack or minor stroke associated with high-grade carotid stenosis and who received carotid endarterectomy, compared with similar patients who did not receive carotid endarterectomy.

TABLE 2–4   Meta-analysis Options Discussed in the Cochrane Reviewers' Handbook

Type of Data	Summary Statistic	Model	Method of Analysis
Dichotomous	Odds ratio (O-E)	Fixed effect	Peto and Mantel-Haenszel
		Random effects	DerSimonian and Laird
	Relative risk	Fixed effect	Mantel-Haenszel
		Random effects	DerSimonian and Laird
	Risk difference	Fixed effect	Mantel-Haenszel
		Random effects	DerSimonian and Laird
Continuous	Weighted mean difference	Fixed effect	Inverse variance
		Random effects	DerSimonian and Laird
	Standardized mean difference	Fixed effect	Inverse variance
		Random effects	DerSimonian and Laird
Individual patient data	Odds ratio (O-E)	Fixed effect	Peto

From Clarke M, Oxman A, eds. Cochrane reviewers' handbook 4.1.4 [updated March 2003]. In: *The Cochrane Library*. Section 8. Issue 4, Chichester, UK: John Wiley & Sons, 2003, with permission (37).

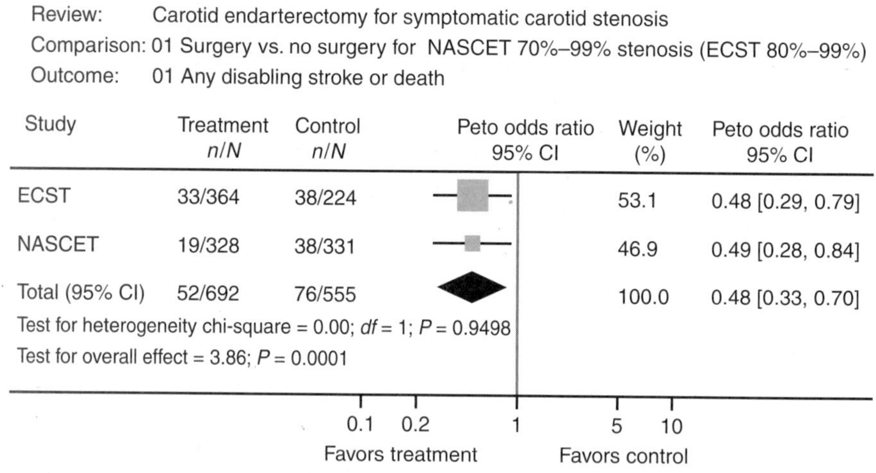

Review: Carotid endarterectomy for symptomatic carotid stenosis
Comparison: 01 Surgery vs. no surgery for NASCET 70%–99% stenosis (ECST 80%–99%)
Outcome: 01 Any disabling stroke or death

Study	Treatment n/N	Control n/N	Peto odds ratio 95% CI	Weight (%)	Peto odds ratio 95% CI
ECST	33/364	38/224		53.1	0.48 [0.29, 0.79]
NASCET	19/328	38/331		46.9	0.49 [0.28, 0.84]
Total (95% CI)	52/692	76/555		100.0	0.48 [0.33, 0.70]

Test for heterogeneity chi-square = 0.00; df = 1; P = 0.9498
Test for overall effect = 3.86; P = 0.0001

```
            0.1   0.2        1      5    10
         Favors treatment       Favors control
```

FIGURE 2–2   Meta-analysis from a Cochrane review comparing results of trials of carotid endarterectomy for symptomatic carotid stenosis (39). From Cina CS, Clase CM, Haynes RB. Carotid endarterectomy for symptomatic carotid stenosis. *The Cochrane Library*. Issue 4, Chichester, UK: John Wiley & Sons, 2003, with permission.

The conduct of the two trials in the analysis was very similar, and the results were combined using a fixed effects model and analyzed using the Peto test, based on the odds ratio. The weight given to each trial in the meta-analysis is determined by the number of outcome events in each and is reflected by the size of the "blob" accorded to each in the graph, commonly called a "blobogram" (or somewhat more formally, a "forest plot"). The blobs for both trials are on the "favors treatment" side of the "no difference" line (an odds ratio of one represents no difference), and the "whiskers" extending on either side of the blobs, representing the 95% confidence intervals for their odds ratios, also do not overlap the "no difference" line. This indicates that both studies had statistically significant results favoring carotid endarterectomy.

It may seem to you to be an impossible leap to produce a table like this from your current state of knowledge. However, if you have followed all the steps in this chapter, you understand the basic elements that are needed. The hard work, in fact, is not in the graph itself, but in getting to the point where the graph can be created. Once you have justified comparing studies on the basis of similar questions, settings, participants, interventions, and outcome measures, and then extracted the number of events for each group (as shown in Figure 2–2 in the columns titled Treatment and Control, where n = the number of events and N = the number of participants), the Cochrane software [Review Manager (REVMAN)] takes over and generates the rest of the graph. REVMAN is free from the Cochrane Collaboration, but you must join a Cochrane Review Group if you want any help using it beyond what's in the manual that comes with it. Descriptions and contact information for Cochrane Review Groups are included in the Cochrane Library. Other software for SRs can be found through a review of meta-analysis software by Matthias Egger et al. (*http://bmj.bmjjournals.com/archive/7126/7126ed9.htm*). Special considerations apply to the meta-analysis of data from cluster randomized trials, as discussed by Alan Donner et al. (40).

The "ultimate" in data extraction from studies is an "individual patient data (IPD)" review, in which investigators of all pertinent studies agree to provide their original data. If the studies were conducted in a highly similar way, with virtually identical protocols, this permits pooling of data (as if all data were from one large project) for much more precise analyses, often within subgroups of patients (e.g., men versus women, older versus younger, and more severely affected versus less severely affected). A limitation of such reviews is that it is often impossible to collect the data from all potentially eligible studies, violating the fundamental principle of SRs to include all eligible studies. One likely consequence of this is to exaggerate the effects of "publication bias," in which smaller negative studies are less likely to be published, leading to inflated estimates of effect sizes (e.g., overestimates of how large an effect CDSSs have on patient outcomes). Other methodological and practical challenges are inherent in the combination of different datasets and databases, including differing definitions of baseline and outcome variables, differing definitions and timing of assessments, and differing data software packages (41). Nevertheless, when feasible, IPD meta-analyses represent the most powerful way to extract findings from multiple studies on the same topic.

The impact of a meta-analysis can be enhanced by plotting the results of trials cumulatively, starting with the first trial published, then adding the results of subsequent trials in sequence (42). If we were to do this for the studies in Figure 2–2, the first trial, European Carotid Surgery Trial (ECST), would appear as is. For the second "box and whiskers" plotted in the graph, the North American Symptomatic Carotid Endarterectomy Trial (NASCET) results would be pooled with the ECST results to give a combined result, instead of the NASCET findings alone. In this case, because the findings for the two studies are very similar, the plot would look about the same except that the center box would be larger (indicating the combined populations of the two studies rather than just the population of NASCET) and the "whiskers" of the box (i.e., 95% confidence intervals) would be shorter (indicating the increased precision of the estimate of effect due to the increased sample size). Pooling data like this is justified only when all features of the studies being merged are very similar.

Finally, it is important to translate the results of a meta-analysis into clinically useful terms. For statistical purposes, a meta-analysis provides results of an intervention relative to a comparison group, using statistics such as odds ratios or relative risk. Both odds ratios and relative risks are difficult for clinicians to interpret. When they indicate a statistically significant effect, both can, and should, be reported along with absolute risk reductions (ARRs) and the number needed to treat (NNT). For example, the authors of the review from which Figure 2–2 is drawn reported their results as shown in Table 2–5, with adjustments for the differences in the measurement of carotid stenosis in the ECST and NASCET studies. All the information needed for these calculations is in Figure 2–2, and the definitions and procedures for doing the calculation are on the ACP Journal Club Web site at *http://www.acpjc.org/shared/glossary.htm*.

TABLE 2–5 **Details of Risk Reductions and Number Needed to Treat (NNT)**[a]

% Carotid Stenosis				
ECST	NASCET	RRR/I (95% CI)	ARR/I (95% CI)	NNT/H (95% CI)
82–99	70–99	RRR 48% (27%–63%)	ARR 6.7% (3.2%–10%)	NNT 15 (10–31)
70–81	50–69	RRR 27% (5%–44%)	ARR 4.7% (0.8%–8.7%)	NNT 21 (11–125)
<70	<50	RRI 20% (0%–44%)	ARI 2.2% (0%–4.4%)	NNH 45 (22–infinity)

[a]ECST, European Carotid Surgery Trial; NASCET, North American Symptomatic Carotid Endarterectomy Trial; RRR, relative risk reduction; RRI, relative risk increase; 95% CI, 95% confidence interval; ARR, absolute risk reduction; ARI, absolute risk increase; NNT, number needed to treat; NNH, number needed to harm.

✓ Choose your sample size.

Generally, SRs include all accessible studies. Therefore, there is no need to sample from available trials, just include them all. If, however, hordes of studies exist on the topic of your review (say >50), it is theoretically reasonable to take a random sample of these studies for detailed analysis rather than the whole lot (43). Doing so will limit your ability to analyze reasons for heterogeneity or to provide precise estimates for subgroups, but this loss may be acceptable if what you want and can afford is a general estimate of the summary effect size. If you will be sampling available studies, indicate the sampling method and provide the assumptions and calculations for the number of studies to be sampled. The principles and details for calculating sample sizes are discussed in several chapters, including Chapters 5, 6, and 7.

An arguably better way to limit the number of studies you need to analyze in detail is to set criteria for methodological excellence. Therefore, if there are few studies of a health care intervention, you could include all studies of all design types (randomized trials, nonrandomized trials, before-after studies, etc.), but if there are many randomized trials, limit the review to these. If there are many randomized trials, you can take this to the next level by limiting the review to higher quality trials, especially if the criteria you apply are based on methodological features that can be reproducibly assessed and that are known to reduce bias, such as randomization, concealment of allocation, and blinding (44), concepts that will be explored in detail in Chapters 5 and 6.

✓ Plan your budget.

Many, perhaps most, SRs are "labors of love" or part of the preparation for grant applications for original research. Engaging students in initiating or updating an SR is also an excellent way for them to learn the principles and practice of applied research and for investigators to do reviews on a slim budget. Many academic institutions and funding agencies have start-up funds for research that can be acquired for doing reviews without the bureaucratic rigmarole of a full-bore grant competition. These honorable traditions will no doubt continue.

Reviews are a lot of work, however, and it is desirable to seek adequate funds to train and pay research staff to do much of this. Few grant competitions exist for investigator-initiated SRs, but an increasing number of funding agencies commission reviews for topics of interest to them. The first step in seeking external funds to do SRs is therefore to find a funding source that wants a review that you want to do. An additional advantage of doing such reviews is that they often signal priorities of the funding agencies for original research—what better way to prepare!

Bearing in mind the amount available from funding sources that you plan to apply to, prepare a budget for the work needed to complete the review, including staff, literature searching and photocopying costs, software for handling references and meta-analysis, any needed computer hardware, mail or telephone costs to contact primary authors, travel costs for presentation of your findings, and publication costs. We won't go into the details here because the scope of reviews, the amount of funds available for doing reviews, and the allowability of various expenses are so variable that the best guide will be the detailed instructions of the funding agency. For example, reviews funded by agencies in Canada are often in the range of about Can $30,000, whereas US Agency for Healthcare Research and Quality (AHRQ) brokers reviews of the order of US $250,000. The quality of the review should be the same in either case, but the scope of AHRQ reviews is generally much broader than those in Canada. AHRQ reviews also require intensive interaction and negotiation with the organizations (such as the American Heart Association) that commission AHRQ reviews.

2.4 HOW MANY SYSTEMATIC REVIEWS SHOULD YOU DO?

We hope you will do lots of SRs! We end this chapter as we began it, with a reminder that SRs are an essential component of research translation, bridging the gaps between past and future research, and between research and health care. They are research projects in their own right and are the best way to begin any research project. The latest version of our CDSS review has now been published (48) and its findings have been incorporated into our latest clinical trial.

If you find that you are doing a lot of reviews, we suggest that you read a definitive resource for more options and ultimate means of achieving SR nirvana (45). And for reviews of diagnostic tests, a brief paper by Pai et al. (46) leads to a wealth of resources.

REFERENCES

1. Hunt DL, Haynes RB. Using old technology to implement modern computer-aided decision support for primary diabetes care. *Proc AMIA Annu Fall Symp* 2001;274–278.
2. Taylor FC, Cohen H, Ebrahim S. Systematic review of long term anticoagulation or antiplatelet treatment in patients with non-rheumatic atrial fibrillation. *BMJ* 2001;322:321–326.
3. Antithrombotic Trialists' Collaboration. Collaborative meta-analysis of randomised trials of antiplatelet therapy for prevention of death, myocardial infarction, and stroke in high risk patients. *BMJ* 2002;324:71–86.
4. Attia J, Hatala R, Cook DJ, et al. Does this adult patient have acute meningitis? *JAMA* 1999;282:175–181.
5. Garg AX, Suri RS, Barrowman N, et al. The long-term renal prognosis of diarrhea associated hemolytic uremic syndrome: a systematic review, meta-analysis and meta-regression of 3476 children from 49 studies. *JAMA* 2003;290:1360–1370.
6. Pearce N, Douwes J, Beasley R. Is allergen exposure the major primary cause of asthma? *Thorax* 2000;55:424–431.
7. Bunker SJ, Colquhoun DM, Esler MD, et al. Stress and coronary heart disease: psychosocial risk factors. *Med J Aust* 2003;178:272–276.
8. Deeks JJ. Systematic reviews in health care: systematic reviews of evaluations of diagnostic and screening tests. *BMJ* 2001;323:157–162.
9. Devillé WL, Buntinx F, Bouter LM, et al. Conducting systematic reviews of diagnostic studies: didactic guidelines. *BMC Med Res Methodol* 2002;2:9. *http://www.biomedcentral.com/1471-2288/2/9*
10. Shojania KG, Bero LA. Taking advantage of the explosion of systematic reviews: an efficient MEDLINE search strategy. *Eff Clin Pract* 2001;4:157–162.

11. Montori V, Wilczynski N, Morgan D, et al. for the Hedges Team. Optimal search strategies for retrieving systematic reviews from MEDLINE. *BMJ* 2005;330:68–73.

12. Hunt DL, Haynes RB, Hanna SE, et al. Effects of computer-based clinical decision support systems on physician performance and patient outcomes: a systematic review. *JAMA* 1998;280:1339–1346.

13. Dickersin K, Min Y-I, Meinert CL. Factors influencing publication of research results. Follow-up of applications submitted to two institutional review boards. *JAMA* 1992;267:374–378.

14. Easterbrook PJ, Berlin JA, Gopalan R, et al. Publication bias in clinical research. *Lancet* 1991;337:867–872.

15. Pham B, Platt R, McAuley L, et al. Is there a "best" way to detect and minimize publication bias? An empirical evaluation. *Eval Health Prof* 2001;24:109–125.

16. Begg CB, Mazumdar M. Operating characteristics of a rank correlation test for publication bias. *Biomertrics* 1994;50:1088–1101.

17. Egger M, Smith GD, Schneider M, et al. Bias in meta-analysis detected by a simple, graphical test. *BMJ* 1997;315:629–634.

18. Duval S, Tweedie R. Trim and fill: a simple funnel-plot-based method of testing and adjusting for publication bias in meta-analysis. *Biometrics* 2000;56:455–463.

19. Higgins JP, Thompson SG, Deeks JJ, et al. Measuring inconsistency in meta-analyses. *BMJ* 2003;327:557–560.

20. Moher D, Fortin P, Jadad AR, et al. Completeness of reporting of trials published in languages other than English: implications for conduct and reporting of systematic reviews. *Lancet* 1996;347:363–366.

21. Gregoire G, Derderian F, Le Lorier J. Selecting the language of the publications included in a meta-analysis: is there a tower of babel bias? *J Clin Epidemiol* 1995;48:159–163.

22. Egger M, Zellweger-Zahner T, Schneider M, et al. Language bias in randomised controlled trials published in English and German. *Lancet* 1997;350:326–329.

23. Moher D, Pham B, Klassen TP, et al. What contributions do languages other than English make on the results of meta-analyses? *J Clin Epidemiol* 2000;53:964–972.

24. Altman DG. *Practical statistics for medical research.* London: Chapman & Hall, 1991:404–409.

25. Fleiss JL, Levin B, Paik MC. Statistical methods for rates and proportions. *Wiley series in probability and statistics*, Chapter 18. New York: John Wiley & Sons, 2003.

26. Jadad AR, Moore RA, Carroll D, et al. Assessing the quality of reports of randomized clinical trials: is blinding necessary? *Control Clin Trials* 1996;17:1–12.

27. Schulz KF. Assessing allocation concealment and blinding in randomized controlled trials: why bother? *ACP J Club* 2000;132:A11–A13.

28. Moher D, Jadad A, Nichol G, et al. Assessing the quality of randomized controlled trials: an annotated bibliography of scales and checklists. *Control Clin Trials* 1995;16:62–73.

29. Moher D, Jadad AR, Tugwell P. Assessing the quality of randomized controlled trials: current issues and future directions. *Int J Tech Assess in Health Care* 1996;12:195–208.

30. Moher D, Pham B, Jones A, et al. Does quality of reports of randomised trials affect estimates of intervention efficacy reported in meta-analyses? *Lancet* 1998;352:609–613.

31. Juni P, Witschi A, Bloch R, et al. The hazards of scoring the quality of clinical trials for meta-analysis. *JAMA* 1999;282:1054–1060.

32. Schulz KF, Chalmers I, Hayes RJ, et al. Empirical evidence of bias. Dimensions of methodological quality associated with estimates on treatment effects in controlled trials. *JAMA* 1995;273:408–412.

33. Lazar HL, Chipkin S, Philippides G, et al. Glucose-insulin-potassium solutions improve outcomes in diabetics who have coronary artery operations. *Ann Thorac Surg* 2000;70:145–150.

34. Lazar HL, Chipkin SR, Fitzgerald CA, et al. Tight glycemic control in diabetic coronary artery bypass graft patients improves perioperative outcomes and decreases recurrent ischemic events. *Circulation* 2004;109:1497–1502.

35. Haynes RB, McDonald H, Garg AX. Interventions for helping patients to follow prescriptions for medications. (Cochrane Review). *The Cochrane Library*, Issue 2, Oxford: Update Software, 2002.

36. Cohen J. *Statistical power analysis for the behavioural sciences*. Hillsdale, NJ: Erlbaum, 1988.

37. Clarke M, Oxman A, eds. Cochrane reviewers' handbook [updated March 2003]. In: *The Cochrane Library*. Section 8. Issue 4, Chichester, UK: John Wiley & Sons, 2003.

38. Alderson P, Green S, Higgins JPT, eds. Glossary. Cochrane reviewers' handbook 4.2.2 [updated December 2003]. In: *The Cochrane Library*. Issue 1, 2004. Chichester, UK: John Wiley & Sons, 2003.

39. Cina CS, Clase CM, Haynes RB. Carotid endarterectomy for symptomatic carotid stenosis. *The Cochrane Library*. Issue 4, Chichester, UK: John Wiley & Sons, 2003.

40. Donner A, Piaggio G, Villar J. Meta-analyses of cluster randomization trials. Power considerations. *Eval Health Prof* 2003;26:340–351.

41. Schmid CH, Landa M, Jafar TH, et al. Constructing a database of individual clinical trials for longitudinal analysis. *Control Clin Trials* 2003;24:324–340.

42. Lau J, Antman EM, Jimenez-Silva J, et al. Cumulative meta-analysis of therapeutic trials for myocardial infarction. *N Engl J Med* 1992;327:248–254.

43. Morton SC, MacLean CH, Ofman J, et al. Different sampling strategies for identifying eligible studies: the effect on outcome of a meta-analysis of nonsteroidal antiinflammatory drug-associated dyspepsia. 7th Annual Cochrane Colloquium Abstracts, Rome, Oct. 1999.

44. Schulz KF. Assessing allocation concealment and blinding in randomized controlled trials: why bother? *ACP J Club* 2000;132:A11.

45. Egger M, Davey Smith G, Altman D, eds. *Systematic reviews in health care. Meta-analysis in context*, 2nd ed. London: BMJ Publishing Group, 2001. *http://www. systematicreviews.com*

46. Pai M, McCulloch M, Enanoria W, et al. Systematic reviews of diagnostic test evaluations: what's behind the scenes? *ACP Journal Club* 2004;141:A11.

47. Lobach DF. Electronically distributed, computer-generated, individualized feedback enhances the use of a computerized practice guideline. *Proc AMIA Annu Fall Symp* 1996;493–497.

48. Garg AX, Adhikari N, McDonald H, Rosas-Arellano MP, Devereaux PJ, Beyene J, Sam J, Haynes RB. Effects of computerized clinical decision support systems on practitioner performance and patient outcomes: a systematic review. *JAMA* 2005;293:1323-38.

APPENDIX 2.1 SEARCH STRATEGIES

Initial MEDLINE search strategy:

1. explode artificial intelligence and not robotics
2. decision making, computer-assisted
3. diagnosis, computer-assisted
4. therapy, computer-assisted
5. drug therapy, computer-assisted
6. explode evaluation studies
7. explode E5.318.760
8. (1 or 2 or 3 or 4 or 5) and (6 or 7)

Second MEDLINE search strategy (and number of articles retrieved):

1. explode decision making, computer-assisted (2548)
2. explode artificial intelligence and not robotics (1561)
3. 1 or 2 (3747)

4. 3 and explode evaluation studies (495)
5. 3 and explode longitudinal studies (159)
6. 3 and explode research design (35)
7. 3 and explode e5.318.760 (361)
8. 3 and randomized controlled trials (59)
9. 4 or 5 or 6 or 7 or 8 (816)
10. explode *decision making, computer-assisted or exp * artificial intelligence (2639)
11. 9 and 10 (548)
12. 11 and not for (la) (509)

Additional MEDLINE search strategy:

1. explode hospital information systems
2. limit to clinical trials

EMBASE search strategy:

1. DECISION MAKING (5278)
2. DC = E5.75.440? (14148)
3. 1 and 2 (291)
4. DECISION MAKING (5278)
5. INFORMATION SYSTEMS! (0)
6. DECISION MAKING AND INFORMATION SYSTEMS! (0)
7. DC = J2.40.10? (571892)
8. DC = J2.40.10.25? (77791)
9. DC = J2.40.10? OR DC = J2.40.10.25? (571892)
10. CLINICAL STUDY! (1107)
11. CLINICAL TRIAL! (74809)
12. CLINICAL STUDY! OR CLINICAL TRIAL! (75861)
13. 3 AND 9 (37)
14. PY = 1992 (348578)
15. PY = 1993 (362580)
16. PY = 1994 (363580)
17. PY = 1995 (172799)
18. 13 and (14 or 15 or 16 or 17) (30)
19. 18/ENG (29)

INSPEC search strategy:

1. EXPERT (33764)
2. SYSTEM? (981344)
3. 1 and 2 (29767)
4. EVALUAT? (180937)
5. 3 AND 4 (3135)
6. PY = 1992: 1995 (846969)
7. 5 AND 6 (929)
8. LA = ENGLISH (2760493)
9. 7 AND 8 (877)
10. MEDICAL (36305)

11. CLINICAL (11662)
12. MEDIC? (41400)
13. MEDICAL OR CLINICAL OR MEDIC? (46749)
14. 9AND13 (170)

APPENDIX 2.2 INSTRUCTIONS FOR REVIEWING CITATIONS (E-MAIL NOTE FOR OUR CDSS REVIEW)

To:
CDSS Review Team

From:
Brian Haynes

In a few minutes I will e-mail a large attachment containing half of the remaining search hits from the CDSS search. After downloading the document (may take a few minutes), and when you are ready to start rating, please carefully follow these instructions:

1. Open the large attachment into WORD.
2. Read and rate each article for relevance: R = relevant, N = not relevant, and PR = possibly relevant.
3. Mark your rating (preferably in red) directly on the document in WORD.
4. Attach your marked, completed document to an e-mail addressed to me at: anders@mcmaster.ca
5. Feel free to include notes, if any, with your rating.

Remember these caveats (from our last meeting):

1. We decided that all neural network studies are out (there is no knowledge base).
2. When in doubt about an article's relevance, put Possibly Relevant (PR).
3. Since we're only reviewing RCTs, if there is no evidence of evaluation, flunk it, and if there is an evaluation, it is still okay to flunk it if you can tell for certain that it is NOT an RCT; if it is unclear whether the CDSS was evaluated by an RCT, then rate as a PR.

APPENDIX 2.3 SAMPLE CDSS REVIEW DATA ABSTRACTION FORM (47)

Reviewer's initials: __BH____

Validity Criteria Scoring

1. Formation of groups
   2   random allocation
   1   quasi-random allocation
   0   selected controls
   •   not stated, follow-up with author

2. Experimental confounders: any baseline differences between groups potentially related to outcome?
   2   no, or yes, but statistically adjusted
   1   yes, no statistical adjustment
   0   can't tell

3. Unit of allocation
   2   practice, clinic, hospital
   1   physician
   0   patient

4. Outcome measure
   2   objective (not open to interpretation), or subjective with raters blind to allocation
   1   subjective outcome with raters not blind to allocation, but explicit criteria for defining outcome
   0   subjective outcome with raters not blind, no mention of explicit criteria

5. Follow-up
   2   outcome reported for 90% or more of participants
   1   outcome reported for 80% to 90% of participants
   0   outcome reported for less than 80% of participants

   Total: 9

1. Abstract (edited)

... The purpose of this study was to determine whether clinician use of a clinical practice guideline would increase in response to having, at the patient visit, a decision support system ... that generates customized management protocols for the individual patient. ... In a six-month controlled trial, 58 primary care clinicians were randomized to receive either a special encounter form with the computer-generated guideline recommendations, or a standard form. ... Availability of patient management recommendations resulted in a twofold increase in clinician compliance ...

2. CDSS

Program is linked to an electronic medical record system. It draws on routinely collected data from the record system and generates a list of recommendations for the care of individual diabetic patients, based on established primary care protocols for diabetes mellitus (DM). These recommendations are printed on encounter forms used by clinicians to record consultation results. The CDSS is automatically invoked when a request for an encounter form is submitted.

3. Setting

Primary care clinic and outpatient clinic.

4. Participants

All 58 primary care clinicians at the clinic (doctors, nurse practitioners, physician's assistants, residents) participated. Data from 28 (48.3%) of the clinicians was excluded because they did not meet predefined criteria for the minimum exposure to diabetes cases during the study. Each clinician must have seen a minimum of 6 different diabetic patients, and have assessed diabetes care in at least 12 encounters.

5. Allocation

The unit of allocation is the clinician. 58 clinicians were randomly assigned to receive encounter forms with CDSS generated recommendations or standard encounter forms. Of the 30 who remained eligible at the end of the study, 16 were in the CDSS group and 14 were in the control group.

6. Intervention and Procedure

See section 2.

7. Outcome Data

Provider outcomes focused on rates of compliance with DM care guidelines. Compliance was determined by audits of lab tests and paper-based medical records. A single clinician judged compliance by explicit criteria; it is not clear that he was blind to each clinician's allocation, but at least some of the criteria were objective.

8. Analysis and Results

Compliance rates were calculated as the percentage of "recommendations due" during an encounter that were followed by the clinicians. A measure of global adherence with the care guidelines was calculated as the percentage of the total number of recommendations for the patient to date (due or not) that had been implemented by the clinician.

8a. Results for provider behavior

	N	Median compliance rates (% of recommendations due)	Median global adherence rates (% of all recommendations)
CDSS	16	32.0	65.0
Control	14	15.6	40.5
Wilcoxon rank-sum		$P = 0.01$	$P < 0.01$

8b. Results for patient health outcomes

None reported.

FINDING INFORMATION ABOUT
THE BURDEN OF DISEASE

Peter Tugwell

When proposing a new study, it is essential to place the research in context by objectively documenting the magnitude of the misery and suffering from the condition of interest. This will provide a firm foundation for planning the study and also impress reviewers about the importance of the research.

CLINICAL RESEARCH SCENARIO

I had a recent opportunity to be a member of an interagency working group composed of investigators from the University of Ottawa (led by George Wells and Karin Kallander), the Karolinska Institute, the United Nations Children's Fund (UNICEF), and the World Health Organization (WHO) to develop a protocol to evaluate home management by mothers to reduce the mortality from malaria and pneumonia in children under five years of age in endemic low-income countries. Malaria and pneumonia cause more than 20% of all childhood deaths in sub-Saharan Africa (1–3). Delayed therapy is thought to be a major remediable factor for reducing this mortality (4). Fever and an increased respiratory rate is the commonest clinical presentation for both malaria and pneumonia, and these two conditions are frequently indistinguishable by mothers and other caregivers. For malaria, the WHO Roll Back Malaria (RBM) strategy recommends prompt administration of an effective antimalarial, preferably on the first day of fever (5). In Ethiopia, a controlled trial of teaching mothers to provide home treatment of malaria demonstrated a 40% decrease in mortality (6).

This does not solve the challenge of the residual mortality from pneumonia. In view of the impossibility of mothers reliably distinguishing between malaria and pneumonia, it is logical for the mother to give both the antimalarial and an antibiotic. However, there is reluctance to give mothers a supply of antibiotics because of the concern that excessive prescribing will lead to increased antibiotic resistance. This concern could be countered if it can be shown that home therapy does more good than harm compared to continuing to rely on local health care workers.

49

A two-arm controlled trial in six countries is being proposed to assess the impact that a program that educates families/community groups and provides sustainable drug supply of antimalarials and antibiotics will have on child survival. In the "malaria-only" arm, mothers will receive family/community access to antimalarials but will have to get antibiotics from health facilities. In the "combined" arm, the mothers will have access to both antimalarials and antibiotics.

Justifying such a trial, especially when resources for carrying it out are likely to be scarce, requires documenting the "burden of disease."

3.1 FINDING AND USING BURDEN OF DISEASE EVIDENCE IN JUSTIFYING AND PLANNING HEALTH CARE TRIALS

One of the most important ingredients of justifying a research study is the accurate portrayal of mortality risks, distressing symptoms, disability (i.e., mental and physical), and the economic burden of diseases that your study will seek to prevent or treat. These ingredients fall under the rubric "burden of disease," which can be defined as the effects of disease on the physical, emotional, and social well-being of the individual. Although some semblance of this information can be retrieved from many sources, including the studies in systematic reviews (Chapter 2), it is often obtained from selected populations or passed along from author to author, with the original source being lost or poorly justified. In this brief chapter, we will delve into the intricacies and mysteries of finding solid information about the burden of disease.

Surprisingly little work has been done on defining how to best search for this information, how much detail to include in a grant submission, and how to avoid bias. This last issue may seem surprising to those of us who glibly or gullibly cite dry and often inflated population statistics from the introductory section of a standard text in our applications for research funding. However, there is an understandable temptation to be selective in using data to justify the importance of the problem you wish to study. Most individuals have more than one disease in their later years—just look at all the conditions listed on a death certificate—but the champions for each disease try to attribute all of the morbidity and mortality to the disorder in which they are interested. One trouble with this is that when a study includes those individuals with only the one condition of interest, the risk for adverse outcomes often falls dramatically, so that the ensuing investigation ends up being hoisted on its own justification and underpowered for comparing interventions or exploring other hypotheses. Furthermore, even if all comers are accepted into an investigation, if the intervention is directed to only one condition, the effect will be diluted or drowned because of the competing conditions that can contribute to a given patient's demise. So what data should one include in justifying a study and planning its execution?

Although the WHO adopted an enlightened, inclusive definition of health in 1948 as "a state of physical, mental, and psychological well-being, and not merely the absence of disease," for many years the focus in assessing burden of illness was on premature mortality. Mere enlightenment is usually not enough to quickly change the way we do things, so it took quite awhile after the announcement of the WHO's holistic definition for the burden of illness statistics to reflect this. Until the 1990s, conventional measures of health status included life expectancy, infant mortality rate, and disease specific morbidity events (e.g., number of myocardial ischemic events). These individual measures were universally used to provide the basic framework of indicators of health status even though they could not be used for comparisons of one disease condition with another or be summed across disease conditions for comparing one group of people with another. Lack of a common measure for health status made direct comparisons over time or of one group with another impossible despite the dramatic changes occurring due to the "Epidemiologic transition" in countries from high to low premature mortality rates; this was characterized by changes in disease profile and age composition, that is, (a) reduced incidence or prevalence of infectious diseases, (b) increased prevalence of noncommunicable and degenerative diseases, and (c) increase in the proportion of elderly and geriatric individuals in a population.

At the end of the 20th century, 52 years after its founding, the WHO established the Global Burden of Disease initiative and adopted a set of summary measures of population health status and reported these in its annual World Health Report (1), including a set of health status measurements for different countries using the "disability-adjusted life-year" (DALY) as the unifying metric that combines the impact of diseases on mortality as well as morbidity. This is the number of fully healthy life-years lost to a particular disease or condition or risk factor. It incorporates the age at which the death occurs and the duration and severity of any disability created. Note in the figures that disabling conditions such as mental health and musculoskeletal diseases are missing from the mortality tables (see Figure 3–1) but dominate the disability measures (see Figure 3–2 and Table 3–1). These data are also available by condition for most clinical conditions, such as those in Table 3–1 summarized by country.

A major strength of the DALY is that it provides a standardized metric so that the sum of mortality and morbidity can be compared across conditions. This combination allows conditions with different mixes of mortality and morbidity to be compared. This metric also handles "competing risks": it allows each individual to die only once! Previously, if a person died with two diseases such as diabetes and cardiac decompensation, the diabetes and cardiovascular advocacy groups each claimed the death.

This Global Burden of Disease initiative has been extremely controversial, mainly because the data were unavailable for most lower- and middle-income countries and, therefore, had to be estimated (8).

Inequity or unfairness in the distribution of the burden of disease must also be considered. In most cases, disease is more prevalent among the poor and disadvantaged. Conversely, if the relative benefits of intervention are stable across populations, the poor and disadvantaged will have greater absolute benefit from a prevention or cure than the more privileged (9)—providing, of course, that they receive the intervention.

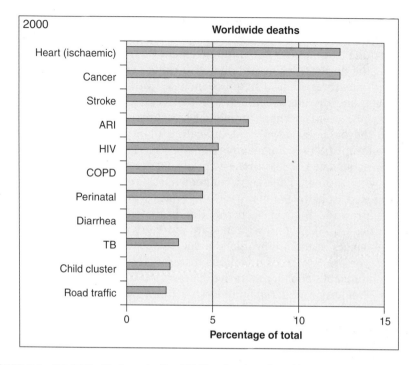

FIGURE 3-1 World Health Organization (WHO) estimates of worldwide deaths by cause for the year 2000 as a percentage of total mortality. ARI, acute respiratory illness; HIV, human immunodeficiency virus; TB, tuberculosis; COPD, chronic obstructive pulmonary disease; Child Cluster, childhood illnesses.

Let's take the Home and Community Management of Malaria and Pneumonia project described at the beginning of the chapter and look at how we went about assessing the burden of disease from these conditions and how we might have done better.

> Search strategy. We searched MEDLINE using the key words "malaria and burden and review," retrieving 55 hits of which 11 were relevant, and we searched with the terms "pneumonia and Africa and burden and review," yielding 5 hits of which 2 were relevant with useful references although not comprehensive.

This could clearly have been done better, by searching for original articles as well as reviews and by using a powerful search strategy, such as the one for systematic reviews in PubMed (*http://web.ncbi.nlm.nih.gov/entrez/query/static/clinical.shtml*). Amends will be made later in this chapter.

Another generic approach to finding information on the burden of disease is to Google it. In this case, a search on Google for "malaria burden of disease" produces a first page link to the malaria part of the Web site

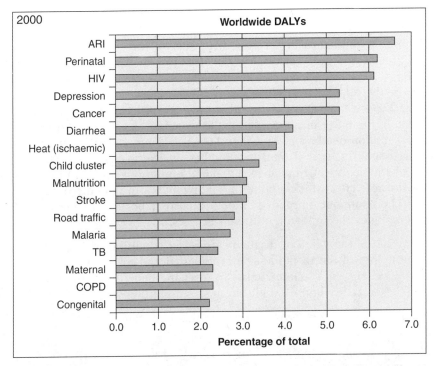

FIGURE 3–2 World Health Organization (WHO) estimates of disability-adjusted life-years (DALY) by cause for the year 2000 as percentage of total disability. ARI, acute respiratory illness; HIV, human immunodeficiency virus; Child Cluster, childhood illnesses; TB, tuberculosis; COPD, chronic obstructive pulmonary disease.

TABLE 3–1 The Leading Causes of Years Lived with Disability, Worldwide, 1990 (7)

Condition	Total (millions)	Percentage of total
All causes	472.7	100
Unipolar major depression	50.8	10.7
Iron deficiency anemia	22.0	2.7
Falls	22.0	2.6
Alcohol use	15.8	3.3
Chronic obstructive pulmonary disease	14.7	3.1
Bipolar disorder	14.1	3.0
Congenital anomalies	13.5	2.9
Osteoarthritis	13.3	2.8
Schizophrenia	12.1	2.6
Obsessive compulsive disorders	10.2	2.2

From Lopez AD. A comprehensive assessment of mortality and disability from diseases, injuries, and risk factors in 1990 and projected to 2020. In: Murray CJL, Lopez AD, eds. *The global burden of disease.* Boston, MA: Harvard University Press, 1996, with permission.

of the World Health Report described above: *http://www.who.int/rbm/ Presentations/MIP-RBM-final/tsld002.htm*. This Web site cites 300 to 500 million clinical cases per year, with 80% of these cases in Africa, and a million deaths per year, with 90% of deaths in Africa, and substantial disability, 40 million DALYs lost annually.

In the appendices of the main WHO report (*http://www.who.int/ whr/2002/en/*), we can also find that lower respiratory infections were responsible for 6.8% of all deaths in the world at all ages. In Africa, there were 1 million deaths and 31 billion DALYs. The methodology in the main report reassures us that the total number of deaths could not exceed the sum of the deaths attributed to individual conditions and that these numbers do not reflect double counting—individuals can only die once.

The economic burden of illness is also important to include. This term includes the following different aspects.

1. What is the value of disability from the condition of interest and of the loss of life to the affected individual and to society?
2. What are the economic costs in foregone benefits arising because of the mortality and disability from this condition?

Here is an example of how to look for this information:

> To check on the economic burden, we searched MEDLINE (via Ovid) using the keywords "malaria and economic burden" (46 hits; 11 useful) and "pneumonia and economic burden" (45 hits; 10 useful). Again, Google came up with some complementary hits, including, for malaria and economic burden, one of the seminal articles by Gallup and Sachs (10).

Our searches produced some useful citations, but for a research proposal it is important to be comprehensive. Clinical investigators are not usually adept literature searchers, so it is wise to seek the assistance of a medical librarian who can help you ensure that you are searching the appropriate databases and information sources as well as using the best strategies (11). We asked an experienced librarian colleague at the University of Ottawa, Jessie McGowan, for help and to tell us how she went about this search. Here's a blow-by-blow account, with a view to showing you "expert-level" searching, allowing you to follow along, illustrating that searching is an iterative process, and providing a few tips that you may be able to use yourself or negotiate with a librarian.

Jessie's approach begins with reviewing the search question, separating it into concepts or elements that can be searched separately, making sure to identify the patient, intervention/comparison, and outcome (remember PICOT from Chapter 1?). When searching in any database, she uses the controlled vocabulary of indexing terms for that database. In MEDLINE, the indexing terms are called MeSH (Medical Subject Heading), and this is the most efficient way to begin searching this database.

Filters can be used depending on the type of clinical or research question being addressed. Some examples of filters include limiting articles to publication types (i.e., meta-analyses, clinical practice guidelines, animal types, or language) (12,13). In this case, Jessie added in a filter for burden of illness. The concept of burden of illness is indexed in both the MEDLINE and EMBASE databases with the subject heading "cost of illness." Although the definition in MEDLINE has "cost" in it, the emphasis is meant to be on social costs (to society or the individuals concerned) rather than monetary costs. The MeSH term "burden of illness" was introduced in 1993. From 1966 to 1992 it was indexed under "costs and cost analysis."

To increase the comprehensiveness of the search, it is useful here to include the following text words: burden of illness, burden of disease, health burden, global burden, quality of life, DALY, mortality, disease cost, sickness cost, and illness cost. A textword search will identify the occurrence of a word or phrase in the title (TI) and abstract (AB) fields of the citation. She notes that when textword searching, one must be careful to account for variations in spelling and synonyms and to use truncation to identify different endings to terms (e.g., singular versus plural). Therefore, when using the term "burden$" in MEDLINE, the truncation symbol "$" means that the search engine would retrieve any citations that contain the words "burden," "burdens," "burdened" and so on.

Searching the current literature about the burden of illness for childhood malaria and pneumonia, Jessie developed the following basic search for MEDLINE using subject headings and textword terms for malaria and pneumonia.

DATABASE: OVID MEDLINE

1. exp Malaria/
2. (plasmodium infection$ or malaria).tw.
3. exp Pneumonia/
4. (pulmonary inflammation or lung inflammation or pneumon$).tw
5. or/1-4
6. cost of illness/
7. (burden adj2 (illness or disease$)).tw.
8. ((health or global) adj2 burden).tw.
9. ((disease$ or sickness or illness) adj2 cost$).tw.
10. quality-adjusted life years/
11. (daly or Disability Adjusted Life Year).tw.
12. or/6-11
13. 5 and 12
14. limit 13 to yr = 2000–2004
15. limit 14 to all child <0 to 18 years>
16. from 15 keep 8 (105)

This search resulted in 105 articles from MEDLINE (1998 to July 2003), 88 of which were relevant—much better than what we found ourselves. This allowed us to be reasonably certain that the search strategy has good specificity (so few irrelevant articles will be retrieved)—but what about sensitivity? We'll return to this in a moment.

This search of MEDLINE was performed using Ovid as an interface. The number in parenthesis in the last line of the search is the number of citations retrieved. The terms with a backslash (/) indicate MeSH terms. The terms with .tw. after them are textwords. [Remember, the textword function searches the title (TI) and abstract (AB) fields]. You can use this search when a MeSH term is not available or to be more thorough in the searching. When searching for textwords where the prefix, suffix, or other such variations need to be taken into account, you can also truncate the term you are searching for by adding the truncation symbol "$." Proximity terms like "adj" are used to indicate that one term needs to be near another term. For example, "ADJ2" indicates that the terms can be two words apart anywhere in a title or the abstract of the article.

However, Jessie notes that in the above search she did not add terms for mortality, morbidity, incidence, or prevalence, which are also part of the burden of disease profile. She was concerned that some relevant studies might be missed. Adding in these terms will make the search strategy more inclusive. In the following strategy, she added lines 12 to 16 to include these concepts in the controlled vocabulary and with textword terms.

DATABASE: OVID MEDLINE

Search Strategy:

1. exp Malaria/
2. (plasmodium infection$ or malaria).tw.
3. exp Pneumonia/
4. (pulmonary inflammation or lung inflammation or pneumon$).tw.
5. or/1-4
6. cost of illness/
7. (burden adj2 (illness or disease$)).tw.
8. ((health or global) adj2 burden).tw.
9. ((disease$ or sickness or illness) adj2 cost$).tw.
10. quality-adjusted life years/
11. (daly or Disability Adjusted Life Year).tw.
12. exp Morbidity/
13. exp Mortality/
14. Life Expectancy/
15. (incidence or morbidity or mortality prevalence).tw.
16. mo.fs.
17. or/6-16
18. 5 and 17
19. limit 18 to yr = 2000–2004
20. limit 19 to all child <0 to 18 years> (2426)

The retrieval now jumps to 2,426 citations for the same period as the preceding search. If this approach is taken, Jessie suggests that the researcher consider the types of studies that she or he wishes to retrieve. To retrieve studies that focus on literature review articles and health surveys, Jessie added lines 21 through 24 to limit the search:

21. review.pt.
22. health surveys/
23. or/21-23
24. 20 and 24 (295)

This reduces the second search set from 2,426 to 295 citations.

Jessie notes that this broader strategy retrieves additional relevant articles that were not included in the first search—and also many citations that were not relevant to the question in this strategy (specificity and precision have fallen)—but, overall, the recall was better (i.e., higher sensitivity, the ability of the search to retrieve all relevant studies).

The bottom line is that from the search outlined above we were able to reassure ourselves that the WHO Burden of Illness study was by far the most comprehensive and authoritative source for the burden of disease from malaria and acute respiratory infections. Despite the variable quality of the data sources such that the exact numbers may not be totally accurate, no one contests the high rankings of these conditions. Thus, the case was relatively easy to make by using the World Health Report 2002 material in the introduction to the research proposal.

This information is also extremely useful for sample size estimation—for example, two references give the baseline mortality rates for malaria (14) and acute respiratory infections (15) that are needed for calculating the sample size required to detect a 25% reduction in mortality with the appropriate adjustment for a cluster design.

REFERENCES

1. Prentice T, ed. *The World Health Report 2002*. Geneva: World Health Organization, 2002.

2. Williams BG, Gouws E, Boschi-Pinto C, et al. Estimates of world-wide distribution of child deaths from acute respiratory infections. *Lancet Infect Dis* 2002;2:25–32.

3. Greenwood B. Malaria mortality and morbidity in Africa. *Bull World Health Organ* 1999;77:91–99.

4. Tupasi TE. Determinants of morbidity and mortality due to acute respiratory infections: implications for intervention. *J Infect Dis* 1988;157:615–623.

5. Delacollette C, ed. *Roll back malaria: global threat against infectious disease*. Geneva: World Health Organization, 2002. *http://www.doh.gov.za/issues/malaria/red_reference/epidemics/epi3.pdf*

6. Kidane G, Morrow RH. Teaching mothers to provide home treatment of malaria in Tigray, Ethiopia: a randomised trial. *Lancet* 2000;356:550–555.

7. Lopez AD. A comprehensive assessment of mortality and disability from diseases, injuries, and risk factors in 1990 and projected to 2020. In: Murray CJL, Lopez AD, eds. *The global burden of disease*. Boston, MA: Harvard University Press, 1996.

8. Almeida C, Braveman P, Gold MR, et al. Methodological concerns and recommendations on policy consequences of the World Health Report 2000. *Lancet* 2001;357: 1692–1697.

9. McAlister FA. Commentary: relative treatment effects are consistent across the spectrum of underlying risks ... usually. *Int J Epidemiol* 2002;31:76–77.

10. Gallup JL, Sachs JD. The economic burden of malaria. *Am J Trop Med Hyg* 2001;64(Suppl. 1–2):85–96.

11. McGowan J. For expert literature searching, call a librarian. *CMAJ* 2001;165:1301–1302.

12. Hunt DL, McKibbon KA. Locating and appraising systematic reviews. *Ann Intern Med* 1997;126:532–538.

13. Haynes RB, Wilczynski N, McKibbon KA, et al. Developing optimal search strategies for detecting clinically sound studies in MEDLINE. *J Am Med Inform Assoc* 1994;1:447–458.

14. Korenromp EL, Williams BG, Gouws E, et al. Measurement of trends in childhood malaria mortality in Africa: an assessment of progress toward targets based on verbal autopsy. *Lancet Infect Dis* 2003;3:349–358.

15. Mulholland K. Global burden of acute respiratory infections in children: implications for interventions. *Pediatr Pulmonol* 2003;36:469–474.

AN INTRODUCTION TO PERFORMING THERAPEUTIC TRIALS

Dave Sackett

Chapter Outline

CLINICAL RESEARCH SCENARIO

In 1969, two methodologists met with a senior neurologist and a basic scientist. The neurologist, Henry Barnett, was a clinical expert in the diagnosis and management of cerebrovascular disease. The basic scientist, Fraser Mustard, was an expert in blood platelet function. One of the methodologists was Mike Gent, a biostatistician with substantial prior experience in randomized controlled trials (RCTs). The other was me, a novice clinical epidemiologist contemplating his first-ever RCT. The hospital that later housed our Department of Clinical Epidemiology and Biostatistics was still under construction, so we met in the tub and shower room of our temporary quarters at a tuberculosis sanatorium.

We met because we shared the idea that drugs that affect platelet function in the laboratory [sulfinpyrazone (brand name: Anturan) and aspirin] might be beneficial to patients with transient ischemic attacks. These strokelike episodes strike suddenly, and last just a few minutes or hours. However, they are the harbingers of permanent and fatal strokes. In 1969, the only RCT-validated treatment for transient ischemic attacks was treating associated severe hypertension (i.e., diastolic blood pressures of 115 mm Hg or more) (1).

Could we design and execute a study that would determine whether the drugs that worked so well at the bench, on blood platelets, did more good than harm, in the clinic, to patients with transient ischemic attacks? Our tactics for doing so, plus the principles on which these tactics were based will provide the framework for Chapters 5 and 6, respectively. Although we performed this "Phase 3" RCT almost four decades ago, its fundamental concept, strategies, and tactics remain relevant today. We will describe many refinements as well.

We named our study long before the fad of euphonious acronyms, and simply called it the "Recent Recurrent Presumed Cerebral Emboli" or RRPCE Study (might we name it the "Aspirin and/or Sulfinpyrazone for Stroke" study today?). We admitted our first patient in November 1971, and our last one in June 1976. We treated and followed all survivors for one more year and closed out the trial on 30 June 1977. Our primary results were published in July 1978 (2).

If you can imagine yourself as a player in that scenario (ignoring the dates!), the next three chapters may be worth your while. They are about a particular set of strategies and tactics for determining whether a pill, an operation, or any other health care intervention does more good than harm to those who receive it: the RCT.

4.1 AREN'T THERE EASIER WAYS TO DETERMINE THE VALUE OF A TREATMENT?

There are plenty of other ways to decide about the value of a treatment, ranging from asking the best-dressed and loudest (and, therefore, most expert) clinician in the room (3) to carrying out a systematic review of all relevant RCTs. The former, "expert" approach is so fallible as to be the butt of jokes and lawsuits (HRT, anyone?) (4). And Chapter 2 in this book has shown you how to carry out the latter, even more powerful systematic review.

On the other hand, interventions that lead to survival in illnesses that were universally fatal till then (say, the first time streptomycin was used for tuberculous meningitis) don't need RCTs to confirm their worth (this "all-or-none" notion is discussed in Section 5.9 (Special Ethical Issues In RCTs).

But what about observational studies, such as cohort-analytic studies of treated and untreated patients or case–control studies of patients who do and don't have certain outcomes? As you'll learn in Section 5.6 (in the discussion on harm), these observational studies are vastly superior to RCTs in detecting rare but awful adverse effects of treatments. However, when observational studies are employed in searching for moderate treatment benefits, they too often mislead us. This generalization, discussed in some detail in Section 6.1, "Confounding, and How To Break It," is supported by systematic reviews that compared observational studies with RCTs of the same treatments for the same conditions and found the former to be simply unreliable (5,6).

For a personal example, we've long known that patients undergoing carotid endarterectomy were at risk of perioperative stroke and death. In searching for ways to reduce these complications, we wondered whether high-dose aspirin might be beneficial (it looked better than low-dose aspirin at the bench). Because we already had some observational data in hand, we compared the perioperative stroke and death rates between a cohort receiving little or no aspirin at the time of their endarterectomies versus an otherwise identical second cohort receiving high-dose aspirin. We found that the cohort of patients who received 0 to 325 mg of aspirin had almost four times the risk of perioperative stroke and death as the cohort receiving 650 to 1,300 mg of aspirin daily.

Despite the large advantage from high-dose aspirin in this observational study, we remained uncertain and decided that we had to test high-versus low-dose aspirin in an RCT. Some of our surgical colleagues were so certain that high-dose aspirin was preferable that they refused to join our trial. However, to everyone's surprise, the trial proved that our observational conclusion was dead wrong. Patients randomized to low-dose aspirin had 26% *fewer* strokes, heart attacks, and deaths than patients randomized to high-dose aspirin (7).

4.2 FOR WHOM WAS THIS CHAPTER WRITTEN?

I selected the content, vocabulary, depth, and style of this chapter to serve a specific audience, and I hope you are in it. First, I wrote it for clinical-practice researchers (8) at any stage in your careers (i.e., from beginning students to seasoned investigators). Thus, I assume that you are competent in the relevant clinical or health care discipline and in the target disorder you want to treat, or are working with others in a team who have these clinical competencies. Second, I wrote it under the assumption that, although you want to carry out RCTs, you don't know much about mathematics or biostatistics. I don't assume that you have any math beyond secondary school nor any but the vaguest recall of any biostatistics courses you may have taken since then.

That's not to say that others might also find this chapter useful, perhaps including some of the real biostatisticians who are trying to teach the rest of us how to do RCTs (and I apologize in advance to these real methodologists for any of the bits of it that make them cringe).

Finally, if you need your RCT to generate a positive result, regardless of the truth, and don't want to wade through this chapter before you carry it out, you can skip all this methodology stuff and hire our team at HARLOT, plc to guide your every step (9).

4.3 HOW IS THIS CHAPTER ORGANIZED?

This chapter is organized like the others in this book:

- It starts with a scenario (you've just read it) describing the conception of an actual study.
- It then carries that scenario through each step in planning, executing, analyzing, and interpreting such a study. Each step includes a

tactical checklist and a highly practical explanation of how you can execute each of these tactics in your own study.

• For those of you who want to expand your understanding of the *principles* behind the tactics, these in-depth discussions are included in Chapter 6. As promised above, these discussions stick to simple math and employ lots of pictures.

4.4 SOME DEFINITIONS: WHAT DO I MEAN BY "EFFICACY" AND "EFFECTIVENESS"?

Several theoretical concepts and practical situations will recur throughout Chapters 4 to 6. To minimize your confusion, I have assigned specific names to each of them, and will define these names the first time I employ them. Here are the first three:

> To denote *both* the beneficial *and* harmful effects of an intervention when it is applied under ideal circumstances, I'll use the term: *efficacy*

> To denote *both* the beneficial *and* harmful effects of an intervention when it is applied under the usual circumstances that apply in health care, I'll use the term: *effectiveness*

> When speaking in general terms about the consequences of treatment, either good or bad or both, I'll use the term: *effects*.

4.5 SOME SIMPLE (BUT OFTEN UNRECOGNIZED) TRUTHS ABOUT RANDOMIZED CONTROLLED TRIALS

After working for 35 years trying to get the strategies and tactics of RCTs right, I've reached two sets of conclusions. Both sets underpin much of Chapters 5 and 6, and you deserve to see them at the start of it. The first set, shown in Table 4–1, comprise simple but profound truths that took me several years to recognize. I hope to save you that time.

4.6 SOME OF MY BIASES ABOUT RANDOMIZED CONTROLLED TRIALS

The second set of conclusions, shown in Table 4–2, are strong personal opinions about how trialists ought to behave. In an era in which lots of trialists and their institutions are for sale to the highest bidder (10), these opinions may be seen either as useful guides to behavior or simply as the anachronistic prejudices of an old fart.

You might find three excursions into RCT principles relevant to this introduction. The first of them (Section 6.1, "Confounding and How To Break It") will explain more fully why subexperiments are an insufficient basis for determining whether a treatment is beneficial. The second

(Section 6.2, "A Tiny Bit of History") will give you a tiny taste of the history of RCTs. And the third (Section 6.3,"Phase I–IV Trials") will walk you through the different stages that a promising treatment might pass through on its way to becoming established, effective therapy.

TABLE 4–1　**Some Simple Truths About Randomized Trials**

	Simple Truth	Explained
1	The important number in your RCT is the number of events you observe, not the number of participants you recruit.	Section 6.6, "Determinants of the signal, and how they can be manipulated to maximize it"
2	The proportion of eligible patients who are randomized is irrelevant to decisions about efficacy unless the patients systematically differ in their responsiveness to experimental treatment.	Section 5.3, "Participant Selection"
3	If you consider an RCT as a diagnostic test for whether a treatment is beneficial, its sensitivity is represented by its power.	Section 5.8, "Calculate your sample size requirement"
4	To halve the confidence interval around your treatment effect, you have to recruit four times as many participants.	Section 5.8, "Sample Size"
5	You should routinely observe "quantitative" differences in the degree (a lot or a little) to which different subgroups of study patients respond to treatments.	Section 6.11, "Large, Simple Trials"
6	You should (almost) never observe "qualitative" differences in the direction (good for some, harmful or powerfully useless in others) in which different subgroups of study patients respond to treatments.	Section 6.11 "Large, Simple Trials"
7	There is no such thing as a "negative" RCT nor one that "proves" that there is "no difference" between two treatments.	Section 5.7, Analysis: "Never describe your indeterminate trial "negative," or as showing "no difference"
8	The number of patients you needed to convert your indeterminate trial into an informative one depends on what you found at the end of the trial, not on your sample size calculations at its beginning.	Section 5.7, Analysis: "Never describe your indeterminate trial "negative," or as showing "no difference"
9	"End-of-study" tests for blindness of patients and clinicians don't test for blindness; they test for hunches about efficacy.	Section 5.5, "Should you test for blindness during and after your trial?"

RCT, randomized controlled trial.

TABLE 4–2 **Some Personal Opinions About Randomized Trials**

1 If you don't start looking for a biostatistician co-principal investigator the same day that you start formulating your study question, you are a fool, and deserve neither funding nor a valid answer.
2 Once a treatment has been shown to be effective in a systematic review of high-quality RCTs, you are both stupid and unethical if you test its promising challenger against a placebo among patients who would otherwise be taking it.
3 Consider the possibility that the Secretariat of the "International Conference on Harmonization of Technical Requirements for Registration of Pharmaceuticals for Human Use" just might be heavily influenced by big pharmaceutical companies.
4 Never mistake uncertainty for theoretical equipoise.
5 Field data should never be channeled through or controlled by an RCT's sponsor, regardless of whether it's a benevolent government, a voluntary health organization, or a manufacturer out to make a profit.
6 Nobody who works for or holds stock in the sponsor should sit on an RCT's Data Safety and Monitoring Board.
7 Research ethics committees delay effective treatments, and their claims that their ever-growing regulations will actually serve patients are rarely evidence-based.
8 No RCT should be approved until it has been registered in an international all-comers registry that assigns unique numbers (such as Controlled Clinical Trials' meta-Register or the ISRCTN).
9 Untested expensive technologies should only be available within RCTs.

RCT, randomized controlled trial; ISRCTN, International Standard Randomized Controlled Trial Number.

If you have a question or comment about any of this chapter (or if you've caught us in a typo!) go to the book's Web site at *http://hiru. mcmaster.ca/CLEP3*. There you also will find comments from us and other readers, chapter updates, and examples of how the authors and others use the book in teaching.

REFERENCES

1. Veterans Administration Cooperative Study Group on Antihypertensive Agents. Results in patients with diastolic blood pressures averaging 115 through 129 mm Hg. *JAMA* 1967;202:1028–1034.
2. The Canadian Cooperative Study Group. A randomized trial of aspirin and sulfinpyrazone in threatened stroke. *N Engl J Med* 1978;299:53–59.
3. Oxman AD, Chalmers I, Liberati A, on behalf of the World Artifexology Group. A field guide to experts. *BMJ* 2004;329:1460–1463.
4. Sackett DL. The sins of expertness and a proposal for redemption. *BMJ* 2000;320:1283.

5. Britton A, McKee M, Black N, et al. Choosing between randomised and non-randomised studies: a systematic review. *Health Technol Assess* 1998;2:13.

6. Kunz R, Vist G, Oxman AD. Randomisation to protect against selection bias in health care trials (Cochrane Methodology Review). Updated 22 Aug 2001. In: *The Cochrane Library*. Issue 3, Chichester, UK: John Wiley & Sons, 2004.

7. Taylor DW, Barnett HJM, Haynes RB, et al. ASA and Carotid Endarterectomy (ACE) trial collaborators. Low-dose and high-dose acetylsalicylic acid for patients undergoing carotid endarterectomy: a randomised controlled trial. *Lancet* 1999;353:2179–2184.

8. Sackett DL. The fall of "clinical" research and the rise of "clinical-practice research". *Clin Invest Med* 2000;23:331–333.

9. Sackett DL, Oxman AD. HARLOT plc: an amalgamation of the world's two oldest professions. *BMJ* 2003;327:1442–1445.

10. Horton R. The clinical trial: deceitful, disputable, unbelievable, unhelpful, and shameful–What next? *Control Clin Trials* 2001;22:593–604.

THE TACTICS OF PERFORMING THERAPEUTIC TRIALS

Dave Sackett

Chapter Outline

5.1 LITERATURE REVIEW

When we designed the Recent Recurrent Presumed Cerebral Emboli (RRPCE) trial in 1969, the bibliographic database called "Index Medicus" was available only in print. Moreover, the personal computers that we use so casually today for searching the literature wouldn't even exist for another decade. Our literature review therefore consisted of hand-searching annual and monthly issues of Index Medicus, plus our recall of relevant articles, and a search of our personal files. The result, as it appeared in our original grant application to the Canadian Medical Research Council (MRC), summarized just 39 clinical papers. No randomized control trials (RCTs) had been carried out yet, so we cited a single cohort study, a community-based incidence survey, several case-series, and a host of expert opinions. Our application also cited 13 papers describing bench research into the effects of our proposed drugs on platelets and platelet-function (and more than 60% of these had been written by our colleagues at McMaster). This primitive review reinforced our optimistic uncertainty about the value of aspirin and sulfinpyrazone for transient ischemic attacks (TIA). Fortunately, the MRC agreed and funded our trial.

Twenty-three years later, another review, on the same topic but different in almost every other way, was published. This review (to which we'd contributed our RRPCE results) summarized individual patient data from 197 antiplatelet trials involving over 135,000 patients.

This scenario illustrates not only the extremes of the depth of literature reviews, but also how they have evolved over the past three decades. The decade following the publication of the RRPCE trial witnessed a flurry of "antiplatelet" RCTs. To make better sense of them, Richard Peto and Colin Baigent at the Clinical Trial Service Unit in Oxford invited their investigators to collaborate in carrying out systematic reviews of the accumulating evidence (1). The resulting "Antithrombotic Trialists' Collaboration" has updated its initial review about every 5 years, most recently in 2002 (2), applying the following tactics. Rather than belabor our primitive efforts of 35 years, let's take a look at the current state of the art, set by this group.

The Review Question

Among patients at high risk of stroke, myocardial infarction, and other occlusive vascular events, can antiplatelet therapy reduce the occurrence of these events?

Identification of Trials

The Antithrombotic Trialists' Collaboration used several strategies for finding possibly relevant trials:

- Electronic search of a growing number of bibliographic databases: Medline, Embase, Derwent, Scisearch, Biosis, and trials registers of the Cochrane Stroke and Peripheral Vascular Disease Groups.
- Hand-search of relevant journals, abstracts, and proceedings of meetings.
- Scrutiny of reference lists of trials and review articles.
- Inquiry among colleagues and pharmaceutical companies.

Eligibility of Trials

They unearthed 448 apparently randomized trials comparing an antiplatelet regimen with a control or other antiplatelet regimen in an "unconfounded" fashion; that is, the patients in these trials differed only in their antiplatelet therapy. The entry characteristics of the patients in these trials suggested a greater than 3% annual risk of vascular events (either because of their risk factors or because they already had suffered an event). After rigorous review of these trials (including direct contact with study coordinators), they excluded 166 trials: 52 were not properly randomized, 24 had confounded antiplatelet therapy with other interventions,

3 had large losses-to-follow-up, 13 had been abandoned before collecting any outcome data, 20 had a crossover design, and 54 had not systematically recorded any of the relevant events. They also excluded 66 trials restricted to dementia or occluded retinal veins. Finally, 19 trials were never able to provide essential information for meta-analyses. Although these rigorous criteria excluded more than half of the studies they unearthed, 197 trials, involving over 135,000 patients, were available for their most recent systematic review.

Data Gathered for the Systematic Review

Besides the published results of these trials, the reviewers gathered two additional sets of data for more refined analyses. First, they asked trialists with less than 200 patients in their RCTs to provide *summary tables* of patients and events in a standard format. Second, they asked trialists with 200 or more patients to provide both summary tables and *individual patient data* on baseline characteristics (age, sex, blood pressure, and medical history), follow-up, and vascular events. Finally, they gathered data on major complications of antithrombotic therapy

Analysis .

Accordingly, the Antithrombotic Trialists' Collaboration could enter three levels of data into their analysis: published results, standard tables, and individual patient data. These three levels nicely illustrate the double-edged sword of meta-analysis: evermore-informative data are evermore difficult and expensive to obtain.

As described in their 2002 report, they began by creating 2×2 tables showing outcomes by treatments for each individual trial. Then, for each treatment in each trial, they calculated the observed minus expected number of events (O-E), and its variance (V). By dividing each (O-E) by the square root of its variance, they could calculate the statistical significance (z) of any treatment effects. They then looked to see whether the same treatment had the same or different effectiveness from trial to trial (a test for "heterogeneity"), and where appropriate, combined the trial results for different treatments and different vascular outcomes. They expressed the impact of treatment in the form of odds ratios plus confidence intervals (so that odds ratios less than 1.0 suggested that the antiplatelet therapy was effective). Finally, they expressed the practical health impact of treatment in terms of the number of thrombotic events it would prevent per thousand patients treated with it for a given time.

Results and Interpretation

Antiplatelet therapy reduced the odds of any serious vascular event by about one fourth; nonfatal myocardial infarction by one third; nonfatal stroke by one fourth, and vascular mortality by one sixth. The "number of patients needed to be treated" (NNT) for 2 years to prevent one more serious vascular event was 28 for patients with prior myocardial infarction, previous stroke, or TIA. Finally, the absolute benefits of antiplatelet therapy substantially outweighed the absolute risks of major extracranial bleeding.

The results of this systematic review provide a firm basis for prescribing antiplatelet drugs for a number of clinical problems and also provide a foundation for new trials, with treatments that have not been tested adequately to date. I close this section of the chapter with the happy expectation that, like the Collaborative Review Groups of the Cochrane Collaboration, the Antithrombotic Trialists' Collaboration will continue to update this review on a regular basis. We now return to the RRPCE study that set the stage for lengthy series of investigations summarized by the Antithrombotic Trialists' Collaboration.

5.2 THE RESEARCH QUESTION

The RRPCE study was designed 3 decades before trialists began asking research questions in the "PICOT" format: what *Persons*, receiving what experimental *Intervention*, compared with what *Comparison* intervention, experienced which *Outcomes*, over what period of *Time*? Nonetheless, all these elements were there in 1969, and they can be stated as follows: "Among highly compliant out-patients with TIAs or minor completed strokes, can aspirin (325 mg. four times a day) or sulfinpyrazone (200 mg. four times a day), singly or in combination, when administered by expert neurologists, reduce the risk of subsequent stroke or death better than placebos (and with an acceptably low rate of adverse drug effects) over the subsequent 2 years?"

However, this was the first RCT designed by our team and submitted to the Canadian Medical Research Council. To convince them that we could pull off this first-ever multicenter Canadian trial, we proposed a two-stage trial. The first stage added a more frequent but less serious outcome, continuing TIAs, so that our PICOT question ended: "…. can these drugs reduce subsequent *TIA*, stroke, or death?"

Once we convinced the MRC that we were capable of running the trial, we shifted to the second stage and restricted our question to the outcomes to stroke or death. In one of life's ironies, we graciously shared our protocol with a Texan who used it to test just aspirin and published (before us!) a positive result for TIAs but an indeterminate one for stroke or death.

As it happened, the first draft of our PICOT question confined the intervention to a single drug, sulfinpyrazone. But, Mike Gent and I argued that a *factorial design* could test two drugs in the same trial. When the other PIs and participating neurologists finally accepted our argument, we added aspirin to the trial. (Imagine our disappointment if we'd stuck with our initial, single-drug RCT of sulfinpyrazone, which turned out not to benefit our patients.)

Research question checklist:

To help you focus on the tactics of designing and executing an RCT, I'll open each section with a "checklist" of issues you'll need to consider and resolve. Here is the checklist for generating the trial question:

> ✓ **Choose your collaborators. Involve every potential collaborator (plus some critics and consumers) in hammering out your trial question. Don't rush it.**
>
> ✓ **Position your question. Decide where to site your question along the explanatory—management continuum.**
>
> ✓ **Specify your PICOT. Make sure that your question includes the relevant Persons, the Intervention, the Comparison intervention, the key Outcomes, and the Timing of their measurement in the trial = "PICOT."**
>
> ✓ **Identify your question's methodological impacts. Consider the impact of your question upon each subsequent step in your trial's design and execution.**

This Is the Most Important Section in This Chapter

That's because the question drives the entire trial. As you will see throughout this chapter, it is the question that specifies which types of individuals will receive which types of interventions (and ancillary care), at which types of sites (primary or tertiary care), from which types of clinicians (average ones or experts), with what sort, length and intensity of follow-up, and with what sorts of mechanisms for identifying which types of events (both good and bad).

As you may already have recognized, the RRPCE question describes an *explanatory* trial: "When given by experts to highly compliant patients, *can* these drugs do more good than harm?" (NOTE: if the terms "explanatory" and "management" are new to you, take a side-trip right now to Section 6.4 (on "Explanatory versus Management Trials"). As you'll see throughout the rest of this chapter, the fact that we were posing an explanatory question dictated our decisions at every subsequent stage of the trial's design, planning, execution, analysis, and interpretation.

I'll now take you through each item on the checklist.

✓ *Choose your collaborators. Involve every potential collaborator (plus some critics and consumers) in hammering out your trial question. Don't rush it.*

In hammering out your PICOT question, you should begin by involving every potential collaborator, whether methodologist, relevant bench scientist, clinician, or potential collaborator at a distant study center. You also should show early drafts of your question to potential critics who will help you sharpen it by disagreeing with it. Two other groups whose input is vital are the patients who would have to accept the treatment shown to be superior, and the policy-makers who will have to implement and pay for it.

By not rushing prematurely to your question's final wording, you will reap five benefits before you start your trial. First, as you saw in the RRPCE scenario, you can avoid the indeterminate result that would occur if you studied the wrong treatment, or just one of several promising treatments. Although many innovations that show great promise at the bench turn out to be useless or harmful, you need to be sure that you give them the best possible opportunity to display their efficacy in your trial.

Furthermore, your basic-research colleagues can help you decide whether and how to incorporate the latest developments in the "genomic era" (3). Advances here hold promise of identifying genomic subgroups of highly responsive patients. For example, the question posed in a trial of an inhaled beta-agonist in mild asthma asked whether patients with two different amino acid residues in their beta-2-adrenergic receptors responded differently to albutalol (4); they did.

(2) Second, when potential clinical collaborators join the process of hammering out the study question, the study becomes "theirs," not just "yours." As a result, they are much more likely to expend the time and energy necessary for recruiting, caring for, and following sufficient numbers of study patients.

(3) Third, it's wise to discuss your question with those who think you're asking the wrong one, or one that's already been answered. They may be right, in which case you need to revise your question. In doing so, you can convert your critics into your supporters. And if your critics are wrong, you can build the refutation of their criticisms into the way you conduct and report your trial.

(4) Fourth, discussing your question with patients who would be offered your experimental treatment if it proved efficacious will help you make it as palatable, painless, and convenient as possible. Even more important, patients may suggest some outcome measures—especially around function and quality of life—that will add greatly to the power and persuasiveness of your results. In fact, you may want to extend your collaboration with patients to include the initial identification of high-priority questions they'd like to see answered. For example, a collaboration between patients and clinicians in the United Kingdom has been created to confront important uncertainties about the effects of health care and to promote RCTs that can help reduce these uncertainties. It is named the James Lind Alliance (*http://www.lindalliance.org*).

(5) Fifth and final, most positive trials call for changes in facilities, staff, drug budgets, and clinical organizations. Accordingly, you'd do well to discuss your question with the relevant managers and organizations and seek their support before, not just after, your trial.

✓ *Position your question. Decide where to site your question along the explanatory–management continuum.*

As I stress in Section 6.4, and as summarized in 6–3, whether you ask your question in an explanatory mode ("Can the intervention do more good than harm under ideal circumstances?" = efficacy) or a pragmatic one ("Does the intervention do more good than harm under the usual circumstances?" = effectiveness) *determines every subsequent step in the design, execution, analysis, and interpretation of your trial.* It determines not only your approach to the recruitment of both patients and clinicians, but also your choice of regimens, events, analyses, and interpretations (5). If you haven't already read Section 6.4 on "Explanatory versus Management Trials," I urge you to do so before you go any further.

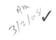

✓ *Specify your PICOT. Make sure that your question includes the relevant Persons, the Intervention, the Comparison intervention, the key Outcomes, and the Timing of their measurement in the trial = "PICOT."*

Forcing yourself and your collaborators to specify each of the PICOT elements refines the process of translating an initial idea into a viable study:

Persons: what sort of patients or other persons, from which sources, with what qualifying features, and undergoing which preadmission determinations of things such as compliance with health recommendations?

Interventions: of what sorts, at what doses, administered by whom, with what level of expertise, where, and with what sorts of monitoring for compliance and side effects?

Comparison intervention: again, of what sort (placebo or active), at what doses, administered by whom, with what level of expertise, where, and with what sorts of monitoring for compliance and side effects?

Outcomes: both good and bad, of what sort, determined when, defined how, and ascertained and adjudicated by whom?

Time: at what time following your intervention do you intend to decide whether it does more good than harm? To be sure, you will follow the persons in your trial from the moment they are recruited. But the timing of your ultimate decision about the benefits and risks of your intervention will be determined by the natural history of disease, the latency in the effects of interventions, the need to overcome the short-term harms of surgery or aggressive chemotherapy, and the like.

It's at this time that you should also begin deciding the smallest difference in outcomes between experimental and control patients, which, if observed at the end of the trial, your patients and (we trust) you would consider humanly important (often called the Minimally Important Difference or *MID*). We'll return to the MID several times in this chapter.

Almost all collaborators in our RCTs start out disagreeing with us and with each other about at least one of these PICOT elements and about the proper size of the MID. So will yours. The earlier you expose these differing opinions, the sooner you will achieve a thoughtful "buy-in" and consensus about "our" trial. This process both deserves and requires a great deal of time. Although my coauthors claim I'm exaggerating, I hold that a third of all the intellectual effort that goes into an RCT (from the germ of an idea to the publication of its results) should go to hammering out the question it is supposed to answer. Along the way, a quick way to tell whether your question remains sensible is to confirm that it (still) can be answered "yes," "no," or with a specific number.

PICOT questions usually ask whether an experimental intervention is "superior" to its control intervention. However, other PICOT questions ask whether the experimental intervention is as good as, or "noninferior" to, its comparison intervention, but preferable for some other reason (such as safety or cost). In case these terms are new to you, I'll define them here; Section 6.5 discusses them in detail.

Superiority and Noninferiority Trials

Consider the question we posed in the RRPCE study: " ... can aspirin or sulfinpyrazone reduce the risk of subsequent stroke or death *better than placebos*?" We asked whether either or both drugs were *superior* to placebos, and the direction posed by this sort of question gives it its name: *a superiority trial*. After our positive RRPCE trial, other investigators conducted a superiority trial to see whether a newer drug (ticlopidine) was superior to placebo (6). Again, the answer was yes, but ticlopidine caused some rare but serious side effects [it wasn't until later that an arguably more appropriate "head-to-head" superiority trial found that ticlopidine was superior to aspirin (7)].

It then made sense to look for a drug that was *as good as* (equivalent), or at least *not inferior to* ticlopidine, but avoided its dangerous side effects.

Some RCTs ask both questions in the same trial. First, they ask, "Is the new experimental treatment *superior* to established treatment?" If not, they ask the second question, "Can it at least be shown to be "no worse" than established treatment (*noninferior*)?" For example, some cardiologists thought that a combination of antithrombotics might be better, or at least no worse but preferable for other reasons, to a single antithrombotic in acute myocardial infarction (8). Sure enough, you needed to treat approximately 333 patients with the combination to save one more life at 30 days than you'd save with the single antithrombotic drug (the combination wasn't superior to the single drug), but it satisfied their criterion for noninferiority. Moreover, the combination reduced the occurrence of reinfarction and some other complications.

Unless this brief superiority/noninferiority discussion has told you all that (or more than) you wanted to know about these ideas, you can find more about them, including a graphical way of thinking about them in Section 6.5 (on "Superiority and Noninferiority Trials").

✓ *Identify your question's methodological impacts. Consider the impact of your question upon each subsequent step in your trial's design and execution.*

It is at this stage that methodologic purity begins to confront reality. For example:

1. In recruitment: "Ideal" patients are highly compliant, have only the disease of interest and none other, and can be found in ordinary clinical settings. On the other hand, they may be so scarce, so atypical in their risk or responsiveness, or so difficult and expensive to identify that it doesn't make sense to plan an RCT just around them.
2. In applying the intervention: You don't want to attempt a pragmatic, primary care trial of an intervention that is so complex and tricky that generalists can't or won't apply it.
3. In choosing outcomes: Will the outcomes you've chosen require rare or expensive investigations that are not available to most patients?

These confrontations between purity and reality have arisen in the planning stages of every RCT we've ever done. Once again, their discussion and resolution are central to hammering out the study question.

A Parting Shot: Checklists Must Be Read in Both Directions

Finally, remember that the research question checklist reads in both directions. Not only does the question determine the methodology at later steps in a trial, so too, the conclusions at each of these later steps should cause you to reverse course and revisit the question you posed at the outset. When there is a mismatch between your question and your methods, then you'll have to revise one (or both) of them. At the end of the day, you will succeed only if you couple the question that you really want to answer to a set of methods that will really answer it.

5.3 PARTICIPANT SELECTION

Canvassing 26 centers across Canada, we recruited stroke-neurologists who were genuinely uncertain whether aspirin or sulfinpyrazone was efficacious for TIAs. Patients with TIAs referred to them were eligible for our trial if they had experienced at least one transient cerebral or retinal ischemic attack in the 3 months before entry (during the first year of the trial, only patients with multiple attacks were admitted, and the protocol was then revised to include patients with single attacks). We developed definitions for symptoms of TIA that were agreed upon by all participating neurologists. Certain symptoms were sufficient for entry when they constituted the only manifestations of an attack, whereas others had to occur in predefined combinations (see text). Patients with residual symptoms beyond the 24-hour limit were eligible only if the symptoms were both stable and capable of subsequent observable further deterioration. Neurologically stable patients were nonetheless excluded if they had coexisting morbid conditions that could explain their symptoms, if they were likely to die from other illnesses within 12 months, or if they were unable to take the test drugs. Participating neurologists were asked to submit information on all patients excluded from the trial.

Participants checklist:

- ✓ Define your RCT's inclusions. Draft patient eligibility criteria that match your study question.
- ✓ Define your RCT's exclusions. Make sure you'll exclude patients who cannot help you answer your study question.
- ✓ Make sure your clinical collaborators can employ these definitions. Make sure your inclusion and exclusion criteria are objective and unambiguous by achieving "very good" agreement when they are applied by different clinicians to the same patients.
- ✓ Start thinking about sample size. Anticipate your sample size requirements and begin to consider strategies for achieving them.
- ✓ Define your collaborators' eligibility criteria. Generate the criteria that would have to be met by your potential clinical collaborators.
- ✓ Create patient-entry forms.
- ✓ Decide how to handle "eligible-but-not-randomized" patients.
- ✓ Decide how to handle patients whose ineligibility is not discovered until after they are randomized.
- ✓ Decide whether and how to carry out a "dry run" of forms and systems.
- ✓ Revisit your study question. See whether what you've done so far is consistent with your study question.
- ✓ Create a patient-flow diagram.

The first three steps describe the iterative process of successive attempts to describe, with even greater precision, the sorts of patients who will permit you to answer your study question. If they are ever to apply the results of your trial, clinicians must know how to identify exactly which patients should be offered the better treatment.

✓ *Define your RCT's inclusions. Draft patient eligibility criteria that match your study question.*

In the RRPCE study, we devoted considerable time and energy to hammering out exactly what, for purposes of our trial, a transient ischemic attack was. I interviewed several stroke-neurologists and pestered them until they specified which signs or symptoms, singly or in combination, constituted TIA, and from what vascular territory (carotid or vertebrobasilar) they arose. For example, weakness of an extremity was sufficient all by itself. Diplopia had to be accompanied by dysphagia, hearing loss, mental change, or vertigo. Drowsiness, headache, tinnitus, or vertigo were acceptable components of a transient ischemic attack, but insufficient for its diagnosis by themselves. As they discussed and debated these points, our neurologist colleagues began to take over the "ownership" of the trial.

During the first year of the trial, we documented large numbers of patients who were otherwise eligible for the study, but had been referred to participating neurologists following just one, initial TIA. We decided that, despite their slightly less firm diagnoses, they would be obvious candidates for any therapy found effective in patients with multiple attacks, so we altered the eligibility criteria to admit them thereafter.

We carefully discussed and debated this protocol change, as we needed to be sure that the answers it generated wouldn't interfere with our primary question. In a similar fashion, you should discuss any protocol changes in your trial with colleagues and your trial monitor. Remember that you'll need to describe and justify any protocol changes in publications arising from your trial.

✓ *Define your RCT's exclusions. Make sure you'll exclude patients who cannot help you answer your study question.*

Your exclusion criteria must prevent the admission of three sorts of patients who will obscure the answer to your study question. First, you need to exclude patients with "mimicking" disorders that arise from, or respond to, other causes or cures. Therefore, the RRPCE study excluded patients with severe aortic stenosis, an unrelated illness that could cause identical symptoms but called for surgical, not medical, intervention.

Second, patients who succumb to other illnesses during the study period obscure your answer in two ways. Not only won't they survive long enough to display a benefit from experimental therapy, but they also will add statistical "noise" to any analysis that includes death as an outcome event. Thus, the RRPCE study excluded patients likely to die from other illnesses within 12 months.

The third sorts of patients who cannot answer your question are those in whom it is already known, at entry, that they *must* or *must not* receive one of your study treatments. An example of the former would be when an otherwise eligible patient has to take your drug (or another drug from the same class) for an extraneous comorbid condition. An example of the latter is an otherwise eligible patient who has previously suffered an adverse reaction to your drug (or one that cross-reacts with it).

✓ Make sure your clinical collaborators can employ these definitions.

Make sure your inclusion and exclusion criteria are objective and unambiguous by achieving "very good" agreement when they are applied by different clinicians to the same patients.

After a few meetings with your collaborators (who may number as few as one [your statistician co-principal Investigator (PI)] or as many as a hundred or more), you will begin to reach consensus about your study question and, from it, your eligibility and noneligibility criteria. As soon as you start roughing them out, start creating increasingly subtle paper scenarios describing patients who do and don't (and don't quite) meet your criteria. Ask your clinical collaborators to judge them, discuss any mistakes and discrepancies, and repeat the process until you have "very good" agreement (i.e., kappa >0.8) (9). If the criteria include subtle clinical findings, replace the paper scenarios with volunteer patients who exhibit them.

You can consume lots of time and energy carrying out the first three items on this checklist. Moreover, your efforts can result in lengthy, complicated patient-entry forms. But lengthy entry forms discourage patient accrual, so you may want to explore a radical approach to simplifying your eligibility criteria. For example, you could replace most of your eligibility criteria with an all-inclusive "uncertainty" decision between potential study patients and their clinicians (10). When either or both of them feel certain, for any reason, that they know which treatment is better for them, they receive that treatment and do not enter the trial. Only when both the patient and their clinician are uncertain about which treatment is preferable is the patient invited to enter the trial. I discuss this "uncertainty principle" and its use in large, simple trials in Section 6.7.

In Section 5.5, under "deciding what to do about monitoring (and, if necessary, improving) patient compliance," I describe a pretrial "faintness-of-heart" period in which you would ask potential study patients to comply with tasks similar to those they'd face if they entered the trial. Because stratification for compliance in the analysis is valid only if it's determined *before* randomization, you need to decide whether low compliance could severely hamper your ability to answer your study question. If it will, you may need some prerandomization filter for it, such as the Sikhar Banerjee design illustrated in Figure 6-1.

✓ Start thinking about sample size. Anticipate your sample size requirements and begin to consider strategies for achieving them.

During the discussions that led to specifying the exact sorts of patients you do and don't want in your trial, you should have begun to get a sense of how many such patients you would need and where you might find them. There are several rules of thumb for estimating the availability of eligible patients for RCTs, and all of them are pessimistic (e.g., "The best way to make a disease disappear is to start an RCT about it."). Although I postpone discussing sample size determinations until Section 5.8, you should start thinking realistically right now about how many, where, and how you will find patients for your trial. For example, some trialists ask potential collaborators to start keeping logs of potentially eligible patients they encounter as soon as they consider joining the trial.

✓ *Define you collaborators' eligibility criteria. Generate the criteria that would have to be met by your potential clinical collaborators.*

Your early estimates of your sample size requirements often will reveal the necessity to recruit several clinical collaborators and perhaps even several centers. You need to involve them early on if they are to adopt the trial as "theirs" and make it succeed. Accordingly, you need to develop objective, unambiguous eligibility criteria for deciding whether a potential collaborator or center is eligible for joining your RCT. For one thing, they should be genuinely uncertain about the efficacy of the experimental treatment in the target illness. A point to remember is that initially "certain" clinicians may become "uncertain" (and eligible for the trial) when they realize how many of their colleagues are uncertain.

A second major criterion for the eligibility of clinical collaborators concerns their level of expertise in applying the study treatments. In the RRPCE trial, most of the small family of Canadian stroke-neurologists had trained at the same institutions, were already known to be of high caliber, and were uncertain about the efficacy of aspirin and sulfinpyrazone in TIAs. Accordingly, we invited all of them to join. In other explanatory trials, however, you will want to go beyond pedigree, professed interest, reputation, pledges, and good will, and make sure they are expert clinicians. In the latter case your criteria may require potential collaborating clinicians to document not only their volume of eligible patients but also the quality of care provided to them. For example, in the North American Symptomatic Carotid Endarterectomy Trial (NASCET) we asked the "explanatory" or "efficacy" PICOT question: "Among patients with symptomatic carotid stenosis, does the performance of carotid endarterectomy *by an expert neurosurgeon or vascular surgeon* lower the overall risk of subsequent severe stroke or death (due both to their underlying diseases and to perioperative complications in patients randomized to surgery)?" We therefore set up a panel of surgical co-PIs, and they reviewed the past surgical performance (with special attention to complication rates) of potential surgical collaborators, offering participation to just the best of them.

✓ *Create patient-entry forms.*

Two issues are important here, substance and style, and each presents challenges to trialists. The substance challenge is how to ask for enough primary entry data to permit a thoughtful trial analysis, but not to ask for so much entry data of secondary importance (regardless of how "interesting" it might be) that the effort required for its collection discourages patients and clinicians from entering or continuing in the trial.

The Long and Short of Patient-entry Forms

There is no unanimity on this issue, and the United States and the United Kingdom trialists populate its extremes. Entry forms for the National Institutes of Health (NIH)-sponsored NASCET of surgery versus no surgery for symptomatic carotid stenosis were 33 pages long; for the simultaneous European Carotid Endarterectomy Trial that asked the same question and got the same answer, the entry forms were two pages long. Proponents of the more extensive entry (and follow-up) data gathered in the NASCET trial point out that they permitted a number of ancillary studies and 44 additional publications.

The RRPCE entry forms were 17 pages long. The shortest entry form I've encountered is the ATLAS (Adjuvant Tamoxifen—Longer Against Shorter) trial, randomizing women who appear to be disease-free following any type of curative surgery for their breast cancer, to stop or continue their adjuvant tamoxifen (*http://www.ctsu.ox.ac.uk/~atlas*) from the Clinical Trial Service Unit of Oxford University. Its entry form is a single page and its investigators state the reason on their Web site: "To encourage wide participation, the ATLAS study involves virtually no extra work for collaborators, so that even the busiest clinicians can take part. The entry procedure is quick and easy, no examinations are required beyond those given as part of routine care, and minimal, annual follow-up information is requested."

Vital and Nonvital Entry Data

I suggest that you create two lists of entry data, one for the vital data and one for data that, although they might be interesting, are not vital, as shown in Table 5-1:

TABLE 5-1 Item Generation for Randomized Controlled Trial Patient-entry Forms

Data that are *vital*:

1. To uniquely identify the patient (and how to keep track of them)
2. To confirm that the patient has the target disorder
3. To confirm that the patient meets all the other eligibility criteria
4. To permit stratification into the risk-response categories that will be used for stratifying patients both prior to allocation and during analysis
5. To describe other baseline (preintervention) variables that will be used in the *primary* hypothesis-testing analysis (including sociodemographic information if relevant)
6. To permit combining the results with those of previous trials in systematic reviews.

Data that may be *interesting, but are not vital*:

1. To capture additional clinical, biochemical, physiologic, or imaging data that might be interesting to explore in a hypothesis-forming analysis
2. To document comorbid conditions not already known to affect responses to treatment

The first, "vital" list begins with data required to uniquely identify the patient. In addition, if yours is a long-term trial you should consider getting contact information for someone "who will always know your whereabouts." This should be one or more of their younger relatives or close friends who do not live with them. These contacts can prove invaluable in preventing study patients from becoming lost to follow-up.

The second set of vital-entry data are those that confirm the patient's diagnosis, and the third, their eligibility for the trial. The fourth set of vital-entry data are derived from prior evidence (or suspicion) that subsets of eligible patients differ to important degrees in their risk of an outcome event and/or their responsiveness to experimental therapy. Suppose that, by the play of chance, patients receiving your experimental treatment were at much higher risk of an outcome event than control patients at entry to your trial. They might make even a very effective treatment appear useless, mightn't they? The same misinterpretation would occur if, by chance, patients receiving your experimental treatment were much less responsive to your experimental treatment. The effects of these differences in risk and responsiveness are described in Section 6.6 on "Physiological Statistics."

If you decide you need to allocate different "risk-response" subgroups in precisely equal proportions to experimental and control treatments (rather than leave it to simple randomization), you must identify them at entry. In addition, because some study patients may not respond at all to (or might even be harmed by) an otherwise efficacious experimental treatment, you will also want to be able to identify any special features about them in your analysis. In the RRPCE study, we suspected that a number of subgroups might differ in their risk of an outcome event and/or their responsiveness to our study drugs. Accordingly, we gathered entry data on the site of their TIA, how many they had suffered, whether they displayed any permanent neurologic damage, their age, sex, blood pressure, cholesterol level, and cigarette use, and whether they had diabetes or a history of myocardial infarction.

The third vital data set is determined not by you, but by the funding agencies and licensing authorities who have their own requirements for data on RCT patients. You need to find out their requirements in plenty of time to build them into your data forms.

Interesting but Not Vital Data

Items are far too often nominated to the second, "interesting, but not vital" list for no better reason (especially in North America) than "it would be nice to have them." These "interesting but not vital" data create a three-edged sword. On the one hand, their analysis can generate important, exciting hypotheses for testing in other, independent investigations or in the next logical RCT. Second, however, their sheer volume can discourage busy investigators and patients from going through the trouble of joining your trial. Similarly, documenting them can add considerable expense to your trial (and to the patient, their insurer, or the institution where they are enrolled).

The third sword edge produced by collecting "interesting but not vital" data is the most damaging one. The potential for damage occurs when they become fodder for "exploratory subgroup analyses" (read "data-dredging exercises"), some of which *must* generate statistically significant results by chance alone. The real damage occurs when their conclusions are used, not for hypothesis-generation, but for clinical pronouncements about efficacy. This is particularly so when the primary analysis is indeterminate or underpowered and fails to find the hypothesized benefit of the experimental treatment. The temptation to carry out extensive subgroup analysis in the hope of identifying at least one responsive subgroup can be overwhelming. I discuss the pitfalls of "looking for the pony" in Section 5.7. For now I simply refer you to Richard Horton's Commentary on star signs and trial guidelines (11). In it, he describes how he negotiated with the ISIS-2 investigators (who demonstrated the benefits of aspirin and streptokinase for suspected heart attacks) to include a nonsensical subgroup analysis, the patient's astrological birth sign, in their primary paper. Thus, it was "revealed" that aspirin is ineffective in Geminis and Libras with heart attacks.

The RRPCE study is another case in point. We got into trouble even with our "vital" entry data on sex and comorbidity. Our subgroup analyses on these "vital" data led us to conclude that aspirin probably didn't benefit women, diabetics, or those with prior myocardial infarctions. Our publication of these cautions caused confusion among treating physicians and it took a few years and several more RCTs to refute our false-negative conclusions about the benefit of aspirin in these subgroups.

Having considered the content of the patient-entry form, you should turn your attention to its format and appearance. Both elements can have major impacts on the completeness and accuracy of both vital and merely interesting data. The strategies and tactics for generating effective forms have been well described elsewhere, and we recommend these resources to you (12–14).

✓ Decide how to handle "eligible-but-not-randomized" patients.

As you can see from the RRPCE patient-flow diagram in Figure 5–1, 141 patients were eligible for the trial but refused randomization. Whether they received neither, one or both of the study drugs was not determined by random allocation. Rather, it resulted from an unblind, joint decision with their clinicians. We took the view that they could not contribute to a valid efficacy analysis. Therefore, we did not engage in the expensive and labor-intensive task of keeping track of them and their outcomes.

We had four reasons not to follow the "eligible-but-not-randomized" patients (besides the huge amounts of time and money required to do that). First and foremost was the proposition that following cohorts of nonrandomized patients couldn't tell us whether sulfinpyrazone and aspirin were efficacious, useless, or harmful. Indeed, if nonrandomized patients could have answered that question, we wouldn't have needed the RRPCE or any other RCTs! Jumping ahead 30 years, this claim was most recently validated by Regina Kunz et al. They carried out a Cochrane systematic review that compared the estimates of efficacy that were found

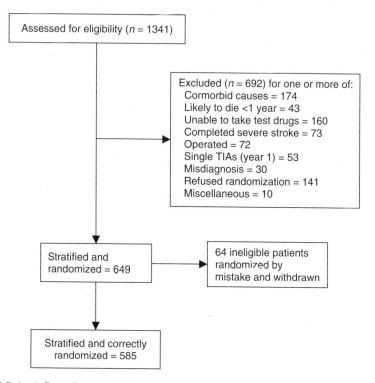

FIGURE 5–1 A flow diagram of the recruitment phase of the RRPCE (Recent Recurrent Presumed Cerebral Emboli) trial.

in nonrandomized and randomized studies (15). Their bottom line: "On average, nonrandomized trials and randomized trials with inadequate concealment of allocation tend to result in larger estimates of effect than randomized trials with adequately concealed allocation. However, it is not generally possible to predict the magnitude, or even the direction, of possible selection biases and consequent distortions of treatment effects."

Second, we realized that the *proportion* of eligible patients who are randomized into a trial is irrelevant to decisions about efficacy, unless they have importantly different risks or responsiveness to the experimental treatment. For example, only a small minority of children with leukemia were joining RCTs back then, but the results among that minority had already started to save the lives of most leukemic children. This fact has been repeatedly demonstrated since.

Third, we expected an "inclusion benefit" for TIA patients inside the trial compared with TIA patients cared for outside it. That is, we anticipated that trial patients would be more likely to receive aspirin and sulfinpyrazone, to be more closely followed up, and more likely to receive high-quality care for other, related conditions. As it happened, our anticipation was borne out 3 decades later when David Braunholtz and his colleagues concluded: "While the evidence is not conclusive, it is more likely that clinical trials have a positive rather than a negative effect on the outcome of patients" (16).

Finally, we believed that patients in RCTs received as good or better care than similar patients treated outside of trials. We didn't buy the popular press image of RCT patients as "guinea pigs," "sacrificed" to help future generations. Thus, we had little to learn from "eligible-but-not-randomized" patients. And, once again, this view was validated in a later Cochrane review carried out by a team led by Gunn Vist. They found that the outcomes of patients who participate in RCTs are just as good as those of similar patients receiving these same treatments outside of trials (17).

Taking all this into consideration, you'd have to have pretty convincing evidence that the low-reliability data you could obtain from following "eligible-but-not-randomized" patients in your RCT could ever justify the expense or effort required to generate it.

✓ Decide how to handle patients whose ineligibility is not discovered until after they are randomized.

Early in an RCT, despite all your planning, collaborating clinicians and centers often err in applying your eligibility criteria. The result is a few ineligible patients in your trial. Accordingly, you need to decide in the trial's planning stage how to handle such patients. As demonstrated in Section 6.6 (on "Physiological Statistics"), including patients with the wrong diagnosis, other terminal illnesses, and a prior allergy to a study drug will add noise to your analysis and decrease its power (5,18). Accordingly, you'd better establish a bias-free means for removing them right now (some trialists apply the funny term "de-randomization" to such removal). I recommend reviewing the eligibility of *all* randomized patients, *blind* to their allocated treatment, as soon as their entry data are verified and "clean." For example, early in the RRPCE study the routine, blind review of all randomized patients discovered that 64 of them were actually ineligible for the trial. They didn't have TIA; they had brain tumors, aortic stenosis, migraine, and the like. Or, they had a second disease likely to kill them within a few months, or already were known to be allergic to aspirin. We didn't know their treatment group assignment when we decided their eligibility, so removing them was unbiased. Note, however, that this strategy is valid only when there is blind, equally intensive review of all patients in all treatment groups.

A large number of such postrandomization exclusions can detract from the credibility, if not the validity, of your trial. The best way to deal with them is to reject them prior to randomization. You can accomplish this by training your research staff (e.g., with test cases) and by giving rapid feedback to centers when they enter a patient who proves to be ineligible. Alternatively, you can use one of the automated data systems that "reads" and rejects entry forms of ineligible patients. Finally, you can send bulletins to all study investigators, outlining common mistakes. This sort of "quality assurance" program is exceptionally important at the beginning of your trial, so that everyone learns quickly from their mistakes and those of others.

The foregoing strategies apply when patient eligibility can be unambiguously determined from data obtained before they are invited to join the trial. In other trials, it may take weeks to process the eligibility evidence (e.g., when you need to create and review special pathologic preparations). In this latter situation, your proper course of action is, as usual, determined by the question you posed. Suppose, for example, that you are conducting a management trial to test a treatment policy among patients whose eligibility cannot be ascertained prior to their treatment, both inside the trial and in routine practice. In that case, it makes sense to include the "late" ineligible patients in your intention-to-treat analysis. This policy is especially sensible when your treatment is "permanent," such as an operation, rather than a medication with negligible adverse effects. Either way, when you report your results you'll need to include the numbers, types, and justifications for excluding every patient you remove from your trial. Finally, your RCT's results will be the most credible when the reintroduction of *all* ineligible patients makes no difference to its conclusion.

✓ Decide whether and how to carry out a "dry-run" of forms and systems.

If this is your first trial, or it is the initial trial for a particular clinical condition, most or all of your forms and systems for recruiting, investigating, and determining the eligibility of your study patients will be new. It would be a shame (in terms of both validity and credibility) to discover important flaws in them only after you've started the trial. Accordingly, you would be wise to perform a "dry-run" of your forms and systems before you start the formal trial (I prefer "dry-run" to the more ambiguous "pilot" or "feasibility" terms that address other issues such as the availability of study patients or the skills of a trial's clinicians).

You can use the "dry-run" to correct errors of omission, commission, and ambiguity in your data forms. It will also let you identify and solve problems in the flow of study patients and study data. In our trials, we test, revise, and retest draft forms until our study patients, interviewers, clinicians, and data managers are satisfied that the data coming from the field are accurate.

What sorts of study patients should you use in "dry-runs?" It would be vital not to "use up" eligible patients for this. We usually put members of our study staff through first because they are already tuned into potential problems and aren't shy about pointing them out. After fixing those problems, we often perform a second "dry-run" with consenting patients who, although they have the target condition, are already known to be ineligible for our trial.

✓ Revisit your study question. See whether what you've done so far is consistent with your study question.

In executing the first nine items on the checklist, you may have made decisions that unintentionally damage your ability to answer your PICOT question. For example, if you're asking a pragmatic question (can the treatment work among typical patients?), did you wind up with eligibility criteria that excluded otherwise typical patients because they have comorbid conditions, have a track record of low compliance, or are older than your arbitrary age cutoff? If so, you're going to have to change either your question or your eligibility criteria. Reiterate, reiterate, reiterate.

The sorts of patients you do and don't admit to your trial, the extent to which they comply with your study treatment, how well you keep track of them, and how accurately you ascertain their events all can have huge effects on how confident you (and your readers) will be about the answer you get. The relations between these factors are complex, and are the bread and butter of sophisticated biostatisticians. Many clinician trialists are bewildered and intimidated by the formulas and statistics used to determine and control these factors. However, if clinicians contemplate these relationships in physiological, rather than mathematical, terms, they can not only understand them, but also manipulate them. Accordingly, a discussion of "Physiological Statistics" can be found in Section 6.6. Before going there, however, you need to start your patient-flow diagram.

✓ Create a patient-flow diagram.

We agree with the revised CONSORT statement (19) that the flow of participants through each stage of an RCT ought to be described, preferably in the form of a diagram. Accordingly, we'll provide an updated patient-flow diagram for the RRPCE study at the end of each section of this chapter. Figure 5–1 shows what the RRPCE Study looked like at this stage.

5.4 ALLOCATION OF PATIENTS TO TREATMENTS

After a participating neurologist in the RRPCE trial completed an eligible and consenting patient's admission forms, he telephoned our central office, identified himself and the patient, and told us the vascular territory for the patient's TIAs (carotid, vertebrobasilar, or both) and whether they had any neurologic residua. Our central office staff then consulted a previously generated (by computer) randomization schedule for that neurologist and those clinical features (balanced every four patients within each stratum), and gave the neurologist a randomly generated four-digit number that identified prepackaged supplies of the two study drugs or their corresponding placebos already on hand in his hospital's pharmacy. We asked patients to avoid nontrial aspirin, and made arrangements with the clinical laboratories at each center to withhold telltale laboratory results (because sulfinpyrazone lowers serum uric acid).

Allocation checklist:

✓ Create an audit-trail. Double-check your system for registering and keeping track of every eligible consenting patient as soon as you identify them.
✓ Identify and (maybe) use prognostic information.
✓ Select an allocation method (e.g., stratified randomized blocks, minimization, factorial, etc.).

✓ Pick, train, and monitor your allocators.
✓ Establish allocation concealment at the start of your trial.
✓ Decide whether, who, and how to blind.

Note that the set of tactics in our RRPCE trial achieved four important objectives:

1. The neurologist could not influence the patient's assignment to a specific treatment, because we had concealed our allocation scheme.
2. We could guarantee a good *prognostic factor balance* between the treatment groups by stratification before randomization.
3. We set the stage for *blinding* both the neurologists and their patients as to who was receiving which of the four treatment regimens.
4. We established an *audit trail* for every randomized patient.

Because of their interconnectedness, I won't try to consider these items one-by-one. Instead, I will integrate them as I answer some important questions about allocation in RCTs. The objective in all this is to help you collaborate with your statistician-coinvestigator in making decisions about how to allocate your trial patients to their treatments.

Why It Is Vital to Conceal the Assignment of Patients to Treatments

Systematic reviews of RCTs have shown that when clinicians know ahead of time which treatment their next eligible and consenting patient will receive, they may (consciously or unconsciously) enter patients with lower risk and/or higher responsiveness into the experimental treatment group. As a result, the trial can become biased in favor of experimental therapy from the start. For example, Ken Schulz has led empirical studies showing that trials that failed to conceal their assignment schemes tended to exaggerate treatment effects (although with scope for bias in either direction) (20). However, this assignment of highly responsive patients to experimental treatment is not universal. The previously noted systematic review by Regina Kunz, Gunn Vist, Andrew Oxman et al. uncovered examples of underestimating as well as overestimating treatment effects in RCTs with inadequate concealment.

How to Conceal the Assignment of the Next Patient

The mechanics of concealing patient allocation to treatment vary widely, but all of them rely on assignment by an external source that neither clinicians nor patients can influence or even know about (alas, locally held allocation lists can be leaked or burgled, and "sealed" envelopes can be opened prematurely or held up to a strong light). The allocation strategy could be as simple as a coin-toss by a third party (but remember that 100 coin tosses usually contain six heads or tails in a row at some point in the sequence!).

Nowadays allocation is often performed by a central randomization service (such as a 24/7 telephone number) that employs a computer-based randomization algorithm, with or without provisions for the prognostic stratification and minimization approaches discussed here. Many statistics texts contain random number tables, and statistical software often includes random number generators. Your choice of the specific strategy to use in your trial should arise out of discussion with your principal statistician.

Trials of emergency treatments can't wait around while a central service reviews a critically ill patient's eligibility and randomizes her or him. In these situations, treatment can be assigned by some bias-free (you hope!) method such as odd-versus-even day of the month, or by handling caregivers as "clusters." Alternatively, trial clinicians can simply tear open the next-of-a-sequence of prepackaged, prerandomized treatment "boxes" and administer its contents.

When the dust settles, blind adjudication might find that several patients in an emergency trial were, in fact, ineligible for it. For this reason, the postrandomization exclusion tactics described in Section 5.4 [sometimes called "de-randomization" (21)] will be required.

In drug trials, it is usual for the allocation system to safeguard concealment by assigning patients to specific previously assembled and identical pill containers kept in stock at the study sites. You should label each of these containers in a fashion that defies identification of their contents. For example, we "numbered" each container in the RRPCE trial with four random digits.

Allocating roughly equal numbers of patients to experimental and control therapy, both overall and in subgroups, boosts the power of the RCT [confidence intervals around, say, absolute risk reductions (ARRs) are smallest when treatment groups are identical in size (22)—but not too identical]. Ken Schulz and his colleagues examined 206 obstetrical and gynecological RCTs and found that differences in the numbers of treatment and control patients were far smaller than would be expected by the play of chance, raising suspicions that some investigators were interfering with randomization.

Roughly equal-sized groups also increase the study's credibility before clinical audiences. Accordingly, randomization schemes typically employ "balancing" or "blocking" exceptions to strict random allocation. For example, suppose you want to balance the numbers of experimental and control patients at the end of every four who are entered (a "block" of four). Then, if both the first and second patients in your block of four were randomly assigned to control therapy, you would not randomize the third and fourth patients, but would assign both of them to experimental therapy. Although blocking is tidy, it can be risky. If you were "blocking" within admitting teams or sites and they got wind of your blocking scheme and kept track of patient assignments, concealment would be lost and they could determine the next patient's treatment. For this reason, you should keep your blocking plan secret from study clinicians, some investigators randomly switching between blocks of varying numbers of patients.

When clinicians or patients are only slightly uncertain that a new treatment does more good than harm, some authors suggest changing the allocation ratio of experimental to control assignments from 1:1 to 2:1 or even 3:1. If you decide to do this, you must remember that, to obtain the same confidence interval around the treatment effect, a 2:1 trial requires 12% more patients overall and a 3:1 trial requires 33% more patients. Thus, at the end of the day a 3:1 trial doesn't reduce the number of control patients by half, but only by one third (Altman D. Personal communication, 2002).

Why Prognostic Factor Balance Is Important

Just as *Figure 1* of any RCT report typically provides a "flow-chart" of patients as they progress through the trial, *Table 1* of any RCT report typically provides a "baseline" comparison of experimental and control patients upon admission to the trial. The key entries in this table are factors known to affect study patients' risks of the outcomes of interest or their likely responsiveness to the experimental treatment. You will enhance readers' confidence in your trial result when you achieve a close balance in these prognostic factors.

Many RCT reports make the mistake of testing the statistical significance of any difference in each prognostic factor between experimental and control patients. This is neither wise nor informative. In small trials, biologically important differences will often be statistically nonsignificant; in large trials, biologically trivial differences will often be statistically significant. As the following example will show, the issue is more one of credibility than of validity.

Example of a Threats to Trial Credibility from Prognostic Factor Imbalances

By its very nature, randomization must inevitably occasionally lead to random but big differences between treatment groups in randomized trials. The results on the credibility of the affected trials can be devastating. For example, an excellent team of trialists designed and executed an RCT (23) that, among other objectives, asked the question: "Among patients with type 2 diabetes, does an oral hypoglycemic agent (tolbutamide), when compared with placebo, reduce the occurrence of nonfatal vascular complications and death?" They employed simple random allocation (with no prior stratification), and a comparison of vascular risk factors between the tolbutamide and control groups at the start of the trial looked like Table 5–2.

That all five of these risk factors were more common in the tolbutamide group is unusual in an individual trial (sign-test $P = 0.0625$), but must happen sooner or later in a large group of trials. Nonetheless, this nonstatistically significant imbalance became a key target for the drug's manufacturer [and its hired consultants (24)] when it was found that the active drug produced a 44% *increase* in total mortality on the raw data. In truth, however, this baseline imbalance didn't affect the study's conclusions. Multivariate modeling with logistic regression (to control for these imbalances) reduced this increase by just 2% to 42%. Moreover, an independent team of the best

TABLE 5-2 **Risk Factors for Vascular Complications and Death at the Start of the University Group Diabetes Program Trial**

Risk Factor	Placebo Group (%)	Tolbutamide Group (%)
Definite hypertension	30	37
History of digitalis use	4.5	7.6
History of angina pectoris	5.0	7.0
Significant ECG abnormality	3.0	4.0
Elevated cholesterol	8.6	15

ECG, electrocardiogram.

statisticians in the land "adjusted" for important baseline differences and upheld the study conclusion (25). For some readers, however, the damage had already been done, and the credibility of this important RCT suffered.

Achieving Prognostic Factor Balance by Stratification Prior to Randomization

Our research groups usually employ one of two "mixed" allocation strategies to prevent this distracting situation from happening. The first of them employs prognostic stratification before randomization. It begins by stratifying each patient for the presence or absence of important prognostic factors, or for whether they lie above or below a guesstimate of the median value for a continuous prognostic factor (such as blood pressure) or effect modifier (such as age). Or, if we are performing a simultaneous explanatory-pragmatic trial, we stratify by whatever prerandomization evaluation identified as whether a patient should go in the explanatory or management arm. Then, allocation occurs separately within each stratum.

For example, in the RRPCE trial we stratified for three presumed sites of ischemia (carotid, vertebrobasilar, or both) and for the presence or absence of residual signs and symptoms following the qualifying TIA. We thus had 3 × 2 or 6 strata from which we randomized patients to their study regimens. We employed a separate randomization schedule, and balanced every four patients, for each stratum (with an independent randomization schedule for each center). The resulting baseline balance in these prognostic factors for men in our trial appears in Table 5-3.

If you run your eye along the rows, you'll see good balance for these two prognostic factors. Every treatment group had the highest percentage for one factor, and no group had the highest rate for more than two of them. No wonder, then, that baseline balance was never an issue in the interpretation of this trial, even by its detractors.

Achieving Prognostic Factor Balance by Minimization

The second "mixed allocation" strategy we have used to achieve prognostic factor balance is named "minimization" (26). Although sometimes used in mega-trials, it is particularly useful for achieving good balance in small trials.

TABLE 5-3   Baseline Balance for Prognostic Factors among Men in the
Recent Recurrent Presumed Cerebral Emboli Study

Site and Residuum	Sulfinpyrazone (%)	Aspirin (%)	Both (%)	Neither (%)
Carotid, with residua	27	29	28	30
Carotid, no residua	35	37	41	34
V-B, with residua	10	6	8	7
V-B, no residua	15	19	17	13
Both, with residua	9	3	4	2
Both, no residua	4	5	3	13
Totals	100	100	100	100

You begin by identifying the prognostic (or simply cosmetic) factors you want balanced. Then you dichotomize them, either at some estimated mid-point or at some clinically sensible break-point. For example, in one of our compliance trials we had just 38 noncompliant, uncontrolled hypertensive steel workers in whom we wanted to test a set of behavioral strategies for their effects on compliance and blood pressure control (27). We were concerned about balance (for reasons of credibility as well as confounding), so we began by identifying three factors we thought needed balancing:

1. The level of their diastolic blood pressure (upper versus lower halves of their overall distribution of diastolic blood pressures).
2. Their past compliance 6 months into their treatment for hypertension (upper versus lower halves of their distribution of percent compliance by pill-count).
3. Whether they had previously gone through a special education program for hypertensives.

We assigned arbitrary scores of 1 each to the upper half of diastolic blood pressure, the lower half of compliance, and having received education. Thus, a study patient with "upper half" blood pressure, "lower-half" compliance, and who had not received education would score 1 + 1 + 0 = 2 points.

We then allocated patients according to a set of standard minimization rules that minimized the differences in total points between the experimental and control patients. Although we've long since thrown away the actual allocation schedule for this 1974 compliance trial, the schedule shown in Table 5-4 is an accurate representation of how we handled each patient:

- patient no. 1 was randomized (she had a score of 2, and was randomized to the control group),
- patient no. 2 had a score of 1, and to minimize the difference in total scores between the two groups, he was allocated to the experimental group
- patient no. 3 had a score of 2, and minimization allocated him to the experimental group as well and so on, as shown in Table 5-4.

TABLE 5–4   **Allocation by Minimization**

Patient No.	Score	Allocated By	Running Score Totals Experimental	Control
At the start			0	0
1	2	Randomization	0	Randomized here, so running score for control patients = 2
2	1	Minimization	Minimized here, so running score for experimental patients = 1	2
3	2	Minimization	Minimized here again, so 1 + 2 = 3	2
4	1	Minimization	3	Minimized here, so 2 + 1 = 3
5	0	Randomization	Randomized here, but 3 + 0 still = only 3	3
6	3	Randomization	3	Randomized here, so 3 + 3 = 6
7	2	Minimization	Minimized here, so 3 + 2 = 5	6
Etc.	Etc.	Etc.	Etc.	Etc.

Note that every time the running scores are tied, the next patient was randomized.

By employing minimization, we achieved excellent balance for these prognostic factors in our small compliance trial (its execution and positive result appears as the scenario for Section 6.12 on "Small Trials"). Moreover, in part because of the correlation between the factors we chose and age, height, weight, and symptoms, we also achieved excellent balance for these latter features.

There are a few other "chance" methods for assigning patients to treatments, but we won't discuss them here; they are nicely reviewed in the Lancet series from Ken Schulz and David Grimes (28).

Should Minimization Replace Randomization in All Trials?

Although it may sound heretical, a strong argument can be made for choosing minimization over randomization in all RCTs, even the very large ones. This argument rests on a series of realizations. First, randomization serves two purposes: concealment and balance. Second, there are other tactics (such as assignment through a central facility) for achieving concealment.

Third, as we've just shown you, minimization is a better method for achieving balance for *known* prognostic factors.

However, that leaves the *unknown* prognostic factors. They are ignored in minimization, but on average balanced by randomization. Because of this potential imbalance in important but unknown prognostic factors, many methodologists are uncomfortable abandoning the "gold standard" of random allocation for the "platinum standard" of minimization (29).

Allocation of Patients to Multiple Treatments: the Factorial Design

Thus far, we have described allocation to a single experimental group and a single control group. But, what if you want to study two drugs rather than just one, as in the RRPCE trial? Although you could perform a 3-arm trial (Drug A, Drug B, and Placebo) there is another design that gives the same information with fewer patients, and as a bonus may even detect interactions between the two drugs.

This is the factorial design in which patients (following stratification) are randomized (or minimized) to one of *four* groups as shown in Table 5–5.

As long as there is no "interaction" between the two drugs (such that one of them works better or worse in combination with the other than it

TABLE 5–5 A Factorial Design

		Treatment A		Efficacy of S
		Active	Placebo	
Treatment S	Active	a	b	a + b
				vs.
	Placebo	c	d	c + d
	Efficacy of A	a + c vs. b + d		

does when given by itself), the efficacy of both treatments are determined "at the margins." That is, the efficacy of Treatment S is accurately determined by comparing outcomes for the *combined* arms (a + b) versus (c + d), and the efficacy of Treatment A is accurately determined by comparing outcomes for the *combined* arms (a + c) versus (b + d). As a result, it becomes possible to test two drugs for the price (in terms of sample size) of one, which is why the factorial trial is often recommended by methodologists (30) and becoming increasingly popular among trialists. As noted at the start of this paragraph, however, when the drugs interact (such that their effects are not additive) it becomes inappropriate to assess their efficacy at the margins, and the sample size advantage is lost (we'll come back to this issue in Section 5.7 ("Analysis and Interpretation").

Why Blinding Is Important, and How to Initiate It

In an ideal RCT, the experimental treatment is given to everyone in the experimental group and to no one in the control group. Moreover, both groups are treated equally in all other respects. Finally, their outcomes are ascertained and reported with equal vigor and accuracy. These ideals are at risk whenever the treating clinician or patient "breaks the code" and learns who is receiving which treatment. The risks of "unblinding" are three:

1. *Contamination of the control group:*   When either the clinician or the patient is pretty certain that the experimental therapy is superior, one or both of them may take steps to ensure that control patients receive it. The result of this contamination is a decrease in any difference in outcomes between the two groups. The damage done by contamination adds a methodologic justification to the ethical justification for employing the "uncertainty principle" in recruiting patients for RCTs. As discussed in Section 6.7, unless both clinician and patient are genuinely uncertain as to which treatment is better, the patient should not be enrolled in the trial.

2. *Unequal cointervention:*   New treatments are not tested in isolation, and patients in RCTs can (and, in the case of previously validated treatments, must) receive a wide array of other (we'll call them "ancillary") treatments that will, on average, favorably affect their outcomes. If these cointerventions are unequally applied to, or complied with by, experimental and control patients, it may become impossible to decide whether any end-of-study differences in their outcomes are due to the experimental treatment or to unequal cointervention. The problem of cointervention is especially troublesome when it is also an outcome used to assess the efficacy of experimental therapy (such as the decision to hospitalize or operate on a study patient).

3. *Unequal ascertainment of outcomes:*   Some trial outcomes (such as total mortality) are unambiguously "hard." That is, they are easy to ascertain, and even unblinded observers of a given study patient are unlikely to disagree about whether they have occurred. But what

about "softer" but important outcomes (such as mild discreet clinical events, symptoms, function, or quality of life)? When blinding is lost, the ascertainment of these outcomes may be affected by study clinicians' or patients' preconceived notions about efficacy. When study patients or their clinicians know which treatment they are receiving, they may be followed more or less closely for "soft" outcomes, and their symptoms played up or ignored. Moreover, the threshold for carrying out definitive diagnostic testing may differ. Finally, a patient's knowledge of their treatment (a "new and promising drug" or "just a sugar pill") can affect not only their symptoms, but also their quality of life.

As shown in the preceding text, concealed allocation and blinding, if protected throughout the trial, permit you to avoid contamination, cointervention, and unequal ascertainment of outcomes. We'll describe some tactics for maintaining both in later stages of a trial as they arise.

You may have noticed that we never employ the term "double-blind" in this chapter. That's because a team led by PJ Devereaux documented that this term has several meanings for both trialists and clinicians (31). As a consequence, it cannot accurately describe the "blind" status of the (at least) seven sorts of individuals who are involved in any clinical trial (trial patients, their clinicians, data collectors, outcome assessors/adjudicators, data analysts, trial monitoring committee members, and manuscript writers).

We also haven't replaced the term "blinding" with the euphemism "masking." Readers who wonder why or prefer the latter term should ponder whether they've ever seen a Halloween mask that didn't actually prevent blindness by providing holes through which the wearer could see what was really going on.

Should You Test Patients' and Clinicians' Blindness During and After Your Trial?

Some writers about RCTs suggest testing clinicians and patients for "blindness" during and after trials. We don't, for two reasons. First, during the trial, we want our clinicians and patients to focus on following the protocol and taking study medications as prescribed. We don't want them distracted by "games" or detective work that might break the code (20).

Second, asking patients or their clinicians after a trial to guess which treatment each of them received is *not* a test for blindness. In fact, it confounds bad blinding with good hunches about efficacy. If that last sentence is either totally mystifying or terribly tantalizing, skip to the discussion of "Should you test for blindness during and after your trial?" in Section 5.5 ("Intervention, Follow-up, and Protocol Adherence"). In summary, we work very hard before starting a trial to establish and test blindness in its "pilot" phase, but we never test for blindness during or after our trials.

What Should You Do When Blinding Is Impossible?

Finally, blinding is impossible for lots of trials. "Mock" surgery, such as skin incisions alone versus full arthroscopic knee surgery (32), is rarely employed, and its ethics become hotly debated when it occurs (33). Placebo physical or psychologic therapy is difficult to design and apply. As a result, tactics for preventing or minimizing the effects of the absence of blinding in RCTs are very important. They include rigorous, all encompassing ancillary treatment protocols (to prevent unequal cointervention), equally intense follow-up of experimental and control patients, and the employment of blind, external outcome adjudicators (to reduce biased outcome assessment). These tactics will be discussed in subsequent sections of this chapter.

Why an Audit Trial Is Important, and How to Create One

For scientific validity, and even more so for clinical credibility, you must be able to account for every patient who was allocated to treatment in your trial. This accounting has to include patients who refused their treatment allocation or left the trial for any reason, because they remain essential members of any intention-to-treat analysis. Registration of every study patient at allocation also permits you to start an individual patient file. Not only can you add all pertinent follow-up information to this file; you also can employ it to schedule their follow-up visits and to remind their clinicians if they fail to show up.

Alternative Allocation Strategies

There are six other allocation strategies that are employed by some trialists, sometimes. We've never used most of them, so we won't pretend to know their ins and outs. Instead, we will refer you to other sources that describe them in greater detail.

CLUSTER RANDOMIZATION. Study patients don't exist in isolation, nor do the clinicians who offer them experimental treatments. Sometimes you might want to apply your intervention to clinicians, or hospital wards, or entire villages, rather than individual patients. In these situations, it is neither possible nor even sensible to try to allocate individual patients to your intervention. Asking a clinician to apply guidelines for more appropriate diagnostic testing on just a random half of his patients guarantees contamination in how he manages the other, "control" half. Holding facilitated public meetings for improving birth outcomes with just half the women in a village can't avoid contaminating their neighbors.

The solution here is to allocate study individuals in "clusters" such as families, practices, hospital wards, communities, provinces, and the like. For example, 12 pairs of Nepalese villages were randomized in a cluster trial of "facilitated monthly women's discussion groups" (34). A female facilitator made nine visits a month to one of each pair. This low-cost intervention produced striking reductions in both maternal and neonatal mortality.

Because the responses of study individuals within these clusters can be expected to be more similar (or "concordant") than the responses of individuals belonging to different clusters, sample sizes have to be adjusted upwards, as I'll remind you in Section 5.8 (on "Sample Size Calculations").

You can apply a powerful form of cluster randomization when your state, province, or country decides to provide a community-based intervention to all of its citizens. Typically, it doesn't have the resources to start it in every community at once. In that case, why not randomized the *order* in which communities receive the intervention?

ALLOCATION BETWEEN PAIRED ORGANS. Most patients have two eyes, arms, hips, and kidneys. When an experimental treatment acts only locally, a case can be made for randomizing organs within patients, thereby removing a source of between-patient "noise" from the determination of a treatment's effectiveness. For example, an RCT of prophylactic laser treatment admitted patients whose both eyes were at risk of macular degeneration (35). One eye was randomized to undergo laser treatment, and the other to observation only. A similar allocation strategy has been used or suggested for trials of locally acting topical drugs or hip-protectors. The risk in allocation between paired organs, as in other trials, is contamination in the form of a carry-over of the experimental treatment to the control organ of the pair, reducing the difference in outcomes between them. Because this is a conservative bias (leading to the conclusion that treatment is worthless when, in fact, it is beneficial), this design deserves greater use. However, allocation between paired organs can obscure systemic adverse effects.

ALLOCATION IN PAIRED SEQUENTIAL TRIALS. When outcomes occur quickly and eligible patients present in a steady stream, some trialists randomize the first member of a pair (sometimes after matching them for important prognostic factors) and assign the second member to the alternative therapy. The outcomes are assessed within each pair, assigning a "+" to the pair if the experimental patient fared better, a "0" if they fared the same, and a "−" if the control patient fared better. The results for successive pairs are then put into a graph such as shown in Figure 5–2, with enrollment of successive pairs along the *x*-axis and their outcomes along the *y*-axis. A "+" result raises the cumulative results line one unit along the *y*-axis, a "−" result lowers it one unit, and a "0" result keeps it on the level. Statistical boundaries can be constructed such that, when they are crossed, a conclusion can be drawn that experimental therapy is efficacious or harmful, or that it is futile to continue the trial. In the example depicted in Figure 5–2, the experimental therapy ultimately crosses the statistical boundary for efficacy. You can read more about sequential designs in Curt Meinert's book (36).

ADAPTIVE ALLOCATION STRATEGIES BASED ON OUTCOMES. Some trialists have generated methods for altering the allocation ratio based on the outcomes of previously admitted patients. Thus, if the last patient allocated to experimental therapy did well, the probability that the next eligible patient

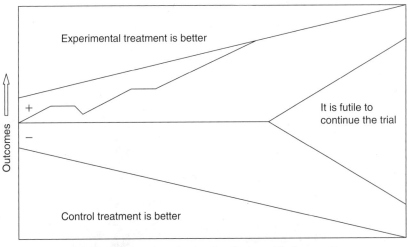

FIGURE 5-2 A sequential trial.

would be allocated to experimental therapy would rise. These "play-the-winner" strategies are appealing to some trialists, but are at risk of revealing the likely allocation of the next patient. In addition, they are not well-suited for long-term trials with substantial delays between entry and outcome. Again, we refer you to one of the RCT texts for more about adaptive allocation strategies (37).

ALLOCATION IN CROSSOVER TRIALS. When the outcomes of interest in a trial are symptoms, functional capacity, or other outcomes that produce no permanent changes in study patients, you can reduce "noise" and your sample size requirement by giving both the experimental and control treatments to every patient, simply randomizing the order in which they are applied (38). Although ideal for some situations, you can't determine whether the treatment given first has any permanent ("carry-over") effects until the trial is over. If it does display this "order effect," the power of the crossover design is reduced to that of a two-group RCT. Moreover, in infertility trials where pregnancy is the outcome, a McMaster team showed that crossover trials overestimated odds ratios for efficacy by 74% (39). Stuart Pocock devotes a chapter to crossover trials in his RCT text (40).

ALLOCATION BY RANDOMIZED CONSENT ("ZELEN" TRIALS). Marvin Zelen introduced an allocation strategy in which eligible patients are randomized to one of two groups *before* seeking their consent (41). Members of Group 1 are offered the experimental treatment and undergo full RCT informed consent. Members of Group 2 are offered current standard therapy and undergo only routine clinical consent. The Zelen "randomized consent" design is preferred by clinicians who are concerned that the informed consent

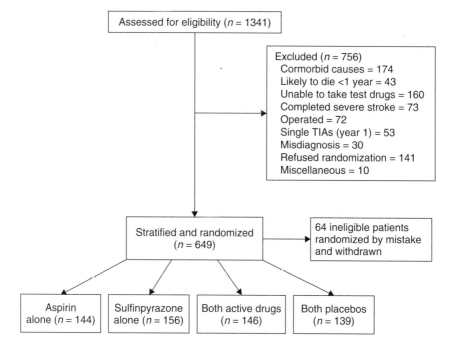

FIGURE 5–3 Recent Recurrent Presumed Cerebral Emboli (RRPCE) patient-flow diagram after allocation.

procedure impairs the physician–patient relationship and patient accrual. They may be right, for the introduction of the Zelen allocation strategy into a flagging breast cancer trial was followed by a sixfold increase in its recruitment rate (42). Not surprisingly, some ethicists are concerned about including outcome and other information from control patients who haven't undergone informed consent to be analyzed.

Once trial patients are allocated, their regimens have to be applied, adhered to, and monitored. The next section of this chapter deals with interventions (including non-drug maneuvers), placebos, compliance, protocol adherence, and compliance. Before we go there, however, we invite you to take a detour to Section 6.7 and consider an absolute prerequisite for allocating any patient to any trial intervention: uncertainty.

The update of our RRPCE patient-flow diagram appears in Figure 5–3.

5.5 INTERVENTION, FOLLOW-UP, AND PROTOCOL ADHERENCE

We randomized study patients to one of four oral regimens. Each was taken four times daily and consisted of, a 200-mg tablet of sulfinpyrazone plus a placebo capsule, a placebo tablet plus a 325-mg capsule of acetylsalicylic acid, both active drugs, or both placebos. Each active drug and its corresponding placebo were identical in size, shape, weight and color and were shipped to the participating centers in identical bottles of 130, labeled with 4-digit random numbers. Neither the patient nor the clinician were told which regimen had been assigned, but both were given a 24-hour telephone number for emergency code-breaking. To prevent participating neurologists from inadvertently breaking the code by discovering the hypouricemia that sulfinpyrazone produces, local laboratories deleted uric acid values from their local reports and sent them directly to the Methods Center. At the end of the trial (but before the code was broken), we asked the neurologists to predict both the overall study results and the regimens for each of their patients.

We asked our patients to return unused medication at each follow-up visit, and we counted their remaining pills to estimate medication compliance. We also measured compliance, contamination, and cointervention by determining changes in serum uric acid, sulfinpyrazone blood levels, and aspirin-specific *in vitro* effects on platelet function (keeping all of these results from patients and their neurologists throughout the trial). Because aspirin-containing compounds were ubiquitous, we urged our patients to avoid cold remedies and other over-the-counter nostrums, and recommended acetaminophen (paracetamol) when they needed an analgesic. Finally, because many psychoactive drugs also affect platelet function, we asked study patients' clinicians to restrict their choice of tranquilizers to diazepam or chlordiazepoxide.

We reevaluated study patients face-to-face at 1 and 3 months and every 3 months thereafter. At each visit we obtained a detailed neurologic history and examination, smoking history, blood chemistries, hematologic measurements, and platelet function tests (we repeated chest films and electrocardiograms annually). At the end of each visit, study staff telephoned the Methods Center and the next bottle of study drugs was assigned.

The treatment code was broken for just one patient, and only one other patient was permanently lost to follow-up.

Intervention, follow-up and protocol adherence checklist:

✓ Specify your precise experimental and comparison regimens.
✓ Identify the source and "packaging" of your regimens.
✓ Set up a system for distributing and maintaining supplies of your regimens.
✓ Set up a system for emergency code-breaking (when patients and/or clinicians are blind).
✓ Set up a system for maintaining blindness (when patients and/or clinicians are blind).
✓ Decide what to do about monitoring (and, if necessary, improving) patient compliance.

✓ Design follow-up procedures.

✓ Set up a system for avoiding (and documenting) contamination and cointervention.

✓ Set up a system for maintaining protocol adherence by your collaborators.

The scenario chronicles how we handled the items on the checklist, and contains, in retrospect, one dumb mistake (see if you can spot it before we get to it in the text below).

✓ *Specify your precise experimental and comparison regimens.*

You should begin by deciding who should do what to your study patients, and when and where this should take place. As with every other item on the intervention checklist, whether your decisions here are "right" or "wrong" depends on how well they match your study question's location along the explanatory–management spectrum. Consistent with the highly explanatory nature of the RRPCE study, expert stroke-neurologists applied its specially prepared treatments in a double-blind fashion during frequent patient-visits to the subspecialty clinics of major university-affiliated hospitals. This specification would have been inappropriate for an extremely pragmatic trial of these drugs in community settings. In the latter case, we might go so far as to recruit general practitioners into a trial of open-label-aspirin versus nothing, carried out in their routine office practices.

We will discuss placebos a lot in Section 6.8 ("Placebos, Placebo Effects, and Placebo Ethics") and, as pointed out there, they can be presented as mock procedures or nontherapeutic patient–clinician interactions as well as by dummy pills. Often it is either impossible or unethical to devise mock-procedures in surgical trials. For example, in our RCT of extracranial-intracranial anastomosis for threatened stroke we never even discussed drilling unnecessary burr holes and carrying out "mock" superficial temporal–middle cerebral artery anastomoses (43). On the other hand, a group of Texas-based investigators, with approval from their ethics committee, carried out skin incisions and simulated debridement of knee joints in the "placebo" group of their RCT of arthroscopic surgery for osteoarthritic knees (44). It's a good thing that they did, because they wound up ruling out any important difference in pain and function following the full and mock procedures.

When the application of experimental treatments requires patients to spend considerable time with those who treat them, it may become difficult to distinguish the effect of the "active ingredient" (psychotherapy, skills training, and the like) from the simple effect of the attention they've received while getting it. If this is an issue in your RCT, you might consider introducing an "attention placebo" in which control patients spend an identical amount of time with their therapists, but receive none of the experimental "active ingredient" along the way. For example, a group of psychologists in North Carolina wanted to see whether a specific maneuver ("eye movement desensitization and reprocessing" or EMDR) would reduce the suffering of patients whose panic disorders included agoraphobia (the fear of open spaces and public places) (45). They randomized patients currently on their waiting list for desensitization and reprocessing to three regimens: immediate EMDR, remaining on the waiting list, or an immediate attention placebo consisting of relaxation training plus "association" therapy, none of which had been shown previously to help such patients. They found that patients undergoing immediate EMDR had less severe symptoms on follow-up than patients randomized to remain on the waiting list. However, EMDR patients fared no better than patients who received the attention placebo, and the authors concluded, "EMDR should not be the first-line treatment for this disorder."

When is it wrong to use placebos? This is discussed in some detail in Section 6.8 on "Placebo Ethics." For now, we'll simply state that we stop using placebos as soon as the totality of evidence (including especially systematic reviews of relevant RCTs) convince the "expert clinical community" that an experimental treatment does more good than harm. This conviction, or reduction of uncertainty (which could also be described as a loss of clinical equipoise), converts the previously experimental treatment into "established effective therapy," (which I will call EET). As soon as an effective therapy is established, we don't think it is either ethical or clinically sensible to test the next promising intervention against placebo. The only exceptions to this rule are when patients can't or won't take the EET, or when the next promising treatment is an "add-on" to it.

By "add-on" I mean a promising, untested "new treatment" (which I will call "NT") that you think might provide further benefit to patients when it is added to EET. In that case, you can determine the "superiority" or incremental benefit of combination therapy by giving your control group the EET plus placebo-NT, and by giving your experimental group EET plus active-NT.

For example, several investigators have carried out RCTs of ACE-inhibitors in the secondary prevention of cardiovascular disease. However, previous trials had already established the effectiveness of aspirin, β blockers, and statins for this condition. As a result, it was neither clinically sensible nor ethical to randomize patients to receive just the ACE-inhibitor or a placebo. Rather, these latter ACE-inhibitor trials compared the effects of aspirin, β blockers, and statins alone (in the control group) with the effects of these EETs plus an ACE-inhibitor (in the experimental group). When drug trials of this sort need to be carried out in a blind fashion, control patients are given EETs plus placebos, resulting in what is often called a "placebo add-on" trial. The key issue here, however, is that all patients in both groups receive EETs.

Suppose, on the other hand, you are not testing an "add-on" to be given at the same time as EET (say it's a new antiplatelet drug that, for safety reasons, can't be given with aspirin). In this case, it's both sensible and ethical to specify your treatment groups as EET (control) versus the new treatment (experimental). Because such "head-to-head" trials withhold EET from the new treatment group, you need plenty of prior evidence (from bench research and Phase 1 and 2 trials) to justify withholding it. Ideally, this prior evidence will strongly suggest that your new treatment is better than EET. Alternatively, it should strongly suggest that your new treatment is as good as EET, but possessing some other advantage such as being safer, cheaper, easier to take, or the like.

✓ Identify the source and "packaging" of your regimens.

As in the RRPCE study, it frequently is possible to obtain free active drugs and indistinguishable placebos from drug manufacturers, especially when the latter stand to gain financially from a positive trial. Clearly, the time for you to test their indistinguishability is before, not during, your trial. You want to be sure, before you begin, that they look, taste, smell, feel, and float the same. Next, you need to be sure that the unblinding of one patient does not unblind any other patients (as would occur if, as in one study we know about, all active containers were labeled "Treatment A" and had black caps and all placebo containers were labeled "Treatment B" and had white caps). "Mock procedure" and "attention" placebos need attention of a rather different sort. The objective there is consistency in applying the mock procedure or attention to every control patient.

✓ Set up a system for distributing and maintaining supplies of your regimens.

Mundane but crucial, you need to be sure that every center has enough of the experimental and control regimen at hand to meet the needs of every new and follow-up patient. Overnight couriers can get you out of trouble, but they eat up your budget.

✓ Set up a system for emergency code-breaking (when patients and/or clinicians are blind).

Patients and their clinicians must have 24/7 access to an emergency code-breaking service. When this service is supplied by the local center's pharmacy, code-breaking may occur for trivial reasons. When feasible, we prefer to provide a central code-breaking service that can study and discuss each specific request. As a general rule, if the subsequent management of a patient who stops the study drug for any reason would be the same whether the patient was on the experimental or control regimens, there is no reason for breaking the code. This policy is especially important if the patient is likely to resume taking the study drug at some later date. Among the 585 patients in the RRPCE trial, we broke the code for just one.

✓ Set up a system for maintaining blindness (when patients and/or clinicians are blind).

Systems for maintaining blindness begin with the provision of identically-appearing active and control treatments. This is easy when both are pills, but can be difficult for non drug regimens. You've already learned in Section 5.5 ("Intervention, Follow-up, and Protocol Adherence") how a surgical trial maintained blindness by performing incisions on both groups. The most intricate I've encountered was a trial on the question: "Among in-patients with proximal vein thrombosis, does a continuous heparin infusion (compared with intermittent subcutaneous heparin) reduce the risk of recurrent venous thromboembolism?" (46) Because the search for outcome-events included clinical suspicion as well as routine surveillance, blinding was vital. We solved this by giving every study patient both infusions and subcutaneous injections, only one of which was real and the other a placebo (some trialists call this a "double-dummy" strategy). We even gave the ward staff regular instructions to change the doses of both the active and placebo regimens.

In some trials, you will need to blind patients and clinicians to telltale "markers" of their treatments as well as to the treatments themselves. As you learned in the scenario, one of the drugs in the RRPCE trial caused a fall in the serum uric acid results that were included in most routine laboratory reports. Special arrangements had to be made with each laboratory to delete these values from routine reports and send them only to the Methods Center (see next checklist item).

Should You Test for Blindness During and After Your Trial?

Should you continue to test for the maintenance of blindness throughout and after your RCT? Although we urge that such tests be routine and rigorous before the trial, as the regimens are being created and debugged, we think testing for blindness should stop there. Our reasons are two. First, we don't want to create a "guessing game" environment during the trial that might render patients and clinicians more interested in guessing their regimen than in following it.

Second, we learned the hard way that "end-of-study" tests for blindness don't really test for blindness (and this is the mistake we alluded to at the start of this section). As noted in the scenario, at the end of the RRPCE trial, but before its results were given to them, study neurologists completed forms in which they predicted both the overall study results and the regimens for each of their patients. With four regimens, we'd expect blind clinicians to guess the correct one for 25% of their patients. We held our breath, hoping that our clinicians wouldn't do better than this, for fear that their "loss of blindness" would damage the credibility of our trial. As it happened, they did statistically significantly *worse* than chance, correctly identifying the regimen for only 18% of their patients! (47) Our faulty reasoning was exposed when we examined their predictions of the overall study results: they tended to predict that sulfinpyrazone was efficacious and aspirin wasn't, precisely the reverse of the actual result. It then dawned on us that we were testing them, not for blindness, but for their hunches about efficacy. When their patient had done well they tended to predict they were on sulfinpyrazone, and when they had done poorly, on placebo or aspirin. How fortunate for us all that their hunches were wrong! If they had been correct, the interpretation of our end-of-study test for blindness would be that they had broken the randomization code. We hope that future trialists won't repeat our mistake.

✓ Decide what to do about monitoring (and, if necessary, improving) patient compliance.

Sometimes you can make a case for omitting ongoing compliance monitoring. For one-shot treatments (operations and the like), compliance monitoring is complete at the start of the trial. In management trials that are testing alternative treatment policies for their real-world effectiveness, you can argue that you should leave patients alone to comply or not as they would if no trials were under way. Even in this latter case, however, readers of your subsequent report will wonder whether study patients followed their assigned regimens. Accordingly, you should consider setting up unobtrusive compliance measurements even in the most pragmatic of trials. These could include monitoring (but not feeding back to patients or clinicians) the extent to which the former kept follow-up appointments, refilled prescriptions, and the like.

It is in performing explanatory (efficacy) trials of repeated or long-term treatments that compliance monitoring and intervention are important. Because your explanatory trial's objective is to show whether your experimental treatment can work under ideal circumstances, you want to be sure that study patients are complying with it. One way to achieve high compliance is to identify and exclude noncompliers before the trial begins. For example, the US Veterans Administration landmark hypertension trials in the 1960s placed all prospective study patients on a riboflavin-laced placebo and gave them a set of clinic appointments, at each of which their urines were tested for riboflavin (48). Only patients who kept their appointments and consistently passed riboflavin were eligible to be randomized.

If such a "faintness-of-heart" strategy is not feasible, you will have to decide how to detect the different forms of noncompliance and what to do when you find them. We've summarized some advice about this in Table 5–6.

You should contact patients who drop-out of your trial and, unless they wish to be left alone, identify the problems that caused this. You can then negotiate solutions to these problems with them (transport to and from the study center, more convenient visits, home visits for delivering

TABLE 5–6 **Types of Noncompliance and What to Do About Them**

Type of Noncompliance	Detection	Strategy for Preventing or Improving
Dropping-out	Stops attending to renew study drugs	Transport, home visits, or at least keeping in touch
Stopping study treatment	Returning full containers	Negotiation
Missing follow-up visits	Partial attendance	Home visits
Low compliance with study treatment	Interviews, pill-counts, electronic pill containers, body fluid measurements	Behavioral strategies, including feedback and incentives

study drugs and monitoring progress, etc.). Study patients who miss occasional follow-up visits may accept home visits. When patients keep their appointments but return full containers or aren't following any of their assigned treatment, problem-solving and negotiation should center on gaining their willingness to take at least some of it. If sensible given their regimen, "drug holidays" can be negotiated, followed by resuming all or at least some of their assigned treatment.

The most common problem for most trials is low compliance with study regimens among otherwise cooperative study patients. The cold, hard fact is that people who are prescribed self-administered medications in routine clinical practice typically take less than half of their prescribed doses (49). In RCTs, however, compliance as measured by pill-counts is usually high (92% in the RRPCE trial). This may be due to the increased attention, information, and supervision trial patients receive. The methods for detecting low compliance, ranked from easiest (but least sensitive) to hardest (but most sensitive) are: asking the patient, counting returned pills, employing electronic pill containers that record whenever they are opened, and (for the most accurate determination of compliance on the day of measurement) determinations of drugs or their metabolites in body fluids.

Once detected, what can be done to improve study patients' compliance with their treatments? Effective strategies identified so far tend to be rather weak, and must be combined and sustained to be helpful. They are combinations of: more convenient care, information, reminders, self-monitoring, reinforcement, counseling, family therapy, and other forms of additional supervision by or attention from a health care provider (physician, nurse, pharmacist or other) (50). We suggest that you periodically consult The Cochrane Library to keep abreast of updated systematic reviews about effective compliance-improving strategies.

✓ Design follow-up procedures.

If yours is a pragmatic trial involving "hard" outcomes such as death, you may plan for no follow-up visits at all, just an end-of-study determination of study patients' outcomes. At the other extreme, an explanatory trial may require frequent follow-up visits and extra attention that would not be provided in ordinary care (in the RRPCE trial we asked patients to come in every 3 months regardless of how they felt they were doing).

How frequently to schedule follow-up visits in an RCT is a balancing act. On the one hand, the increased cost, bother, investigator and patient fatigue, and opportunities for lost or incomplete data all argue against frequent follow-up visits. On the other hand, the need to search for and respond to side effects, the attention required for maintaining high compliance, the need to detect subtle or intermittent outcome events, and the simple necessity for keeping track of study patients may require frequent visits. Blind trials always require identical follow-up schedules for experimental and control patients. Moreover, when outcome-events are mild (fatigue) or "soft" (fleeting sensory TIA), identical follow-up schedules for experimental and control patients will detect them with equal accuracy.

In any case, you want to keep track of every patient in your trial. You laid the groundwork for this by gaining contact information for the patient's younger relative at the time of recruitment, and in long-term trials you may need to update this information periodically. With care at the outset and effort along the way, it is possible to keep track of virtually every patient in your trial (we lost one of our RRPCE patients, but none of 1,495 in the EC/IC Bypass Trial and none of 662 patients in the NASCET trial).

✓ Set up a system for avoiding (and documenting) contamination and cointervention.

You don't want control patients to accidentally (even worse, intentionally) receive the experimental regimen (contamination). This is easy when the experimental regimen is available only within the trial. But when it is available outside the trial you will need to ask patients and study clinicians to avoid it and to use alternative drugs when required. For example, in the RRPCE we asked all study patients to avoid aspirin and other platelet-suppressing drugs, recommending acetaminophen for pain. We monitored aspirin contamination in several centers with a platelet function test specifically affected by aspirin, and sulfinpyrazone contamination with a review of serum urate levels (which are lowered by sulfinpyrazone).

Similarly, you don't want just one of your groups to receive some additional intervention that might affect their risk of an outcome-event (cointervention). When it is possible to keep patients and their clinicians blind to their treatments, this is not a concern. When blinding is impossible or unwarranted, you might ask study clinicians to generate consensus-protocols for all other treatments, including interventions for frequent or perplexing comorbid conditions, in both groups.

✓ Set up a system for maintaining protocol adherence by your collaborators.

We've already described some of the elements of this system (monitoring code-breaking, patient compliance, contamination, and cointervention). You'll want to monitor the timeliness with which follow-up visits are held and reported, as well as the quality and timeliness of the data submitted in these reports. The speedy detection and intervention around protocol violations is important, and although some of this work can be carried out by study staff, one of the most important functions of the PI (and a high priority for their time and talents) is to go out to centers with flagging adherence and help them improve their performance.

Once again The Cochrane Library can provide the trialist with promising strategies that have been shown to improve the rates with which clinicians apply clinical protocols. Chief among these strategies is audit and feedback (51), with marginal additional improvements from interactive (not merely didactic) workshops (52), and educational outreach visits, particularly when "educational influentials" apply "social marketing" strategies (53).

Much of the foregoing is oriented toward drug trials. Placebos often play a central role, so you might want to read about them in Section 6.8

(on "Placebos, Placebo Effects, and Placebo Ethics"). But because many trials don't involve drugs at all, there's a chunk on nondrug trials in Section 6.9 ("Special Issues in Nondrug Trials").

5.6 EVENTS

We examined follow-up data for the three events of TIA, stroke and death, and harm that might have been caused by our treatment.

Transient Ischemic Attacks

We reviewed each follow-up examination for the presence and number of attacks over each period of follow-up. The occurrence of any ischemic attacks during a follow-up period constituted an event. Because patients who go on to stroke may not, and patients who die cannot, have further ischemic attacks, the last two events were included in this analysis of continuing attacks. Among subjects with multiple events, the date of the first relevant event was used for the analysis.

Stroke

From follow-up data, we identified two groups of patients with possible strokes and submitted their "blinded" records for adjudication. The first group consisted of patients in whom neurologists reported a stroke in a follow-up narrative summary. The second group had complained of one or more ischemic events with a residual neurologic deficit lasting for more than 24 hours. Because dead patients cannot proceed to stroke, death was included in these analyses.

Death

Finally, we documented each death and classified its underlying cause (cerebrovascular, coronary, other vascular or nonvascular).

Harm

In addition, at each follow-up visit we carried out standardized searches for side effects and toxicity (vomiting, nausea, upper abdominal pain, hematemesis, melena, heartburn, renal colic or urinary stone, hematuria, hypoglycemic reaction, skin rash, and an open-ended question about any other complications).

Events Checklist:

✓ Choose the events.
✓ Generate event criteria.
✓ Decide how, when, and by whom to ascertain these events.
✓ Consider event-hierarchies.

✓ Set up an event-reporting system.

✓ Set up an event-adjudicating system.

✓ Decide whether any events will be ineligible for the analysis
   (and develop a plan for their bias-free removal).

Glossary Note: I will use the term "event" to describe an occurrence, incident, or experience of a trial patient that is important in answering the
study question about benefit and harm. You will find other words used for
this purpose elsewhere. I won't use the term "endpoint" because of its con-
notation that the study is over when it occurs. I won't use the term "outcome" because it suggests a final, fixed state that cannot change, especially
for the worse. Finally, I will stretch the term "event" to include continuous measures (such as functional capacity or symptom severity) when they
provide important answers to questions about efficacy or safety.

   Events in clinical trials help us document the success of our experimental treatment in achieving one or more of the "5 Ps". Preventing or
Postponing bad events, Promoting good events, Palliating the course of a
relentless disorder, or Poisoning the patient with an adverse effect (54).
The events prevented (or at least postponed) in the RRPCE study were of
the yes/no ("discrete") variety. Other "events" in other trials, such as blood
pressure, number of days of diarrhea in the past month, or quality of life,
are of a matter of degree ("continuous") variety. I'll discuss both sorts in
this section.

   On to the checklist:

✓ *Choose the events.*

As in every other step in your trial, the "right way" to decide on the events
you want to capture is determined by the precise question you hope to answer. Was it about prevention, promotion, postponement, palliation, or poisoning? You could collect dozens of different sorts of events, but the effort
and cost of ascertaining each one of them with accuracy and precision can
be huge. In addition, as you'll learn in the next section (if you don't already
know it), your risk of drawing a false-positive conclusion (that your treatment works when, in fact, it doesn't) rises with the number of different
sorts of events you analyze.

   You should therefore keep the number of different sorts of events to
a minimum. One way to do this is to ask two blunt questions: First, which
events do you need to capture to answer your key questions about benefit and harm? Second, which events will be decisive to a clinician and patient as they discuss whether to use your treatment? If answering the first
question requires a substantially longer list of events than answering the
second, you are overdoing it.

Composite Events

In order to answer your study question, you may need to create a "composite" event made up of several disparate events, any one of which constitutes a

bad result for patients. Sometimes, the components of these composite events are part of the same pathogenetic mechanism. For example, I chaired the Data Safety and Monitoring Committee for a trial of an ACE-inhibitor (ramipril) in a mix of patients who, for one or several reasons, were at increased risk of cardiovascular morbidity and mortality (55). The composite event in that trial was myocardial infarction, stroke, or cardiovascular death. (As it happened, the drug was efficacious enough, and the trial large enough, to generate statistically significant reductions for each of these three events considered individually, but reducing the composite event would have been enough to claim efficacy.)

In other trials, the components of a composite event might be quite independent from each other, resulting from entirely different pathogenetic mechanisms. For example, in carrying out our trials of anticoagulants and antithrombotics among patients with vascular disease, we and our patients were equally concerned about the events we hoped to prevent (e.g., pulmonary embolism) and the "poisonous" adverse events we might cause with our interventions (e.g., life-threatening hemorrhage).

The point here is that the components of the compound event must make sense to readers, and must not simply be a ploy you learned in Section 6.6 on "Physiological Statistics" for increasing the numbers of events in a trial that is too small.

Composite events pose problems in interpretation (56). Just because an experimental treatment reduces the overall occurrence of a composite event, that doesn't mean (and shouldn't be interpreted to mean) that the treatment benefits every individual component of that composite event. The latter conclusion has to wait until several, similar trials have been reported. Only then can we meta-analyze the individual components of a composite event to see whether they benefit from treatment.

There's a special case of composite events in which each succeeding component constitutes a progressively worse manifestation of the same pathogenetic process. Such a "hierarchy" appeared in the scenario as TIA or stroke or death. Hierarchies are important enough to deserve their own entry on the checklist, and I discuss them under the checklist item *Consider event-hierarchies.*

You may want to beef up your composite event by substituting a "biomarker" or "risk-factor" for one or more of your "hard" events. The creation and use of such "surrogate events" is tricky business, as you'll discover in the following paragraphs.

Surrogate Events

Sometimes (always?) you are short on time and patients for your trial. Events, even composite ones, may be so rare, and your treatment may take so long to affect them that you question the wisdom of even attempting a trial. In that situation, you might be tempted to change your "event" from the hard, clinical event itself to a "marker" or "surrogate" one, which, when measured after a few weeks of treatment, predicts the clinical event that won't occur for months or years. Alternatively, you might want to add the surrogate to the clinical event, forming a composite event. For example, in a coronary prevention trial, you might want to add the coronary risk factor levels such as low-density lipoprotein (LDL) cholesterol, or blood pressure (that every study patient has) to the few clinical coronary events (that only a few patients have).

Surrogate events (sometimes called "surrogate biomarkers") possess some real advantages. You can measure surrogates early in your trial. Moreover, they are typically "continuous" events so that every trial patient has a surrogate "event" (remember the "simple truth" back in Table 4–1 that the important number in an RCT is the number of events, not the number of patients?). As a result, the power of your trial (the probability that you'll detect the minimally important difference, if it really exists) soars. No wonder then, that you find surrogate markers such as tumor size in cancer trials, CD-4 lymphocyte counts in HIV-AIDS trials, and bone mineral density in osteoporotic fracture trials. However, markers have to possess certain attributes before they can become valid surrogates for "hard" clinical outcomes. Michael Hughes has thoughtfully described them as a trio (57):

1. They must be prognostic for your "hard" outcomes.
2. Changes in surrogates after starting experimental treatment must retain their prognostic power (i.e., they must predict corresponding changes in the occurrence of your "hard" outcome).
3. Effects of treatments on the surrogate marker should explain, or at least be associated with, effects of treatments on the "hard" outcome.

The problem is that a favorable change in your surrogate marker may not, in fact, guarantee a favorable change in the occurrence of later "hard" events. This can arise in two ways. First, the link between the surrogate marker and the event may be only statistical, not biological. In that case, changing the surrogate "risk-factor" will not change risk. For example, a group of allergists performed an RCT in which they added an oral leukotriene receptor antagonist to a drug regimen for asthma (58). They reported that although the new drug had a favorable effect on some surrogate inflammatory biomarkers, it did not improve lung function. For a second example, various treatments for osteoporosis can increase bone mineral density, a surrogate for fractures. However, a meta-analysis of several trials found no relation between changes in bone mineral density (the surrogate marker) and the risk of nonvertebral fractures (the clinical event) (59).

There is a second way that a favorable change in your surrogate marker may not guarantee a favorable change in later "hard" events. This occurs when your experimental treatment produces some other, harmful effect by a mechanism that is unrelated to your surrogate marker. In that case, the harmful effect could swamp any favorable effect predicted by improvements in your surrogate marker. There are lots of examples (and, tragically, lots of dead patients) that attest to this major drawback of surrogate markers. Several antiarrhythmic drugs have been shown to reduce serious arrhythmias following heart attacks, and several other drugs improve exercise-tolerance in patients with heart failure. Unfortunately, however, both sets of drugs increase mortality. In another "head-to-head" trial, although the newer, sexier antihypertensive drug doxazosin reduced diastolic blood pressure as effectively as "old-fashioned" chlorthalidone, patients randomized to doxazosin were twice as likely to wind up in heart failure (60).

Given these problems with surrogate events, it's wise to avoid relying on them (except perhaps in early Phase II trials). For a more detailed discussion of surrogate events, you could start with the summary of a National Institutes of Health Workshop on this issue (61) or with the excellent discussion led by Heiner Bucher (62). ✓

Harm   *Efficacy vs Toxicity.*

Of 548 new chemical entities approved by the US Food and Drug Administration between 1975 and 2000, 56 (10.2%) were found to cause serious harm (63). As a result, 16 (2.9%) were withdrawn from the market entirely, and 45 (8.2%) had to add a "black box" warning to their packaging to caution prescribers and users of that drug's "special problems that may lead to death or serious injury."

Why do RCTs perform so poorly in detecting this harm? There are two explanations (but no excuses) for this failure. First, we never start an RCT hoping to demonstrate that our experimental treatment does more harm ("Poison") than good. We focus on the other, "positive Ps," and devote most of our brains, time, and resources to their ascertainment.

The second explanation follows from the fact that most "serious unanticipated adverse events" (SUAEs) are rare. By their very nature, Phase III RCTs are insensitive in validating them. Mike Gent and I named the statistical explanation for this the "inverse rule of 3" (64). It simply states that, to be 95% sure of observing at least one adverse event that occurs once per x-many patients, you have to observe $3x$ patients. That is, if your treatment causes one adverse event in every 1,000 patients who receive it, you'll have to follow 3,000 patients to be 95% confident that you'll observe even one of them. Moreover, to conclude that they are occurring significantly more frequently among experimental than control patients, you need to follow several times 3x patients.

Phase III trials are just too small to detect the awful but rare unanticipated adverse events. That's why we've had to employ Phase IV "postmarketing surveillance" studies to detect them and to convince both their manufacturers and regulators to withdraw them.

There are benefits and risks in "lumping" all adverse events together and in "splitting" them into several small categories. Lumping makes for easy summaries, but will hide serious, rare adverse events. Similarly, splitting will provide great detail (e.g., dyspepsia, heart burn, abdominal pain, and cramp), but (like a series of small RCTs) can obscure an overall effect of treatment.

Nonetheless, the fact that SUAEs are rare is no excuse for ignoring them. As you read in the previous section on intervention and follow-up, and as you'll read in the later section on monitoring, you must both respond clinically to them at once and document their occurrence for later incorporation into meta-analyses of sufficient size to determine their importance.

✓ Generate event criteria.

For each type of event, you need to develop criteria that are replicable, not only by your study clinicians, but also by readers of your subsequent trial report. Hammering these criteria out with potential clinical collaborators will not only improve their specification and reproducibility, but also strengthen your collaborators' sense of ownership and cooperation with your trial.

For example, the events in our venous thromboembolism trials included positive venograms as reported by one of two radiologists (65). Before beginning this series of trials, we asked these two experts to read the same set of venograms, and found substantial disagreement (their kappa was only slightly >0.6). We then shut them in a room with a set of venograms and a view-box, and told them not to come out until they resolved their disagreement. To everyone's pleasant surprise, they discovered that they agreed well on the presence or absence of specific venographic features, but disagreed on how they should be combined into an overall interpretation. Once they agreed on how to combine venographic criteria, their agreement soared (their new kappa was almost 0.9).

In a similar fashion, you might want to run workshops in which volunteer patients with and without the target events are examined (and reexamined) by potential study clinicians. In this way you can speed up the generation of both common criteria and high precision in ascertaining them.

When events are continuous measures such as blood pressure, functional status, or quality of life, you need to decide on the appropriate "instruments" with which to measure them. You also need to decide who should apply these instruments. For example, should study clinicians be the ones who measure study patients' blood pressure? If so, do they need hearing tests, training sessions for accuracy and precision (including whether to report muffling or disappearance for diastolic blood pressure, whether to record the nearest lowest 2 mm Hg or the closest 5 mm Hg, and the like) and periodic retesting? Or do you want to measure blood pressure automatically by machine? If so, how often do you want to compare its results with those obtained by a person? Gordon Guyatt and Peter Tugwell discuss the development and validation of questionnaires and interviews for continuous measures in Chapter 11 (on generating measurements).

These tactics apply equally to composite events and surrogate markers. Furthermore, when a composite event includes "judgment call" sorts of clinical interventions, such as the decision to offer revascularization or to hospitalize for heart failure, you need to strive to keep the study-clinicians who make those calls blind to patients' treatments.

✓ Decide how, when, and by whom to ascertain these events.

Some events guarantee ascertainment, such as disabling strokes or deaths, and you need not schedule special appointments to ferret them out. Other events (such as recurrent mild TIAs or upset stomachs from study drugs) may go unrecognized without standardized inquiries during repeated follow-up visits. Regardless of whether events shout for recognition or only murmur, you must first decide *how* to ascertain each of them. Can you wait for patients to spontaneously call or visit your study center? Or, should you carry out standardized searches for them at regularly scheduled follow-up visits? As elsewhere, the right answer to these queries resides in your study question and, in particular, on its location along the explanatory–management axis.

Next you must decide *when* you will ascertain events. Your objective here is to schedule follow-up visits often enough to keep your patients on their trial regimens, ascertain transient events, detect important adverse effects, and keep track of their whereabouts. On the other hand, you don't want to wear out your study patients and their clinicians by insisting on unnecessarily frequent visits. In the RRPCE trial, we needed to ascertain the frequency of continuing TIAs (whose manifestations are transient by definition), so we saw those patients every 3 months. In the Heart Outcomes Prevention Evaluation (HOPE) trial of ramipril among patients at high-risk for dramatic and permanent cardiovascular events, we needed to see patients only twice a year (66).

Finally, you need to decide *who* will ascertain these events. Will clinical laboratories report them as a matter of course? Or, does their recognition require considerable clinical skill, in which case your study clinicians must ascertain them? Or, are they continuous measures from a quality of life questionnaire-interview, in which case trained lay interviewers will outperform most clinicians by a wide margin? Finally, will study patients record them in personal diaries, in which case a friendly, conscientious study clerk could collect them or obtain their contents by telephone? Who does what has major consequences for your trial budget.

Should You Forewarn Trial Patients about Mild Side Effects?

An apparently innocuous decision here can have massive effects on an RCT. It has to do with mild side effects of trial treatments. We discovered its impact in our 3-center trial of aspirin and sulfinpyrazone for patients with unstable angina (a life-threatening illness) (67). Half the patients at each center received aspirin (with or without additional sulfinpyrazone). At two centers (I'll call them A and B), our coinvestigators listed "occasional gastrointestinal irritation and skin rash" as potential side effects in their consent forms. However, in our third center, C, our on-site coinvestigator did not mention these mild side effects in their consent forms. (Yes, local ethics committees had approved both versions of the consent forms.)

During the trial, "informed" patients in centers A and B were far more likely to report mild gastrointestinal (GI) side effects (e.g., nausea, indigestion, heartburn) than "uninformed" patients in center C. Interestingly, however, these side effects were not associated with aspirin; only 56% of symptomatic patients were, in fact, receiving aspirin. The massive effect was that "informed" patients were six times as likely as "uninformed" patients to stop their study drugs because of these mild gastrointestinal side effects. We couldn't blame this huge effect on other differences between "informed" and "uninformed" patients. They were equally likely to develop major side effects such as frank gastrointestinal bleeding. Moreover, none of the patients in centers A and B stopped taking their study drugs because of minor side effects arising outside the GI tract (e.g., weakness, vertigo, or tinnitus). We concluded that we had "sensitized" our study patients, not only to attribute the mild GI complaints we all encounter to the study drugs, but also to stop taking them as a result.

Of course, you should always inform your study patients to be on the lookout for severe side effects and to take immediate action when they occur. However, you should remember that, if you "sensitize" your study patients to potential mild side effects as they enter your trial, they may be both more likely to report them and more likely to stop your study drugs "because" of them.

✓ *Consider event-hierarchies.*

As you can see from the RRPCE scenario, we sought three different events that shared three interesting properties. First, their severity ranged from minor (TIA) to the supremely severe (death). Second, all were manifestations of the same biologic process, the progressive atherosclerotic deterioration of an artery serving part of the brain. Third, and crucially important, the occurrence of a more severe event in the group made it impossible for the affected patient to subsequently display a less severe event. That is, patients with a total loss of sensation and movement in an arm could no longer display the transient sensory or motor deficits in that same arm that we call TIAs, and you can't have a stroke if you're already dead. We therefore had to recognize "event-hierarchies" in which a more severe event along the hierarchy precluded the occurrence of a lesser event. And, as a result, we could never report the lesser event in isolation. Thus, in describing the efficacy of aspirin it would have been nonsensical for us to report the frequency of recurring TIAs all by themselves, because aspirin could have stopped our patients' recurring TIAs by killing them. Similarly, in our subsequent trial of these same two drugs among patients with unstable angina, we never reported myocardial infarctions by themselves, but always as "nonfatal myocardial infarction or cardiac death" (68).

Cause-specific Mortality

I hope you noted in that last example that "cardiac death" is cause-specific mortality, not total mortality. Is that restriction appropriate? After all, patients who get killed by a bus or die from stroke can't have nonfatal myocardial infarctions either. I suggest that it is appropriate for you to designate cause-specific mortality as an event when two conditions are met. First, individuals who are blind to treatment must adjudicate each death and decide its cause. Second, the specific cause should account for most of the deaths that occur among your study patients. In our unstable angina trial, the adjudicators attributed 39 of the 44 deaths (89%) to be cardiac in origin. In fact, this proportion of cause-specific mortality was so high that including all deaths in the analysis led to the same conclusion (that aspirin helped reduce them). We'll talk more about this in the section on analysis and interpretation of trials.

✓ Set up an event-reporting system.

Your follow-up forms need to capture and document all relevant features of the events in your trial. For the first four P's (Prevention, Promotion, Postponement, and Palliation) it is usually appropriate to simply document the event on the follow-up form and submit it with ordinary speed for adjudication and eventual incorporation into the analysis. However, for the fifth P, Poisoning, any major or life-threatening event, especially when it is unexpected, requires immediate action (often including notification of licensing bodies). This is another reason why most RCTs should recruit one or more outsiders (not otherwise involved in the trial) who monitor its progress and respond to just such events. SUAEs can then be reported immediately to the trial's monitor, who breaks the code and decides whether urgent decisions need to be made about modifying the experimental regimen or even stopping the trial.

✓ Set up an event-adjudicating system.

Event-adjudication has become standard practice for any trial in which knowing the patient's treatment group could influence (consciously or subconsciously) the reporting or interpretation (especially for severity) of important events. In the RRPCE trial, we took the records of patients who died or whom we suspected had suffered strokes, and purged them of any information about their study drugs. We then had these purged records reviewed independently by two senior neurologist-adjudicators who were blind to their treatment. Our adjudicators then compared notes, and resolved any disagreements by discussing them in the presence of one of the directors (also blind) of the Methods Center. These adjudicators then ruled on whether the patient had suffered a stroke. If yes, they also ruled whether the stroke was minor (no impairment in activities of daily living), moderate (impairment in activities of daily living, but residing at home and out of bed for all or part of the day), or severe (bedfast or institutionalized for reasons of disability). Although our adjudicators usually agreed with the diagnoses made in study centers, there were important exceptions. Moreover, external adjudication adds to the credibility of any trial result.

Event-adjudication is a lengthy process, and in RCTs in chronic diseases it is not unusual for it to lag behind the occurrence of events by 6 months or more. However, there are two good reasons for striving to shorten this lag time. First, early in your trial, the frequency of true events can be compared with your pretrial estimates. This comparison will tell you whether your sample size is adequate for answering your study question (and, if not, will provide a starting point for reestimating your sample size needs). Second, later in your trial the need to know the number of true events becomes urgent as you apply the statistical warning rules that contribute to your decisions about stopping or continuing your trial.

✓ Decide whether any events will be ineligible for the analysis (and develop a plan for their bias-free removal).

I've already described the exclusion of ineligible patients, both before and soon after randomization. But what about the exclusion of events that occur well into the trial? Here is another excerpt from the RRPCE trial, this time about the eligibility of study events for the efficacy analysis at the explanatory pole:

> Because it was believed that sulfinpyrazone took 1 week to pro-duce a biologically appreciable effect, we decided to exclude any events occurring in the first week of therapy with any of the four regimens. Furthermore, because the withdrawal of patients from the trial might be precipitated by a deterioration in their neurologic status (and thus their exclusion from subsequent analyses might bias the results in favor of their study regimen), we charged any events occurring within the first 6 months after withdrawal against the corresponding study regimen even if the patient stopped taking the study medication at the time of withdrawal. We thought that any bias resulting from this maneuver should be against showing a benefit of treatment.

This strategy was consistent with the explanatory nature of the question we asked in that trial: Can sulfinpyrazone work under ideal circumstances? We derived it from what we knew about the pharmacodynamics of sulfinpyrazone (it took 7 days to exert its effect on platelet function). If sulfinpyrazone were effective, the inclusion, in the efficacy analysis, of events before 7 days of treatment and more than 6 months after its withdrawal would unfairly blame it for events it couldn't control. Their inclusion would raise the sulfinpyrazone event rate and decrease both the relative and absolute risk reductions attributed to it. In our primary analyses, we removed these "ineligible" events from all arms of the trial to prevent biased comparisons between treatment groups. However, we also performed an "intention-to-treat" analysis that included all the "ineligible" events. As it happened, sulfinpyrazone remained ineffective in this pragmatic analysis, but the benefit of aspirin became even greater.

But we risked the credibility, if not the validity, of our trial's conclusion by removing (or "censoring") any events that occur after randomization to eligible study patients. So will you if you censor such events in your trial. Such postrandomization exclusions will (and usually should) increase skepticism about your trial's conclusions. Furthermore, in carrying out postrandomization exclusion of events in a pragmatic trial, you might move your interpretation of a positive result so far away from its pragmatic application that you destroy its clinical usefulness.

Designating any events that occur after randomization "ineligible" is a very risky strategy, and I don't recommend it. Instead, I urge you to recruit enough patients to swamp the negative consequences of including such events in your analysis.

5.7 ANALYSIS AND INTERPRETATION

Preface: Is This Section Really Necessary?

In the opening paragraphs of this chapter, I stressed the importance of recruiting a statistician as co-PI right at the start of formulating the question for your RCT. Why, then, intrude on their turf with a section on the analysis and interpretation of the trial? My reasons are three. First, as you will see in the checklist, several of the issues are not strictly statistical (specifying what to analyze, interpreting your results, and the like). Second, co-PIs are precisely that, and everyone with that title should collaborate in the discussion and debate at every step in the trial. In that spirit, this section's first function is to provide nonstatisticians with a sufficient introduction to RCT analysis to help you contribute to those discussions and debates. Third, when some non-statistician trialists get their feet wet in statistics, they discover (to both their surprise and mine) that they enjoy learning more about it. So, this section's final function is to whet some appetites.

We used parametric (t-test) and nonparametric (chi-squared) tests to analyze baseline differences among study groups, associated hematologic investigations, and compliance. We used the log-rank life-table method suggested by a team of experts led by Richard Peto (69) for our primary analysis. This primary analysis assessed the overall benefit of aspirin and sulfinpyrazone in all patients. However, we also judged it important to examine the relative efficacy of these drugs among some prespecified clinically sensible subgroups. We advised readers to interpret these secondary analyses with caution since true significance levels are affected by repeated challenges of the data.

We also monitored patients who withdrew from our trial to detect possible drug toxicity.

Our first examination of the data for efficacy occurred in April 1976, when we had entered 569 patients into the study. At that time there was a trend favoring aspirin, which was not statistically significant. We decided to continue admitting patients until June 30, 1976, by which time we expected to reach the target of 600 patients. We would then follow all patients for a further 12 months, analyze, and interpret our results.

In our primary analysis, aspirin produced a statistically significant (P <0.05) reduction in the composite hierarchy of TIA, stroke and death. In a secondary analysis that excluded TIAs, aspirin still achieved a statistically significant (P <0.05) reduction in stroke and death. Sulfinpyrazone was not effective.

Aspirin produced a relative risk reduction (RRR) of 31% and an ARR of 7.2% for stroke and death. Thus, the NNT with aspirin for 2 years to prevent another stroke or death was about 14. The Number of Patients one Needed to treat to Harm one of them (NNH) with a major gastrointestinal bleeding over that same period was 48.

I later decided that one of our planned analyses was a bad idea. Can you guess which one that was? Read on.

Analysis and interpretation checklist:

Before you begin your trial, and based on your study question, you should take the following steps:

✓ Draft "Table 1" summarizing the entry characteristics of experimental and control patients.

✓ Specify your primary and secondary data analyses.

✓ Specify any subgroup analyses.

✓ Select your analytic methods (for deciding whether your treatment effect is "real").

✓ Decide how to handle missing data in the analysis.

✓ Decide how to interpret your results for their "importance."

✓ Establish interim analysis plans and statistical warning rules for efficacy, safety, and futility.

After your trial is over, you should take the following additional steps:

✓ Don't exaggerate your conclusions, especially about subgroups.

✓ Never describe your indeterminate study as "negative" or as showing "no difference."

✓ Report your results regardless of their interpretation.

✓ Update the systematic review that justified your trial.

✓ Formulate the question for your next trial.

✓ Draft "Table 1" summarizing the entry characteristics of experimental and control patients.

The first table in your RCT report describes and compares the entry characteristics of your experimental and control patients. We suggest that you show "empty" drafts of this table to potential clinical collaborators, including especially those whom you hope to influence with its results. Typically, such tables include characteristics likely to influence risk or responsiveness to treatment, plus sociodemographic items. We already showed you *Table 1* for men in the RRPCE trial as Table 5–3, and it was accompanied by similar tables for women and for the occurrence and timing of their qualifying TIAs. As we noted back in Table 5–2, a baseline imbalance between treatment groups for important prognostic characteristics can damage a trial's credibility in ways that multivariate statistical adjustments can never rehabilitate. Accordingly, when you create your first draft of your Table 1 before you start the trial, you should decide whether to take steps (such as stratification-before-randomization or minimization) to be sure that your trial is credible as well as valid.

In answer to the question posed at the end of the scenario, I think we erred in applying significance tests to our *Table 1*, and recommend against it. In a small trial, important differences might be statistically nonsignificant. But they should be prevented, not documented after the fact. I've described their preventives (minimization or stratification prior to randomization) in Section 5.4 (on "Allocation of Patients to Treatments"). Conversely, in a large trial, trivial differences will routinely be statistically significant, and will suggest important imbalance when it is absent.

Many trialists seek statistical reassurance that baseline imbalances didn't affect their trial results. They do this by performing multivariate outcome analyses in which they adjust for one or more baseline factors. Some statisticians disagree with this approach (70). When Stuart Pocock's team reviewed 50 RCT reports in general medical journals, 72% of them included such analyses (but gave reasons for doing so only about half the time) (71). When performed, the "covariate adjusted" analyses received more emphasis than the unadjusted analysis about a third of the time. However, only one report changed its conclusion (incorrectly, in the Pocock team's opinion) on the basis of an adjusted analysis.

✓ *Specify your primary and secondary data analyses.*

Which events, at what point or over what period of time, will answer your trial's primary question? If you did a good "PICOT" job of specifying your question back at the beginning, this decision will already have been made. Even if your question addresses equivalence or noninferiority (but greater safety or lesser cost), the issues are the same.

My coauthors and I carry out five sorts of secondary analyses in our RCTs. They deal with determining safety, subdividing a composite primary outcome, assessing secondary outcomes, confirming homogeneity across clinical subgroups and centers, and generating hypotheses for our next RCT. Most of these analyses are straightforward and trustworthy, but others can mislead. Accordingly, I've devoted a subsequent section to the tricky topic of subgroup analysis.

Safety analyses document the magnitude, timing, severity, and outcomes of adverse responses to your experimental therapy. Such "safety" secondary analyses are routine in planning and conducting RCTs, and often must adhere to rigorous external regulations in reporting. The inability of most RCTs to detect rare but awful adverse responses is discussed in Section 5.6.

Subdividing a Composite Primary Outcome

As you learned from Table 4–1, in order to generate enough events to achieve a statistically significant result, many RCTs create composite primary outcomes. Some of these combine primary events (such as death or heart attack), and some may add predicaments (such as the need for hospitalization for unstable angina or heart failure, or the need to perform angioplasty). Others are "hierarchies" that combine frequent mild events with their less common but more severe sequalae. As already reported, in the RRPCE study, our primary outcome was a composite of continuing TIA, stroke, or death. Although TIAs are clinically important, their inclusion in the primary outcome was, in part, a sample-size "hedge." Because they occurred much more frequently than stroke or death, they contributed a lot more events to the primary analysis, and increased the trial's power (i.e., its ability to find, and label as statistically significant, a beneficial effect of aspirin). Once we had our positive primary outcome, we removed patients who only had continuing TIAs and did a secondary analysis on just strokes and deaths. If you're wondering why we didn't analyze TIAs all by themselves, you'd better (re)read about diagnostic hierarchies in the previous section of this chapter.

Assessing Secondary Events

Lots of RCT events are secondary by design. For several of our cerebrovascular trials, Brian Haynes developed measures that captured how well our patients retained their independence in communicating, dressing, eating, toileting, shopping, and the like (72). These measures provided important functional confirmation of the consequences of the clinical events in these RCTs. Because every patient contributes a functional "event" in the analysis, we were confident that we would have ample sample size to demonstrate any MIDs in function, and we were right.

Generating Hypotheses for Your Next Randomized Controlled Trial

You shouldn't hesitate to perform "exploratory data analyses" or "data-dredging" to look for subgroups of patients who display major differences in their responses to therapy. However, the purpose for this search must never be to draw conclusions about subgroup efficacy. Rather, it is to generate questions to ask in your next trial.

For example, in NASCET we let our collaborating surgeons decide the dose of aspirin given to trial patients at the time of their surgery. In dredging our data, we found, to our surprise, that patients taking 650 to 1,300 mg of aspirin daily at the time of surgery were much less likely to suffer perioperative stroke or death (1.8%) than patients taking 0 to 325 mg of aspirin (6.9%). As with any other clinical observation, we could come up with a biologic explanation that would tidily explain this finding (73). But these were only cohort-level data, discovered while looking for a pony. Wayne Taylor decided they weren't a sound enough basis for clinical practice, and led a subsequent RCT that asked: "Among patients undergoing carotid endarterectomy, would giving them 81, 325, 650, or 1,300 mg of aspirin, starting before their surgery and continuing thereafter, reduce their risk of stroke, myocardial infarction or death at 30 and 90 days?" Some surgeons were convinced that high-dose aspirin was efficacious and refused to join this second trial.

However, enough of them and their patients did join to give us the startling and important answer that low-dose aspirin, not high-dose aspirin, was best at preventing stroke and death following surgery (74).

Subgroup analyses are a two-edged sword that you shouldn't wield until you understand their deceptive properties, so I'll take them up here.

✓ Specify any subgroup analyses.

First, you will want to determine whether your primary result is *consistent* across clinically sensible subgroups. Our confidence (and our readers' confidence!) in our positive NASCET result was raised when we found consistent efficacy in clinically sensible subgroups based on sex, site and type of qualifying TIA, and comorbidity.

In multicenter trials, you can look for similar results across centers and countries. For example, in the RRPCE trial we found that 14 of our 24 centers (contributing 75% of our patients) agreed with the overall result, five centers (contributing 10% of our patients) showed no trend, and 5 (contributing 15% of our patients) showed a reverse trend. A test for heterogeneity across centers was not statistically significant, but if it had been, we'd have performed a "sensitivity analysis" to see whether excluding the centers with the most extreme results affected our conclusion about efficacy.

You shouldn't be surprised to find minor differences in the degree of therapeutic responsiveness of different subgroups of patients in your trial. I'll call these "quantitative" interactions, to denote that they represent differences in the *degree* of efficacy, such that one clinical subgroup is slightly more or less responsive to experimental therapy than another. For example, in the NASCET trial the RRR for ipsilateral stroke rose with increasing symptomatic carotid stenosis (from 12% in patients with 70% to 79% stenoses, to 18% in patients with 80% to 89% stenoses, and 26% in patients with 90% to 99% stenoses).

But alarm bells should sound when your secondary analysis suggests a *"qualitative"* difference in efficacy between subgroups. By *"qualitative"* difference, I mean finding that experimental treatment is clearly efficacious in one subgroup and clearly (and statistically significantly) harmful or "confidently ineffective" in another. By "confidently ineffective," I mean that the 95% confidence interval for efficacy in that subgroup excludes any humanly useful benefit.

Secondary analyses among clinical subgroups sooner or later must mislead you, for if you carry out enough of them, you are guaranteed to find one by chance alone. Even when supported by statistical tests for an interaction between efficacy and the presence or absence of a subgroup's identifying characteristic, these sorts of secondary analyses can mislead. Furthermore, the risks of overinterpreting subgroup analyses go beyond mere mischief. They include withholding efficacious treatment from subgroups who need it, forcing useless treatments on subgroups who don't, and wasting millions of dollars on research to cleanup the messes. For example, in the RRPCE trial we concluded that aspirin worked in men but not in women (wrong!), and that it didn't work among diabetics (wrong again!) or in patients with a past history of myocardial infarction (wrong yet again!). The same Christmas story about "looking for the pony" that helped us explain the dangers of performing multiple diagnostic tests on patients in the 2nd edition of this book (75) is useful here:

"Looking for the pony" comes from a Christmas tale of two brothers, one of whom was an incurable pessimist and the other, an incurable optimist. On Christmas day, the pessimist was given a roomful of shiny toys and the optimist, a roomful of horseshit. The pessimist opened the door to his roomful of toys, sighed, and lamented, "A lot of these are motor driven and their batteries will run down; and I suppose I'll have to show them to my cousins, who'll break some and steal others; and their paint will chip; and they'll wear out. All in all, I wish you hadn't given me this roomful of toys." The optimist opened the door to his roomful of horseshit and, with a whoop of glee, threw himself into the muck, and began burrowing through it. When his horrified parents extracted him from the excrement and asked him why on earth he was thrashing about in it, he joyfully cried: "With all this horse shit, there's got to be a pony in here somewhere!"

There are two ways to safeguard against spurious "qualitative interactions." First, you can limit your secondary analyses of subgroups to just one or two, carefully prespecified in the protocol. Second, if you think that you will find an important qualitative interaction between subgroups, you can design separate and simultaneous trials for each of them. Each of these trials should have a sufficient sample size to answer the question.

For example, in NASCET we suspected that there might be a qualitative interaction between the efficacy of surgery and the degree of carotid stenosis. We thought that surgery probably would produce a big net benefit among patients with high-grade stenoses, but that it might be useless or even harmful among patients with only moderate stenoses (where the risk of surgery might outweigh its benefits). We therefore designed and carried out two simultaneous NASCET trials, one each for severed and mild stenosis, but employing the same study staff and follow-up apparatus.

In summary, it's fine to perform "exploratory data analyses" or "data-dredging" to look for a particular pony you might like to ride in your next trial, as long as you don't draw conclusions about subgroup efficacy from any ponies you find in dredging data from the trial you've just completed. If the reasons for this admonition remain unclear, you might want to revisit the trial of differing aspirin doses during carotid surgery I described back at the end of the previous discussion on specifying your primary and secondary analyses.

✓ Select your analytic methods (for deciding whether your treatment effect is "real").

In the following pages, I will provide you with only the "bare bones" of an approach to statistical analysis. No readers in their right minds should undertake RCTs without biostatisticians as co-PIs, and I reckon that most of you already will have taken at least an introductory course in biostatistics. If any of the following ideas and suggestions are unclear, I suggest that you read Chapter 15 (on statistics). If that doesn't help, consult your co-PI and/or your favorite statistical text [mine is Doug Altman's *Practical Statistics for Medical Research* (76)].

Short-term Parallel Trials

As with other steps in executing your trial, the selection of the "right" analytic method depends on the question you posed. If yours is a short-term trial (say a few days or weeks) in which your question calls for a simple comparison of homogenous groups of patients *at the end* of this time period, then simple statistical analyses will do. For short-term parallel trials with events (say, the occurrence of immediate side effects after taking an established drug and its newer, presumably better-tolerated nephew), a straightforward chi-squared test will serve just fine. For short-term parallel trials with continuous measurements (say, which of two bronchodilators produces a better improvement in the ease of breathing [FEV-1] 30 minutes later), your statistician co-PI will probably use an analysis of covariance. When you analyze a result as both an event (such as achieving goal blood pressure) and as a continuous measure (such as average blood pressure reduction), you need to specify up front as to which analysis will take precedence in answering your trial's question. Remember, however, that you will require far more patients to show a real difference in event rates (using the chi-squared family of statistics) than in averages (the t-test family).

Short-term Crossover Trials

Short-term crossover trials would use the analogous paired tests: the McNemar chi-squared or the paired t-test, and we show an example of the latter in Table 5-7, which displays treatment effects (Δ) in patients who have been allocated to receive treatment A or B in the first period and the other treatment in the second period:

However, before you carry out the paired t-test on the data from a crossover trial (Δ all A versus Δ all B) you need to be sure that it is an unbiased analysis, unaffected by "carry-over" or "calendar":

1. You'll need to find out whether there has been any "carry-over" effect of the treatment given in the first period into the second period. This is found by comparing the results within each treatment when it is given first and second: (Δ A1 versus Δ A2 and Δ B1 versus Δ B2); you'll need to show that they are not statistically significantly different in the two periods before you can combine them.

TABLE 5–7   **Treatment Effects (Δ) in a Crossover Trial**

		Effects of Treatment (Δ)	
		Period 1	Period 2
Patient Allocation	A first	Δ A1	Δ B2
	B first	Δ B1	Δ A2

2. You'll need to find out whether there has been any a "calendar" or "temporal" effect in which the patients' underlying illness is getting better (i.e., recovering) or worse with the simple passage of time. You can do this by comparing the differences between treatments in the first and second periods: [(Δ A1 minus Δ B1) and (Δ A2 minus Δ B2)]. Again, you'd need these to be roughly equal before carrying out the paired t-test on the overall result.

If either of these misfortunes has befallen your trial, the appropriate (and probably underpowered) analysis is to compare Δ A1 and Δ B1, excluding Δ A2 and Δ B2.

Long-term Trials

Most of the trials I've carried out have been long-term ones (lasting from two to several years) in which we were hoping to either prevent, or at least postpone, bad outcomes among patients at varying risk for these outcomes. Two special features of these trials have to be taken into account in their analyses, and these are illustrated in Figure 5–4 for experimental patients who enter a trial at point (E), and thereafter may (or may not) go on to minor events (mi), major events (Ma), die (D) or become lost to follow-up (L).

The first of these special features in long-term trials is that patients enter them throughout a recruitment period that can last for years, and finish these trials either at variable times of their terminating event (such as death) or at a common stopping time at the close of the trial. As a result, individual patients are in the trial for widely different periods of time

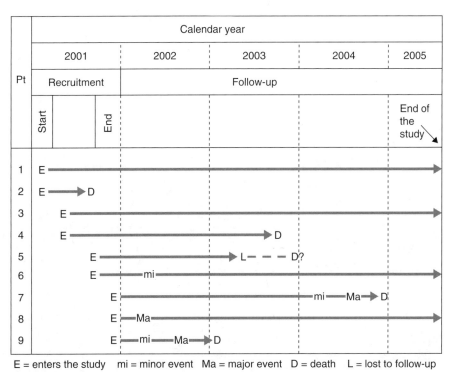

E = enters the study   mi = minor event   Ma = major event   D = death   L = lost to follow-up

FIGURE 5-4   Patients in a long-term trial, in real time.

or "durations of follow-up." In Figure 5–4, Patient 1 survives the entire trial, but Patient 2 is dead even before the end of the recruitment period; Patients 1, 3, 6, and 8 are all present at the end of the study, but their follow-up times differ; Patients 1 and 3 sail through the trial event-free, but Patient 1 is followed for much longer.

The second special feature of long-term trials is that their treatment objectives include postponement of disabling or fatal outcomes (such as severe stroke or death) and not just their prevention (after all, if the trial went on for decades, everyone in it or working on it would eventually die). For example, both Patients 2 and 4 die, but Patient 4 lives event-free much longer. Both Patients 7 and 9 suffer minor, major, and fatal events, but Patient 9 has them in a cluster. Finally, Patient 5 is lost to follow-up, but still has more time in the study than Patients 2 or 9; moreover, a surveillance of the national death registry detects Patient 5's death some time later. Our analyses of such trials have to take these special features of variable length of follow-up and outcome-postponement-as-well-as-prevention into account.

The tactics of doing so begin with ignoring calendar time and thinking of patients as if they all entered the study at the same, common starting point, as shown in Figure 5–5.

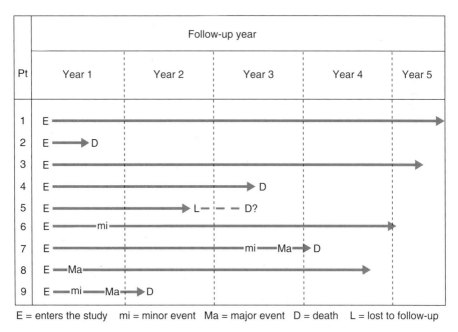

E = enters the study   mi = minor event   Ma = major event   D = death   L = lost to follow-up

FIGURE 5–5   Patients in a long-term trial, taken back to a common starting point.

The result, which is one variant of a "life-table," now more clearly reveals the differences in "survival" and follow-up, as well as the relative timing of events between patients in the trial. From such a table, we can calculate the proportion of experimental patients who are event-free at any given time after entry, and the resulting graph is called a "survival curve." One variant of a survival curve breaks follow-up time into small intervals, say days, and considers the probability that patients alive at the start of each day are likely to survive event-free to the start of the next day. As it happens, the probability of surviving event-free to day no. 120 is the "conditional" probability of surviving on day no. 120, given that you've already survived day no. 119. Survival curves generated in this fashion don't require assumptions about the nature of any theoretical "underlying distribution" of "true" probabilities we are guessing in the trial, and are called "nonparametric" or "distribution-free." The one we've just generated is called a "Kaplan–Meier" survival curve after Edward Kaplan and Paul Meier, the statisticians who described this useful way of thinking about survival (77). By this method we can calculate the probability of "surviving" event-free at any point in the trial or throughout it for experimental and control patients, and can generate a "noise" factor (say, the standard error) for each probability. The Kaplan–Meier curves for any major stroke or death in the surgical and medical arms of the high-grade stenosis NASCET trial are shown in Figure 5–6.

The next step is to compare the survival curves generated for experimental and control patients. The method that my co-PI statistician colleagues

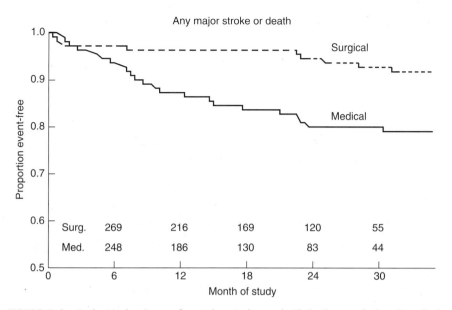

FIGURE 5–6 Kaplan–Meier Curves for major stroke or death in the surgical and medical arms of the high-grade stenosis NASCET trial. (From North American Symptomatic Carotid Endarterectomy Trial Collaborators. Beneficial effect of carotid endarterectomy in symptomatic patients with high-grade carotid stenosis. *N Engl J Med* 1991;325:445–453. Copyright ©1991 Massachusetts Medical Society, with permission.)

routinely use compares the number of events we Observe in each treatment group during any interval (say, any given day) with the number of events we'd Expect to observe if there was no difference in efficacy between the experimental and control treatments. We then cumulate, over each interval of time, the $(O - E)/E$ and the result is our old friend chi-squared, with degrees of freedom equal to (the number of intervals $- 1$). We call this form of analysis the "log-rank life-table" method, and credit for its elegant simplicity goes to Richard Peto (69). It tells us whether any difference in the events we observe between experimental and control patients is *real*; that is, whether that difference in events is "statistically significant."

A final point before we move on. The foregoing discussion is about *whether* an event has occurred. However, it can be carried to a higher statistical plane by considering not just whether an event occurred, but the *time* elapsed between entry and that event. This "time-to-event" analysis is more powerful, but beyond the scope of this chapter. Similarly, many long-term trials include continuous outcome measures such as functional capacity and quality of life. They also present analytic difficulties, especially when patients die or otherwise stop contributing to these measures early in the trial. Analyses of continuous measures are taken up in Chapter 15.

You can read about 1-sided superiority and noninferiority trials in Section 6.5.

Cluster Trials

As you may remember from earlier bits of this chapter, some interventions (e.g., the elimination of insects that transmit a disease, or the introduction of a new way of running a hospital ward) act on groups of people rather than individuals. Other interventions (e.g., teaching clinicians how to tailor drug-taking to daily habits and rituals) are hard to restrict to just half the clinicians' patients without "contaminating" the other half. In these situations we handle the groups of people who receive the same treatment from the same source as "clusters." Cluster trials are excellent for determining the usefulness of interventions directed at groups of patients, practices, villages, and the like. However, because the responses of study individuals within these clusters can be expected to be more similar (or "concordant") than the responses of individuals belonging to different clusters, they require special forms of analysis. A very useful resource for cluster trials is a book by Neil Klar and Alan Donner (78).

✓ Decide how to handle missing data in the analysis.

You need to decide, before the trial begins, how to handle patients like no. 5 in Figure 5–4, who is lost to follow-up part way through the trial. It is tempting to treat them as if they were lost on the final day of the trial, and "censor" anything bad that might have happened afterward. This policy is risky for two reasons. First, if they left the trial because their target condition was deteriorating, ignoring their possible bad outcome would bias your conclusion. Second, ignoring them could lower the credibility of your conclusion.

You can get a "feel" for the seriousness of this problem by examining the ratio of lost patients to events. In the RRPCE trial, the ratio was 1:114, and we concluded that our event rate was valid. On the other hand, in a trial of postmenopausal hormone replacement therapy (HRT) the ratio was 57 lost to 99 cardiac end points, raising concern about the validity of that event rate (79).

Beyond the obvious solutions of not losing any study patients in the first place, and scouring mortality registers for them in the second, what can you do? I suggest that the most convincing way to handle them is a "worst-case scenario" in which you arbitrarily assign them the outcome that will make it hardest for you to answer your study question with a "yes." Suppose you are asking, "In patients of a particular sort, does experimental treatment E, when compared to control treatment C, reduce the risk of death?" In the "worst-case scenario," experimental patients who are lost get assigned the outcome of death, but control patients who are lost are assumed to have survived to the end of the trial. You then present the analysis in two parts. Part 1 "censors" lost patients from the moment they are lost, but in Part 2 they are returned in a "worst-case scenario." After the trial that doesn't lose any patients at all, the trial with the highest credibility is the one in which the Part 2 worst-case scenario analysis reaches the same conclusion as the Part 1 censored analysis.

Many trialists (including some of my coauthors) believe that my "worst-case scenario" approach is too harsh. Various statistical "modeling" procedures have been proposed for assigning "appropriate" (but fictitious) outcomes to lost patients, and I leave it to you to discuss them with your statistician co-PI.

✓ Decide how to interpret your results for their "importance."

For a difference to *be* a difference, it has to *make* a difference (80). Chi-squared, t-tests, and the log-rank test are great at telling you whether your treatment effect is *real* (i.e., unlikely to be due to chance). However, they can't tell you whether your treatment effect is important enough to be useful for patients. Recalling that trivial treatment effects become statistically significant when trials enroll huge numbers of patients, the next step is to determine whether the statistically significant difference your trial generated also exceeds some "MID" that is deemed important by the trial participants (who, as the study "subjects," could comprise patients, providers, teachers, administrators, and others). This is a two-stage process; the first stage is mathematics, and the second stage is a judgment call.

The Mathematics of Minimally Important Differences

I'll begin with how differences are determined, and then move to consider how you might decide whether they are important. The mathematics for determining differences are straightforward for a short-term parallel trial with events as outcomes, as you don't need to adjust for the relative times at which patients entered the trial or had events. In such trials, you simply determine the frequency of events in the control group (the *Control Event Rate* or CER) and in the experimental group (the *Experimental Event Rate* or EER). For example, in our ACE trial of high-dose (experimental) versus low-dose (control) aspirin to prevent stroke, myocardial infarction or death in the month following carotid endarterectomy, the EER among high-dose patients was 8.2% and the CER among low-dose patients was 3.7% ($p = 0.002$) (74).

In a long-term parallel trial with events as outcomes, the same principle holds but we derive the CER and EER as "failure" probabilities from the Kaplan–Meier curves I've already shown you. Kaplan–Meier CERs and EERs take into account both the fact that events are occurring throughout the trial and that their denominators are constantly changing as patients enter and leave the trial. As a result, they are larger than the CERs and EERs you'd calculate (incorrectly) at the end of the trial if you simply divided the numbers of events by the numbers of patients enrolled. In these long-term parallel trials, we generate the Kaplan–Meier CER and EER for some clinically sensible time (we selected 2 years after entry for the NASCET trial), and also generate their accompanying "noise" in the form of, say, a standard error. Thus, in NASCET, the Kaplan–Meier estimates of the CER for major stroke or death at 2 years was 18.1% but the EER was only 8%.

In trials with continuous outcomes, you have two choices. You can stick with the absolute differences between control and experimental groups that you used for determining statistical significance. Alternatively, you can convert these absolute differences into "events" by determining, for example, the rates at which control and experimental patients achieved some preset change in the continuous measure, or the rate at which they achieved a 50% reduction in a continuous measure of symptoms or disability. I refer you to the section on "Continuous Outcome Measures" (in Chapter 15) for a complete discussion of the appropriate approaches.

The Judgments That Determine Which Differences are Minimally Important

In the second, judgment step, you need to decide whether these differences are important. This chapter will provide one example each from the perspectives of clinicians and patients, respectively. Patient's perspectives on their MIDs will receive its major attention in Chapter 11.

A Clinician's Minimally Important Differences

Clinicians' MIDs often are expressed in terms of the number of patients they will need to treat with experimental therapy in order to prevent one more bad outcome or cause one more harmful adverse event. They can be derived for all patients in an RCT by simply generating a CER and EER for the *average* patient in the trial. The resulting *ARR* and *Number Needed to be Treated to prevent one more event* (1/ARR = NNT) also apply to the average patient in the trial. The 95% confidence interval on the ARR translates directly into the confidence interval on the NNT.

For example, in the RRPCE trial, the ARR for major stroke or death (CER–EER) among all patients treated with aspirin for 2 years was 7.2%, and its 95% *Confidence Interval* (CI) ran from 0.8% to 13.6%. Inverting these ARRs produces an NNT of 14 with a confidence interval from 8 to 125.

These same methods apply to judging the importance of harm. The *Absolute Risk Increase* (ARI) and its reciprocal, the *Number needed to be Treated to Harm one more of them* (NNH) can be generated from the side-effect rates in the experimental and control patients. In the RRPCE trial, 2.1% of patients who took aspirin for 2 years had severe gastrointestinal bleeds (with a 95% confidence interval from 0.97% to 4.4%); none of these bleeds were fatal. Thus, the NNH for a severe but nonfatal bleeding episode was 48 with a confidence interval from 23 to 103.

At the time we reported these results, there were no other treatments that had been shown in RCTs to reduce the risk of disabling stroke and death among patients with TIAs. Anything that could reduce these awful consequences was embraced by patients and clinicians alike. No wonder, then, that clinicians decided these results clearly exceeded their MID for stroke reduction, but did not exceed their MID for harm. Aspirin use soared.

But was aspirin for everyone? Might there be subgroups of patients in this or any other trial with important differences in their CERs and EERs? How might their risk and responsiveness be estimated by clinicians for extrapolation to similar groups of patients outside the trial? How might NNTs applicable to subgroups be generated?

For starters, there is growing empirical evidence that in trials of "delaying" treatments, the RRR tends to be constant over a wide range of CERs (81,82). That being so, a case can be made for using the trial's overall RRR and applying it to groups of control patients at different baseline risks to estimate their ARRs and numbers needed to be treated to prevent one more event. The authors of this book disagree with each other (a little, not a lot) about how much credence should be given to the subgroup CERs in a trial. I am less willing to accept them than my coauthors, especially when they have large confidence intervals, and would wait for the meta-analysis (ideally, on individual patient data) of several similar trials before I'd trust them.

Other anecdotal evidence suggests that RRRs might *not* be constant for treatments designed to reverse (as opposed to slow) the progress of disease. I provided one anecdote in an earlier paragraph on subgroup analysis, where I described the rising RRR from carotid endarterectomy as it was performed on patients with progressively more severe carotid stenosis. We don't know enough about the behavior of other RRRs for "reversing" treatments among different subgroups to offer any firm advice on their extrapolation, save to say that you may have to rely on subgroups within the trial.

A Patient's Minimally Important Differences

The patient's MID takes precedence over any other. How might it be determined? This same RRPCE trial can help, by providing patients with information that they can use to determine their own MID. Dr. Sharon Straus has pioneered a strategy for helping patients accomplish this (83). Her method combines the benefits of therapy with its accompanying risks, and then adds the patient's own judgment about the relative severity of the bad outcome prevented by treatment (in this case, the stroke) and the bad outcome caused by treatment (in this case, the bleeding episode).

The key step here is the patient's decision about how much worse or better it would be to have a stroke than a bleeding episode. Suppose a patient was at "average" risk of both the stroke and the bleed. Suppose further that her health preferences and values were such that she considered having a stroke to be four times as bad as having a bleed. With an NNH to cause a bleed of 48, an NNT to prevent a stroke of 14, and her judgment about severity (S) that having a stroke would be four times as bad as having a bleed, we can calculate the likelihood that she would be helped versus harmed *on her own terms* by taking aspirin. The formula for doing this is NNH × S/NNT. In her case, and incorporating her own health preferences and values, she is 48 × 4/14 or over 13 times as likely to be helped versus harmed over the next 2 years if she starts taking aspirin.

For one final wrinkle in this example of creating a patient's MID, we needn't even assume that she is an "average" patient. Suppose that her risk of a stroke was only half that of the average patient in the RRPCE study, but that her risk of a bleed was twice that of the average trial patient. By applying Richard Cook's modification (84) in which these relative risks are expressed as decimal fraction and placed in the denominator of the corresponding NNT or NNH, her NNT to prevent a stroke rises from 14 to 14/0.5 or 28, and her NNH for suffering a bleed falls from 48 to 48/2 or 24. Even then, given that she considers a stroke to be four times as bad as a bleed, the likelihood that she'll be helped versus harmed by taking aspirin for the next 2 years is 24 × 4/28 or over 3 to 1.

Further discussion of the generation and application of these practical indexes for patients' MIDs belong, and are found, in texts devoted to evidence-based health care.

✓ Establish interim analysis plans and statistical warning rules for efficacy, safety, and futility.

Imagine that you are conducting a trial with a 3-year follow-up, but are employing 95% confidence intervals (or P <0.05) to its emerging "interim" results once a month. By doing so, you are at great risk of inappropriately stopping the trial early, for three reasons. In the first place, if your pretrial estimate of efficacy (say, an ARR of 5%) is accurate, then trials of it that stop early will be biased toward overestimating that efficacy, and you certainly don't want to do that. In the second place, trends in the early, unstable portions of trials can flirt with, or even cross, conventional boundaries of statistical significance for harm as well as benefit. Finally, in the eyes (or entrails) of many statisticians, the performance of multiple interim analyses increases the risk of an ultimately false-positive conclusion (that the experimental treatment works, when in fact it doesn't) at the end of the trial. How can you avoid these pitfalls and still stop the trial as soon as your results are both statistically and, more important, clinically convincing?

The first step is to withhold your first interim analysis until you have followed enough patients long enough for the real trends in safety and efficacy to become established. This is a judgment call, based on your patients' likely risk and the timing of their likely responsiveness (good and bad) to your experimental treatment. For example, you might want to perform your first interim analysis when 50% of your projected sample size should have been treated long enough to display the effects of experimental treatment.

The second step is to set the confidence intervals or P values for your interim analyses at quite stringent levels, so that you minimize your risk of wrongly triggering your statistical warning rules. For example, in the HOPE trial we used the original Haybittle–Peto (85,69) approach, and set the interim warning rule to trigger for benefit at two consecutive differences of four standard deviations (one-sided $P \leq 0.00003$) during the first half of the trial and at three standard deviations (one-sided $P \leq 0.002$) in the second half. As you can see, even with penalties for "multiple looks," in which we subtracted the "P" we used up along the way, we retained plenty of "P" for the final analysis ($0.05 - 0.00003 - 0.002 = 0.048$). If these interim P values strike you as absurdly small and unattainable, reducing this "warning rule" exercise to mere window dressing, note that they were, in fact, triggered in the HOPE trial, the PI unblinded, and this trial stopped 8 months before its scheduled close.

We set a less rigorous warning trigger for safety at three standard deviations (one-sided $P \leq 0.002$) in the first half of the HOPE trial and two standard deviations ($P \leq 0.023$) in the second half, retaining our option of unblinding the investigators much sooner if we observed even a few SUAEs.

In a similar fashion, you could set statistical limits for determining when a trial is simply not going to show any minimally important benefit from experimental therapy. You can do this by specifying a very strict confidence interval around your treatment effect and watching to see whether it excludes, on the "ineffective" side, the minimally important benefit.

Statistical Warning Rules, Not Stopping Rules

Note that I've called them statistical warning rules, *not stopping rules*. That's because trialists like me think that decisions to stop a trial should never be based on statistics alone. Accordingly, the third step is to decide what additional information you will use to interpret a statistical warning rule when it is triggered. Typically, this interpretation involves the clinical and biologic sense that might support or refute a decision to stop the trial. For example, in NASCET, we began monthly interim analyses 2 years into the trial, and a recommendation to stop the trial early required a demonstration of efficacy (an RRR of at least 10% for stroke or death) at 3 standard deviations in each of six clinically sensible subgroups, every month for 6 months. Despite these stringent rules, we stopped that trial among patients with high-degree carotid stenosis early. More about how monitors and monitoring committees ought to work begins in Section 5.10 (on monitoring for efficacy, safety, and futility).

Once you've designed your statistical warning rules, you need to make sure that they are understood and accepted by your collaborators and monitor(s) before you start the trial. You can read lots more about warning/stopping rules in Curtis Meinert's heavily referenced RCT text (86).

The final five items on the checklist come into play after you've completed your trial and are polishing off your analysis.

✓ *Don't exaggerate your conclusions, especially about subgroups.*

If you've followed our advice so far, you can carry out a valid RCT. Congratulations! Don't blow it at the end by exaggerating your conclusions in ways that mislead your audience, leave you open to legitimate criticism, and damage your credibility. The three most common exaggerations we encounter are reporting only the "sexiest" efficacy measure, looking for the pony, and calling an indeterminate trial "negative" (the latter is important enough to earn its own heading).

Don't Report Only Your Sexiest Measure of Efficacy

Ironically, the first exaggeration of reporting only the "sexiest" efficacy measure (reporting an impressive RRR rather than a less impressive ARR or number needed to be treated to prevent one more event) is increasingly common in cardiovascular trials, a field that is not only justifiably proud of its past accomplishments, but also a victim of its past successes. A steady progression of positive cardiovascular trials has validated an ever-expanding combination of effective treatments. These combinations thus became "EET." As a result, the question in today's cardiovascular trial is some form of: "Among patients with unstable angina, does the addition of drug X to EET achieve a further reduction in the risk of myocardial infarction or death?" In operational terms, this becomes a "placebo add-on" trial in which both groups receive EET. To do it, we add the promising new drug to the regimen of experimental patients, and add its placebo to the regimen of control patients. As you can learn about in Section 6.6 ("Physiological Statistics"), the EETs pull the CER toward zero, and even new drugs that generate large RRRs will generate only small ARRs and large numbers needed to be treated to prevent one additional event. Thus, in reporting the effect of ramipril on the risk of stroke in the HOPE trial, the investigators confined themselves to the impressive RRR of 32% for all stroke and 61% for fatal stroke (87). It was after several letters of protest (88) that they provided a table of numbers needed to be treated for the entire HOPE trial, including an NNT of 111 to prevent a stroke but a very impressive NNT of only 8 to prevent one of the composite cardiovascular events (89).

This is not academic nit picking. There is increasing evidence that RRRs create higher opinions about efficacy among both physicians (90) and health policy makers (91) than their corresponding ARRs or numbers needed to be treated to prevent one additional event. Moreover, when Stuart Pocock reviewed 45 trials reported in the British Medical Journal, the Lancet, and the New England Journal of Medicine, he concluded: "Overall, the reporting of clinical trials appears to be biased toward an exaggeration of treatment differences" (92). As a safeguard against this exaggeration, the CONSORT recommendation that trialists report "For each primary and secondary outcome, a summary of results for each group, and the estimated effect size and its precision" (*http://www.consort-statement.org/*). Thus, whether trialists focus on relative or absolute risk reductions, they must provide readers with the control and experimental event rates that would permit readers to calculate the efficacy measure they find most informative. This is the editorial policy of our "evidence-based" journals. It is also appropriate, when reliable data are at hand, to report at least the numbers needed to be treated to prevent one additional event for clinically identifiable low, medium, and high-risk subgroups.

Don't Go Looking for the Pony

As you've already read, subgroup analysis is a two-edged sword. In the design phase of the RRPCE trial, I proposed looking for the pony and pushed for subgroup analyses of efficacy based on the nature and location of the qualifying TIAs, age and sex, and several comorbid conditions. This led to more than a dozen subgroup analyses, with some of them further divided by sex. I therefore must take the blame for our statement, based on one of these subgroup analyses, that "Aspirin was of no benefit in reducing stroke or death among women." We didn't base this erroneous statement merely on an effect that was statistically significant in men but not in women. Women were 42% *more* likely to suffer stroke or death on aspirin in our trial, and we showed a statistically significant ($P < 0.003$) difference in the RRRs between the sexes. Despite this extremely large "interaction" and positive subgroup analysis in the first-ever trial of aspirin for preventing stroke, later trials proved it was wrong.

Looking for the pony has caused countless trialists to emerge from subgroup analyses appropriately stercoraceous, even when (as in the RRPCE trial) they demonstrate a statistically significant qualitative interaction. My advice to you is to *never* draw a conclusion (especially in print) about efficacy from any subgroup analysis that produces an unanticipated qualitative interaction (such as a treatment that is effective in one subgroup of patients is either harmful or powerfully useless in another). Rather, I suggest that the only appropriate response to such a finding is replication (in an independent study), not publication. If you're not convinced by this tough stance, revisit our aspirin versus perioperative complications experience described in the introduction to this chapter.

Even if you ignore that admonition, Andrew Oxman and Gordon Guyatt have warned the readers of your RCT report to reject your conclusions about subgroups unless they are big, highly statistically significant, specified before analysis, replicated in other independent trials, and supported by other evidence (93).

✓ Never describe your indeterminate study as "negative" or as showing "no difference."

The third exaggeration is reporting an "indeterminate" trial as "negative"; that is, reporting that an intervention has "no effect" just because the 95% confidence intervals for its RRR and ARR cross 1 and 0.0, respectively. I've illustrated this problem in Figure 6–2, but it deserves attention here as well. This problem is as old as RCTs, and 25 years ago Jenny Freiman et al. examined 71 "negative" trials and found that 94% of them had a greater than 10% risk (power less than 0.9) of missing an RRR of 25% (the sort of effect observed among many efficacious treatments) (94). Alas, 16 years later David Moher and his colleagues documented that this problem had not gone away (95). As previously stressed, whether resulting from a planned "debunking" trial of a treatment thought to be useless, or found as an unexpected result of a superiority trial, the issue is not the (nonsignificant) difference that you found, but the difference, of significance to patients, that you can rule out.

Allan Detsky and I have suggested that there are two appropriate ways to evaluate apparently "negative" trials (96). Both of them reject *a priori* sample size requirements and focus on results ("how many patients you needed depends on what you found"). First, we suggest that you simply generate a confidence interval around the effect that you did observe and see whether it excludes any minimally important effect (as in Figure 6–2). Second, we suggest an alternative in which you test your observed difference against the effect you hypothesized before the trial. Even if you rule out any minimally important effect, I still advise against labeling your result "negative" because you may not have ruled out the effect somebody else considers worthwhile. For this reason, I have expanded Iain Chalmers' earlier proposal to ban the term "negative trial" (97) and have taken the position that the word "negative" should be banned in describing any result from any study (*http://bmj.com/cgi/eletters/325/7373/0/g#27016*). I suggest that far more accurate and useful words are "inconclusive" or, if that is too bitter a pill to swallow in print, "indeterminate."

✓ Report your results regardless of their interpretation.

Failing to report your trial's results, regardless of what they show (or fail to show), is both bad science and bad ethics. Every trial result needs to be included in systematic reviews of that intervention, and avoiding publication bias (especially of trials with indeterminate results) is vital to their validity. Moreover, it is unethical to expose study patients to an RCT environment, with the expectation that they are contributing new knowledge to medical science, and then suppress their contributions to that knowledge.

Even published trials under-report preplanned analyses. For example, An-Wen Chan and colleagues compared the protocols and subsequent publications from 48 Canadian RCTs (98). They concluded that there was incomplete reporting of a third of the efficacy outcomes and over half of the safety outcomes listed in their grant applications. Moreover, efficacy outcomes were almost three times as likely to be reported when they were statistically significant.

In 1997, in recognition of the resistance to submitting and publishing "negative" trials, over 100 editors of medical journals declared an "amnesty for unpublished trials" and provided a free registration service for unpublished trials (99). This offer has been superseded by the creation of the International Standard Randomised Controlled Trial Number, or ISRCTN, from the Current Clinical Trials Web site at *http://www.controlled-trials.com/isrctn/introduction.asp*, and I will describe this in detail later. I think this registration should extend even to fraudulent or "busted" trials in which adherence to the protocol was so awful that they had to be abandoned.

✓ Update the systematic review that justified your trial.

Your work won't be done until you incorporate your trial results (plus any other contemporaneous ones) in an updated systematic review of your intervention. Has your trial provided the necessary confirmation of efficacy or a useful narrowing of the confidence interval around the estimate of effectiveness?

Besides contributing to the science of health care, there are three more personal benefits of updating the systematic review. First, if your trial results were indeterminate, they will nonetheless be incorporated into a systematic review, meeting your scientific and ethical obligations. Second, the updated systematic review contributes another publication to your CV. Finally, it tells you where to go next. Alas, Michael Clarke, Philip Alderson and Iain Chalmers reported that only 3 of 33 RCT reports published in May 2001 in the five major general medical journals even referred to relevant systematic reviews, and none of them presented any systematic attempt to "set the new results in the context of previous trials" (100).

✓ *Formulate the question for your next trial.*

With the possible exception of "debunking" trials that expose the uselessness of established treatments, the interpretation of an RCT result ought to lead to the formulation of the logical question you should ask in your next RCT. Might an effective treatment for your study patients also benefit patients with a different but related disorder? Is the unexpected response of some subgroup of patients that you discovered while data-dredging of such potential importance that you should test it in your next trial? Might a simpler, cheaper, or more easily tolerated regimen be non-inferior to the one you've just validated as efficacious? In addition to formulating a better next, logical question, you should incorporate everything you learned in designing, conducting and analyzing this trial into the design, conduct, and analysis of your next trial.

5.8 SAMPLE SIZE

Preface: Is This Section Really Necessary?

Once again, I stressed the importance of recruiting a statistician as co-PI right at the start of formulating the question for your RCT. Why, then, intrude further on their turf with a section on sample size? As with the previous section on analysis, my reasons are three. First, as you can see in this section's checklist, two of its three entries are not strictly statistical. Second, especially early in thinking about your trial, you may want to do some sample size "doodling" to understand the effects of, for example, recruiting high- versus low-risk patients. Accordingly, this section's function is to provide non-statisticians with sufficient introduction to sample size determinations to be able to roughly estimate them without bugging your statistician co-PI with every new idea. Third, as with data analysis, this section might whet some statistical appetites.

In the RRPCE trial, we estimated that the annual incidence of stroke among our study patients would be 7%, that their annual death rate would be 4%, and that one or both drugs would halve these rates. We decided to limit our risk of concluding that either or both drugs were better than placebo when, in fact, they weren't (the Type I error) to 0.05 (α). We also decided to limit our risk of concluding that neither drug was better than placebo when, in fact, one or both were (the Type II error) to 0.20 (β).

Although a spot survey at our Clinical PI's center predicted that his team would see 52 eligible patients each year, we urged our neurologic collaborators at the other 23 to be very pessimistic in predicting patient availability. Together, they predicted that they could recruit 150 patients per year.

They recruited less than half this number (77) in year 1, and our Clinical PI began to visit every center at frequent intervals. Recruitment rose to 148 patients in year 2 and 164 patients in year 3. Our Clinical PIs' team recruited almost a third of all our study patients.

The scenario nicely describes what happens when collaborators' high-flying, rosy predictions of patient availability come to earth in the swamps where recruitment really happens. In this section, I'll do my best to guide you through these swamps.

Sample size checklist:

✓ Calculate your sample size requirement.
✓ Estimate (with appropriate skepticism) the availability of appropriate patients.
✓ Identify strategies to increase (effective) sample size.

The first part of the sample size checklist applies to the planning stages of your trial.

✓ Calculate your sample size requirement.

Let's begin by considering a superiority trial that uses discrete events as outcomes. You can usefully think about it as a diagnostic test for the truth about efficacy, as shown in Table 5–8.

The rows of this table describe the conclusions you draw at the end of your trial, and the columns describe the truth (that you are trying to "diagnose" with your trial). If your conclusions match the truth, all is well. What you want to avoid is drawing incorrect conclusions. As it happens, you can specify the risks you are willing to run of drawing these wrong conclusions before you start your trial. In a superiority trial, you want to minimize the risk of drawing the false-positive conclusion that your experimental treatment is superior when, in fact, it is not. Statisticians call this a Type I error and trialists prespecify this risk, typically at 0.05, and call it α. After the trial is over, tests for the "statistical significance" between the experimental and control event rates describe the actual risk you ran of drawing the false-positive conclusion, and present it as a P value. If it hasn't already occurred to you, this is why we want P values to be very small.

Similarly, you want to minimize the risk of drawing the false-negative conclusion that your experimental treatment is useless when, in fact, it is superior. Statisticians call this a Type II error and trialists prespecify it, typically at 0.2, and call it β. You are probably more familiar with its complement, $1-\beta$, which we call power. Again, if it hasn't already occurred to you, this is why we want power to be very large. And you may find it useful to think of the power of an RCT the same way that you think about

TABLE 5-8   The Randomized Control Trial as a Diagnostic Test for the Truth About Efficacy

		The truth about efficacy	
		Experimental treatment really is superior	Experimental treatment really is not superior
Results of your RCT	Experimental treatment appears to be superior	$1-\beta$ Power!	Type I error Risk = α P value!
	Experimental treatment appears not to be superior	Type II error Risk = β	

RCT, randomized control trial.

the sensitivity of a diagnostic test. It tells you the probability that you will find superiority, and label it statistically significant, if it really exists.

Sample Size When a Difference in the Occurrence of Events Will Answer Your Question

There are two ways to calculate your sample size requirements here. These are the forward "patients I need" approach and the backward "patients I can get" approach. The "patients I need" approach tells you just that: how many patients you need per treatment group. But the "patients I can get" approach tells you how big a bang (in terms of power) you will get from the patients you can get. I'll describe them in sequence.

The forward "patients I need" approach is the classical, theoretical one that appears in most beginning courses and textbooks. In the "patients I need" approach, you simply pick your α and β, specify the event rates you expect to observe among your experimental and control patients, and calculating your sample size requirement is simple math.

However, I never trust my or my students' hand calculations of sample size (too often they are wildly wrong). Instead, I go to a statistical Web site that will do it right. The one I use is run by Rollin Brant at the University of British Columbia: *http://stat.ubc.ca/~rollin/stats/ssize/index.html* (but in using this site, be sure to pick the option that is labeled "Comparing Proportions for Two Independent Samples"). However, I suggest that you surf until you find the one that's best for you, testing its accuracy against worked sample size calculations from two or more statistics texts.

Regardless of where you get your sample size requirements, you should avoid the common mistake of thinking that they constitute the *total* number of patients you require for your trial. In fact, most of them tell you the number of patients you need *per treatment group*.

Moreover, any way you do it, you shouldn't be satisfied with a single "patients I need" sample size calculation. Just suppose that you've overestimated the true CER and/or the true RRR. As a result, the ARR you'll observe in your trial will be smaller than you'd predicted, and you will have too few patients to generate a statistically significant result with a nice, tight confidence interval. To avoid this pitfall, you should plug in all the clinically sensible CERs and RRRs, as shown in Table 5–9.

Then you can ponder the table and decide what to do. If you could actually recruit the largest ("worst-case") sample size you're likely to require, that would be great insurance. Then, if the actual CER and/or RRR you observe in your trial turn out to be greater than your "worst case," your statistical warning rule should be triggered early.

The crucial mistake you want to avoid is "finishing" your trial and shutting it down, only to discover that it's too small. Imagine your agony if the confidence interval around your moderate but still useful ARR crosses zero. As I'll discuss in Section 5.10, this is another powerful reason why you should get someone to monitor the progress and emerging results of your trial.

Special Cases

You can use this same approach to calculate the "patients I need" to answer one-sided questions about superiority and noninferiority. All that you do differently is to set your α at 0.10 rather than 0.05. In Table 5–9, this reduces the number of patients needed in each cell by about 20%.

You can use this same strategy for 2 × 2 factorial designs if you assume that the effects of the two interventions will be similar and additive (i.e., the response to one of them is unaffected by receiving the other, and there is no "interaction"). This factorial design permits you to "do two trials for the

TABLE 5–9 The Number of "Patients I Need" *Into Each Treatment Group* **if α = 0.05 and β = 0.2 (80% Power) and the Control Event Rates and Relative Risk Reductions are as Shown**

		If the RRR is:				
		20%	25%	30%	35%	40%
	0.60	270	173	120	88	67
	0.55	324	205	148	105	79
If the CER is:	0.50	388	247	170	124	93
	0.45	466	298	203	146	111
	0.40	564	356	244	176	133

price of one," because you use each study patient twice, once for each treatment. The sample size calculation will tell you the numbers of patients you need in the "margins" at the end of each row and column. You can then simply split them between the cells making up that row or column. A note of caution here: this strategy will not give you much power for determining synergy or antagonism between your treatments, as the latter analysis has to be carried out "inside the cells" (101).

I'm warning you right now that your first look at the results of your "patients I need" calculation is likely to chill your blood and bring up your lunch. What you thought was a short and simple single-center RCT can morph before your eyes into a multicenter mega-trial.

For this reason, lots of trialists ignore the forward-looking "patients I need" approach altogether. They reckon it's much more realistic and honest to apply the backward-looking "patients I can get" approach. In this approach, sample-size is an input, not an output. You start by estimating the number of patients you are confident you can enroll in the study. Let's say there are 300 patients "you can get," or 150 per group. As before, you specify a range of reasonable CERs and RRRs, and pick your α. The rest is simple maths, and another visit to Rollin Brant's Web site, *http://stat.ubc.ca/~rollin/stats/ssize/index.html*, will generate Table 5–10.

This time, because you have already specified the number of patients per group, the only thing left for the Web site to calculate is the power ("sensitivity") generated from each pair of CERs and RRRs. The shaded cells in this table spell trouble. They mark those unfortunate combinations of CERs and RRRs in which your 150 patients per group will fail to generate the 80% power (or "sensitivity") that most trialists (and granting agencies) require. What you need to do is get out of the shade and into the clear cells, and a revisit to the section on physiological statistics may help you.

Tables 5.9 and 5.10 are saying the same thing, but in different ways. You can confirm this by noting that the shaded, "underpowered" cells in Table 5–10 correspond to the cells in Table 5–9 that require more than 150 patients per group.

TABLE 5–10 **The Power I Can Generate When the "Patients I Can Get" is 150 Per Group, α = 0.05, and the Control Event Rates and Relative Risk Reductions Are as Shown**

		If the RRR is:				
		20%	25%	30%	35%	40%
	0.60	55%	74%	88%	96%	99%
	0.55	48%	67%	82%	92%	97%
If the CER is:	0.50	41%	59%	75%	87%	95%
	0.45	35%	51%	67%	81%	91%
	0.40	30%	44%	59%	73%	85%

Sample Size When a Difference in Average Values for a Physiologic, Behavioral, or Quality of Life Measure Will Answer Your Question

You decide about α and β as before. Then, you go back to the discussions you had when you were designing your PICOT question and specify the smallest difference in outcomes between experimental and control patients, which, if observed at the end of the trial, your patients and (we trust) you would consider humanly important, the "Minimally Important Difference" or *MID*. Usually, this will take the form of a minimum important difference between the changes in the measure from baseline to the end of the trial in the intervention and control groups. Finally, you need to plug in a description of how these continuous measures vary between patients and repeated measurements, typically in the form of a standard deviation of change. You can then proceed to one of the Web sites and crank out your sample size needs. As before, you should plug in all the reasonable values for the differences you'd like to detect and the standard deviations you're likely to observe.

As Gordon Guyatt and his colleagues have demonstrated, the "minimum important difference" can have tricky properties when applied to quality of life measures (102). Several of the questionnaires they use employ 7-point scales. Patients rate their symptoms, function, or quality of life on these scales by matching their current state with the scale's verbal description. For example, in reporting how short of breath they've been in the last 2 weeks while climbing stairs they can choose from "extremely short of breath" at one end to "not at all short of breath" at the other. Gordon Guyatt's team have documented that the minimum difference that patients consider important (MID) is a change in score of >0.5. However, if some patients benefit greatly from the intervention (change >1.0) and others not at all (change $= 0$), an average MID <0.5 could still be important for the former. An alternative approach here is to assign a favorable "event" to every patient whose scores change by 0.5 or more. By doing this, you convert the analysis (and sample size determination) into the event strategy described earlier. Once again, I refer you to Peter and Gordon's chapter on developing and validating such measures (Chapter 11). They point out that an analysis of covariance may be a more appropriate pathway to follow in determining sample size in trials with "continuous" outcomes. This gets pretty complex pretty fast, and your statistician/co-PI should determine which strategy is more appropriate.

If You Are Planning a Cluster Randomized Trial

As described previously in Section 5.4 (on "Allocation of Patients to Treatments"), the calculations change any time that study patients are allocated to treatments in clusters of two or more, such as families, practices, hospital wards, communities, provinces, and the like. The responses of study individuals within these clusters can be expected to be more similar (or "concordant") than the responses of individuals belonging to different clusters. Because individuals within clusters are not "independent," the traditional methods for determining sample size will underestimate the real sample size requirement (and the traditional methods of analysis may overestimate treatment effects).

Sample size determinations for cluster-randomized trials begin with estimating the degree of concordance within clusters. For continuous outcome measures such as blood pressure, this concordance might be expressed as an intraclass correlation coefficient. For events such as quitting smoking, concordance might be expressed as kappa (103). These concordance factors are then used to determine the appropriate (increased) sample size requirement. Once again I refer you to the writings of Neil Klar and Alan Donner (104), who have developed methods that take concordance nicely into account.

If You Are Planning a Crossover or "Time to Failure" Randomized Control Trial

I won't discuss these less common and more complex RCTs here. If you're doing one of these without a statistician co-PI, you deserve all the trouble you'll get. To talk intelligently with your co-PI, you might want to consult one of the dedicated clinical trials books, such as the third edition of the book *Fundamentals of Clinical Trials* by Lawrence Friedman, Curt Furberg, and David DeMets (105).

A Final Note

Many trialists add, say, 20% to their final sample size estimate to account for patients who don't comply with treatment, drop out, or are lost to follow-up. This is a double-edged sword. On the one hand, it is comforting to have a sample size cushion. On the other hand, losing anywhere close to 20% of your trial's patients will also lose you credibility when you report its results. Moreover, if the risk or responsiveness of the patients you lose differs from that of patients you retain, you will lose validity as well. It is far better to devote the resources required for recruiting another 20% of patients to keeping track of all those whom you've already recruited. I'll come back to this at the end of this section.

✓ *Estimate (with appropriate skepticism) the availability of appropriate patients.*

Four decades ago, we simply asked clinicians at the potential study site(s) to tell us the number of patients they thought they could recruit for the trial. It didn't take us long to realize that this approach led to hopelessly optimistic estimates of available patients. This realization had two effects. First, we adopted the aphorism: "The best way to eliminate a disease is to start an RCT on it." Second, we started applying "rules of thumb," which would divide these rosy estimates by 2, 4, or 8.

Nowadays we ask potential collaborators to make a list or "log" of every potential study patient they encounter over the several weeks or months we spend hammering out the protocol. We ask them to ruthlessly distinguish the minority of patients who meet all the eligibility criteria from the majority who, for one reason or other, don't. If you do this, you'll probably discover that you need a longer recruitment period or more clinical collaborators. This discovery is extremely annoying before a trial begins, but becomes cata-strophic if it only dawns on you after you have started your trial. This leads us nicely into our final suggestion that you read the next bit of this section while you're still in the early planning stage of your RCT.

✓ Identify strategies to increase (effective) sample size.

As with any other potentially fatal disorder, the successful treatment of in-adequate sample size begins with an accurate diagnosis. The reason you can't recruit enough patients may not be because they are rare. It might be the result of clinician- and patient-based barriers to participation. Sue Ross and her UK colleagues systematically reviewed 78 reports of these barriers and I have summarized their findings in Table 5–11 (106).

Based on your diagnosis, you can employ one or more of 12 strate-gies to either increase your sample size or make the most of whatever sam-ple size you do recruit. These interventions come from several sources, including a Cochrane Review (107).

The first seven are general strategies for increasing patient numbers:

1. You can make it easier for clinical collaborators to approach and enter patients into the trial by reducing the entry forms to just those items that are of high and immediate relevance. For example, entry forms for some large, simple trials occupy less than one side of one page.
2. You can reduce the complexity and time spent in deciding whether every patient is eligible for a trial in two ways. First, you can reduce its eligibility criteria to a bare minimum. Second, you can employ the

TABLE 5–11   Barriers to Participation in a Randomized Controlled Trial

Clinician Based	Patient Based
Time constraints	Additional procedures and appointments for patient
Lack of staff and training	Additional travel problems and cost for patient
Worry about the impact on doctor–patient relationship	Patient preferences for a particular treatment (or no treatment)
Concern for patients	Worry about uncertainty of treatment or trials
Loss of professional autonomy	Patient concerns about information and consent
Difficulty with the consent procedure	Protocol causing problem with recruitment
Lack of rewards and recognition	Clinician concerns about information provision to patients

From: Ross S, Grant A, Counsell C, Gillespie W, Russell I, Prescott R. Barriers to participation in randomised controlled trials: a systematic review. *J Clin Epidemiol* 1999;52:1143–1156, with permission.

"uncertainty principle" as the major determinant of an individual patient's eligibility (108). For more about the uncertainty principle, see Section 6.7 (the "Uncertainty Principle and Equipoise").

3. You can reduce the follow-up effort required from busy clinical collaborators by providing Research Assistants to help them with forms, baseline measurements, allocation, and follow-up appointments. Trialists like me vastly prefer this strategy to that of providing "bounties" to clinicians for every patient they enter.

4. You can capture eligible patients who appear at night or on weekends by setting up a 24/7 randomization "hotline," perhaps via your hospital switchboard (109).

5. When a brand new drug or other treatment is not yet available to the public and has never been evaluated in a Phase III trial, many sponsors (especially health care providers who must pay for the innovation) will make the experimental treatment available only within an RCT (110).

6. You can explore collaboration with relevant organizations of patients and families who provide information, support, and advocacy to the victims of the disorder you are studying. Growing numbers of such organizations have become strong and effective advocates for relevant RCTs.

7. You could write directly to your own patients, describing the trial and inviting them to learn more about it. This strategy has often been successful in recruiting patients in primary care.

    The nextthree strategies attack the universal failure of participating centers (including your own!) to approach all eligible patients.

8. You can increase recruitment from your current center(s) by frequently exposing the people in these centers to your most charismatic and respected clinical collaborator. Our cerebrovascular trials succeeded in large part because our principal clinical investigator was willing to devote major time to national and international "circuit-riding" among the centers. His "outreach" visits began with grand rounds and bedside rounds, demonstrating and teaching clinical skills and evidence-based clinical judgment. Valuable in their own right, these sessions also dramatized the clinical relevance and importance of the trial and gained the respect of the front-line clinicians (often in training) who were most likely to encounter eligible patients. Having established and reinforced the credibility of the study and its investigators, he then would turn to issues of recruitment and follow-up, encouraging, instructing, or admonishing as the situation dictated. His visits were almost always followed by dramatic increases in both recruitment and data quality. Equally dramatic are the numbers of trials without peripatetic clinical leaders that failed to recruit even a small portion of their projected numbers of patients.

9. You can increase recruitment by employing strategies that have been shown in other RCTs to change the behavior of clinicians (51,53,111). For example, keeping a "log" of all remotely relevant patients (both eligible and ineligible) at each center provides an audit and feedback

to the individual clinicians who had agreed to approach such patients for the trial.

10. You can increase recruitment by recognizing both the needs and contributions of individual participating centers. Providing continuing education (as well as study clarification) to local staff, recognizing their contributions in final reports, and providing them the opportunity to carry out and publish their own ancillary studies strengthens their commitment to the success of the parent study.

The final two strategies protect against erosion of your effective sample size by making the most of patients you already have enrolled:

11. You can make (or protect) minor gains by keeping the numbers of control and experimental patients approximately equal (but not exactly so if that would threaten allocation concealment). When hunches favoring one of the treatments are strong, it may be tempting to randomize a larger proportion of eligible patients to that arm of the trial. However, there is a price to pay. Randomizing twice as many patients to one of the treatments (2:1 randomization) requires 12% more patients overall; 3:1 randomization requires 33% more patients (Altman D. Personal communication, 2001).

12. The most important admonition throughout this chapter is to protect your sample size by not losing any study patients. Keeping track of all of them serves two related purposes. First, it detects events that otherwise would be missed. Second, it increases your chances of being able to present a convincing "worst-case scenario" (in which all experimental patients lost to follow-up in a trial with a positive conclusion are assigned bad outcomes and all lost control patients a rosy one). When losses-to-follow-up are so few that ARRs and their confidence intervals remain convincing in worst-case scenarios, the credibility of a trial's positive conclusion is enhanced.

This section closes with an admonition. You should be very reluctant to relax your eligibility criteria in order to increase your sample size. This is especially dangerous when you are considering adding patients who are at a lower risk or who are less responsive than your target study population. As you will find in Section 6.6 on "Physiological Statistics," every low-risk, low-response patient you admit to your trial can make your need for additional patients go up, not down.

Strategies 1, 2, and 4 nicely match the tactics employed in large, simple trials, and they are discussed in Section 6.11 ("Large, Simple Trials"). On the other hand, small trials are often big enough to serve several useful purposes, and they are considered in Section 6.12 ("Small Trials").

5.9 SPECIAL ETHICAL ISSUES IN RANDOMIZED CONTROLLED TRIALS

This section will simply identify and expand upon those ethical issues that are of special interest in RCTs, identifying current controversies along the way.

RCT ethics checklist:

Is your RCT ethical at its inception?

✓ Have you carried out a systematic review of all relevant prior trials?

✓ Will your RCT's design and execution move us toward a valid determination of the treatment's efficacy and safety?

✓ Will your RCT withhold "established effective therapy" from any or all of its participants?

Will your RCT remain ethical during its execution?

✓ Will you guarantee potential participants free, informed consent?

✓ Will your participants be free to withdraw without losing care?

✓ Will you preserve participant confidentiality?

✓ Will you identify and act on adverse treatment effects promptly?

✓ Will you stop your RCT as soon as the better treatment is clearly established?

✓ Are your trial close-out procedures ethical?

Will your sponsors and investigators behave ethically during the trial?

✓ Will "bounties" be offered for admitting patients to your RCT?

✓ Will your RCT data be protected from distortion by market considerations?

✓ Will your RCT be terminated for market considerations?

Will your sponsors and investigators behave ethically after the trial is over?

✓ Will you be free to report your RCT, regardless of its results?

✓ Will your RCT publications be "ghost-written"?

✓ Will your RCT's investigators declare their potential conflicts of interest in subsequent speeches, publications, and guideline committee participations?

✓ Will you make the results of your RCT available for updating all relevant systematic reviews?

Note: This section is not about whether ethics committees do more harm than good, although that was a question posed with increasing frequency as this book went to press. The imposition of "ethical" regulations in the absence of credible evidence that they would, in fact, protect patients was reaching epidemic proportions. Clinical researchers in the United Kingdom had just reported that they were finding the procedures used by research ethics committees increasingly damaging to the advancement of evidence-based health care. A single issue of the BMJ contained reports from five separate research groups (112), reporting how an ethics committee impeded, delayed, and sometimes distorted their research.

Is Your Randomized Control Trial Ethical at Its Inception?

✓ *Have you carried out a systematic review of all relevant prior trials?*

Before you design your trial, you should pore over any systematic reviews of previous relevant studies. Has your experimental treatment already been definitively shown to benefit or harm the patients (or some subgroup of them) that you were intending to enroll in your trial? Have the doses and durations of treatment you're considering already been shown to be too much or too little? Have any of the clinical measurements or scales you were intending to use been found wanting or superseded by newer, better ones? Would minor adjustments in your protocol permit the inclusion of your trial results in subsequent, even more informative systematic reviews?

✓ *Will your RCT's design and execution move us toward a valid determination of the treatment's efficacy and safety?*

We (and every trialist we know) agree with the proposition that an RCT is unethical if it is incapable, at the outset, of moving us toward a valid determination of a treatment's efficacy and safety. To meet this ethical requirement of reducing therapeutic ignorance, you have to do two things. First, you must generate a scientifically sound protocol. It must be capable of providing unbiased estimates of efficacy and safety for the patients in your trial.

Second, there has to be a good prospect for combining your results with those of other, similar trials in later systematic reviews. This is especially important if your trial is at risk of being "underpowered" (i.e., too small to generate a usefully narrow confidence interval around the effects of treatment).

Some trialists hold that underpowered (too small) trials are unethical and should not be carried out. We disagree, because that attitude perpetuates therapeutic ignorance. However, everything must be done to maximize the accessibility of every trial's results for systematic reviews. To meet this ethical requirement, you must do two things. First, you must register your trial by the time your protocol is funded and its execution is about to begin (as this edition was being written, the best way to register a trial was to obtain an International Standard Randomised Controlled Trial Number, or ISRCTN, from the Current Clinical Trials Web site at *http://www.controlled-trials.com/isrctn/introduction.asp*. Better still, publish your protocol, preferably at an Open Access Web site, such as that supported by BioMed Central (*http://www.biomedcentral.com*). (Indeed, if you have not yet begun your trial, BMC will send your protocol out for peer review and comment.) Second, you must report the results of your trial in some easily accessible site, regardless of the sample size you achieved. Your report should include a description of the occurrence and reasons for changes that were made in the protocol during the execution of the study.

✓ Will your RCT withhold "established effective therapy" from any or all of its participants?

It's best to introduce this step with two disclaimers and three definitions. The first disclaimer is that withholding EET is not about proper food, clean sheets, and competent, caring nurses and doctors in attendance; those are deserved by any patient, anywhere. The second disclaimer is that this matter is not about "standard" or "traditional" care that is routinely given to patients with the target disorder, regardless of its evidence-base, as long as it is provided equally to experimental and control patients.

The concern here is much more specific, and the first definition promised above is for "EET." The definition used in this chapter is: any intervention, for a specific disorder in a specific group of patients, for which the "totality of evidence" documents that it does more good than harm. Integral to this discussion is a decision on who should define "good" and "harm" here: patients, their clinicians, researchers, regulators, or funders? We favor the patient's perspective, and recognize that individual patients' utilities for "good" and "harm" will lead to some of them accepting very risky treatments and others rejecting fairly safe ones.

This leads us to the second, related definition, this time for the "totality of evidence": either a positive systematic review (epitomized by a Cochrane review) of one or more high-quality RCTs, or the presence of "all or none" evidence.

The third definition, for "all or none" evidence, means two contrasting but convincing situations. In the first of them, *all* patients with the condition died in the days before the therapy was introduced and, afterwards, some of them survived. A nice example here would be tuberculous meningitis, a universally fatal disease before the introduction of streptomycin. Other examples would be choriocarcinoma and testicular cancer before the introduction of chemotherapy, and malignant hypertension before the introduction of antihypertensive drugs. The second convincing situation is when many patients with the condition died in the days before the therapy was introduced but afterwards, *none* (or almost none) of them died. A nice example here would be acute pneumococcal pneumonia in otherwise healthy teenagers, which exhibited a case–fatality rate as high as 30% before the introduction of penicillin.

Withholding Established Effective Therapy in "Me-too" Trials

Trials that propose withholding "EET" are of two sorts, and both are contentious as we write this edition (113,114). The first sort of trial proposes withholding EET to test an alternative (sometimes a "me-too") drug against a placebo. (Here, a "me-too" drug is a promising, new but untested drug, often of the same class as the EET, which requires validation in an RCT to be licensed for sale.) Most often, this sort of RCT is proposed for a condition that is considered "mild" (e.g., acne). Alternatively, the RCT calls for replacing EET with a placebo in more serious conditions, but for just a short time, during which the investigator contends that there will be no serious or permanent damage from its absence (e.g., mild to moderate depression).

Proponents of withholding EET in this situation argue that head-to-head trials (of the new drug versus EET) are just too expensive in view of the tiny risks involved. Opponents of placebo-controlled trials of this sort, including us, argue that they constitute both bad clinical science and bad ethics. We consider them bad clinical science because they ask a dumb question. Patients and clinicians don't want to know whether the new, promising drug is better than nothing (placebo). We want to know whether the new, promising drug is better than EET ("superiority"), or as good as EET ("noninferior") but safer, cheaper, easier to take, or simply providing them a wider choice. The best way to answer this question is with a head-to-head comparison of the new promising drug against the established EET. Second, we find testing a new, promising drug against placebo in this situation is bad ethics because such trials assign half (usually) of their patients to a treatment (placebo) known to be ineffective.

When Established Effective Therapy Is Not Available at the Trial Site

The second situation in which trialists propose to withhold EET is when it is not available in the town, province, or country where the trial would take place. In Canada, for example, this could apply to urgent high-tech treatments that are hours or even days away from the patients who need them (e.g., immediate angioplasty for patients with threatened heart attacks who live in a Newfoundland outport with no roads, or reside above the Arctic Circle). This situation would also apply to entire countries whose economic or political realities may prohibit access to EET (e.g., for AIDS in South Africa).

Proponents of withholding effective but unavailable therapy argue that such trials are good clinical science, and are ethical when three further conditions are met. First, they must be carried out in partnership with researchers, community leaders, and patients at the sites where the RCT is to be done (115). The prerequisites, strategies, and tactics for creating this vital partnership are developing rapidly, and readers might want to catch up with them by following the reports of the Clinical Bioethics group at the US National Institutes of Health.

The second prerequisite follows from the first: such trials must be approved by local ethics committees at the sites where they are carried out, regardless of where their investigators come from (if no local ethics committee exists, this review should be carried out by some other group that is both competent and independent of the trial).

Third, these trials must test new, promising treatments that, if effective, would be available to all other patients in the sites where the RCT will be carried out. Proponents of this view wouldn't hesitate to label as unethical, any RCT carried out to validate expensive drugs for rich folks in Canada by testing them in poor folks overseas who could never afford them.

Opponents of performing RCTs that withhold EET in places that prohibit or can't afford it argue that such trials invoke an ethical "double-standard" (114). For example, when we wrote this edition, the hotly debated fifth revision of the Declaration of Helsinki read: "a placebo may be used as the control treatment in a clinical trial [when] effective treatment is not available to patients due to cost constraints or short supply." That declaration appeared quite clear. However, it then added, in our view, an impossible condition: "This may only be applied when background conditions of justice prevail within the health care system in question; for example, a placebo-controlled trial is not permissible when effective but costly treatment is made available to the rich but remains unavailable to the poor or uninsured." This seemed to us both to deny the former permission and to deny reality. Surely, a major reason for conducting such trials is precisely because EET is available only to the rich. Indeed, one can argue that no country, including Canada, meets this definition of "justice."

A Professor of Pediatrics and Child Health in Pakistan has suggested: "The best way forward is to adopt a more flexible and pragmatic approach that allows existing guidelines to be interpreted in the context of the standards and quality of care available in local or comparable public health systems" (116). Updates on this ongoing debate may be found on the World Medical Association Web site (*http://www.wma.net/e/*), and general developments on the Web site of the international Science and Development Network (*http://www.scidev.net/*).

Will Your Randomized Control Trial Remain Ethical During Its Execution?

The next three items are a familiar but vital trilogy in any research involving human participants:

✓ *Will you guarantee potential participants free, informed consent?*

✓ *Will your participants be free to withdraw without losing care?*

✓ *Will you preserve participant confidentiality?*

You have to tell potential study patients, in ways that they understand, everything that might reasonably be expected to affect their decisions to accept or refuse an invitation to enter your RCT. They must be told who is going to do what to them, when and how often, with what immediate and long-term prospects for good and harm. They must be able to quit the RCT whenever they want without sacrificing their access to care. Moreover, they must be assured that their anonymity will be preserved in any public reporting of the trial or its results.

Trials of emergency treatments for life-threatening conditions often recruit unconscious persons who can neither give informed consent nor actively refuse enrollment. Often there are no family members present to act for them. If you are contemplating such a trial, you should contact your local ethics committee early in the planning process to determine whether, and under what circumstances, they will permit you to proceed.

Two systematic reviews have provided important evidence for informing patients who are considering entering RCTs. Both show that they are not "guinea pigs," sacrificed for the benefit of only later generations. The first of them found that patients with the same disorder had better outcomes, including lower mortality, inside than outside of RCTs (117). The causes for this "trial benefit," (which occasionally extended even to trial patients treated with placebos) are not clear, but probably include a greater likelihood of definitive treatment of their condition, more expert care, more nursing care, closer follow-up, and the detection and treatment of comorbidity. The second systematic review controlled for receiving the same treatment inside and outside a trial, and found no disadvantage to trial participation (118).

The next three items concern the trial once it is under way.

✓ Will you identify and act on adverse treatment effects promptly?

The side effects and toxicity of the EET given in an RCT are usually well-known and even anticipated (bleeding on warfarin and the like). Appropriate responses to their occurrence should be built right into the follow-up protocol. However, the frequency and severity of side effects and toxicity of the experimental treatment often are less well-known. Study patients on these treatments should be monitored for their occurrence and treated accordingly (such as the search for, and treatment of, agranulocytosis among patients assigned to ticlopidine).

Special attention must be given to the serious unanticipated adverse events or "SUAEs" that befall trial patients. If they occur at rates greater than chance, it can become imperative to stop the RCT. A mechanism must be in place for immediately notifying a monitor of their occurrence. For example, when I chair a Data Safety and Monitoring Board, I am informed of SUAEs within 24 hours of their recognition. You may need lots of resources to meet this obligation, especially when sponsors and regulators seek extensive documentation and notification of large numbers of "Not-very-serious-and-already-anticipated" adverse events (NVSAAAAEs).

✓ Will you stop your RCT as soon as the better treatment is clearly established?

In some RCTs, all patients are admitted, treated and complete the study before even minor trends in their outcome-differences emerge. In other

RCTs, however, efficacy or futility become apparent while they are still in their enrollment or long-term treatment phase. This is why we advised statistical warning rules for the latter trials back in the section on analysis. The ethical imperative here is to offer all patients the better treatment as soon as it is clearly identified.

This question is answered slightly differently when an ongoing "non-inferiority" trial is showing equivalence, but with a wide confidence interval, that still includes superiority, inferiority, or both. This trial should continue to a definitive result. I take this topic up again in Section 5.10 (on "Monitoring for Efficacy, Safety, and Futility").

✓ *Are your trial close-out procedures ethical?*

At the end of an RCT, trial patients, their clinicians, and in low-access places, the community should be notified of its results and of the treatment they received during it. In the RRPCE trial, we sent this information to the clinician, who then saw the patient, explained the trial result and their assignment to them, and offered to help them start or stay on aspirin. This is often not the case. Zelda Di Blasi and her colleagues surveyed investigators of placebo-controlled trials published in major journals in 2000 or in a national research register, and found that only 45% of them informed all or most of their participants about their allocation at trial closure (119). Although some justified withholding this information because a further blind follow-up was under way, about half of those who didn't tell patients their treatment stated that they simply never thought to notify them. Fortunately, 75% of this latter group said they would inform their patients in future trials.

After a positive trial, a major ethical problem arises if investigators and sponsors stop supplying the newly established effective experimental therapy to experimental patients and fail to offer it to control patients. It is now common practice to supply drugs at no cost to both groups for 6 to 12 months after a positive trial closes, although a strong ethical case can be made for life-long free treatment. Similarly, in a surgical trial, it is important to offer an efficacious operation to control (unoperated) patients as soon as its efficacy is established. For example, we gave the results of a scheduled interim analysis to the monitors, PI, and Steering Committee for the NASCET endarterectomy trial on a Thursday. All of them decided that afternoon that the trial should be terminated, and a control (unoperated) patient underwent endarterectomy the next day.

Will Your Sponsors and Investigators Behave Ethically During the Trial?

The next three items consider certain actions of trialists and sponsors during the RCT. All deserve and receive prominent negative publicity when they become public.

✓ Will "bounties" be offered for admitting patients to your RCT?

Entering and following trial patients means less time to see other patients. The "opportunity cost" of not seeing, and not billing for, these other patients translates to a loss of clinician income. Furthermore, complex admission and follow-up procedures often require additional laboratory services, specially trained study nurses, and data clerks. Finally, most hospitals insist that all their research costs be recovered. Trialists like us maintain that it is both appropriate and ethical to replace this lost income and pay for these extra services. For this reason, we typically pay our study clinicians a "fee-for-service" when they admit and follow RCT patients. The amount of this fee is set to maintain clinicians' net incomes. Similarly, we pay the salaries of the additional support staff and the local costs of running the trial.

Alas, in many RCTs designed and sponsored by pharmaceutical companies, this "cost recovery fee" is replaced by a "bounty" that vastly exceeds the income lost or other costs of the trial. Bounties of a thousand or more dollars per patient are common, as are bonuses of several thousand additional dollars if some preset number of patients is entered. This means that clinicians in poor countries can earn more in a day from performing a "me-too" trial than they can in a month from caring for the sick.

Bounties can destroy the validity of an RCT when they become a financial incentive to fake the entry of patients and falsify missing follow-up data. Bounties may be harming academic centers as well, where sponsor-initiated trials can buy the talents and efforts of academic staff away from investigator-initiated research and teaching. Sadly, this subversion is often encouraged by the cash-strapped leadership of these academic centers, even to the point of exhorting academic scientists to apply business principles to the conduct of clinical research. One such leader wrote: "Four basic business concepts have been implemented: *viewing the research protocol as a commodity* (italics ours), seeking payment for services rendered, *tracking investments* (italics ours again), and assessing performance" (120).

Trialists like us decry this use of patients for personal financial gain, and regard bounties unethical. The Canadian Medical Association agrees with us and, like many other professional groups, has issued specific policies to govern clinicians who enter and follow their patients in RCTs (121). Replacement of lost income is allowed, as is institutional reimbursement for trial costs. However, they clearly state that "This remuneration should not constitute enticement."

Moreover, to protect against exploitation they require the approval of these financial arrangements by local ethics committees. Finally, they require that "Research subjects must be informed if their physician will receive a fee for enrolling them in a study."

✓ Will your RCT data be protected from distortion by market considerations?

All of my RCTs of drugs have been sponsored in part (but never in whole) by their manufacturers. Their support typically comprises providing the study drug and its placebo, plus a cash grant administered entirely by us. From this grant, we pay for vital activities when their budget-lines are rejected by traditional research agencies. Chief among these are repeated investigators' meetings and visits of our PI and central staff to study centers to solve problems and to maintain accrual rates and protocol adherence. This support has greatly improved the quality of our trials.

Moreover, these manufacturers' pharmacologic expertise has been highly valuable in designing and monitoring trial drug regimens, including alerting study staff to side effects and toxicity. Often, we have invited them to sit on a trial's "Steering Committee," the people who administer the trial while remaining blind to its emerging results.

Note that all of these activities are at arms length from the data. Our industry colleagues never receive raw efficacy data from the field, nor do they carry out any of the primary data analyses. They don't learn the results of our trials until after the TMC has unblinded the PI and that person, in turn, has unblinded the Steering Group.

In our case, keeping data from industry sponsors has never resulted from a lack of trust; we've never worried that our sponsors would distort the data analysis to sell an inferior drug. Rather, we've been concerned about the credibility of the trial result.

However, industries who have sponsored other trials have occasionally been accused of distorting trial data for market considerations. An occasional target of these accusations is a for-profit "Contract Research Organization" (CRO) that runs the trial on a day-to-day basis. In some trials, the field data are held by the CRO or by the sponsoring company itself, and not released to the investigators. Thomas Bodenheimer interviewed a wide array of trialists, pharmaceutical executives, administrators, CRO physicians, and professional medical writers (122). One of the trialists feared that industry control over data allows companies to "provide the spin of the data that favors them." He also pointed out that "In the commercial sector, where most investigators are more concerned with reimbursement than with authorship, industry can easily control clinical trial data." He identified one senior trialist who had refused to place his name on the published results of a study because the sponsor "was attempting to wield undue influence on the nature of the final paper. The effort was so oppressive that we felt it inhibited academic freedom."

Given the risks to validity and credibility arising from sponsors controlling RCT data, major medical journals have issued strict rules of authorship and accountability (123). These are nicely illustrated in *The Lancet*, where the "Role of the Funding Source" must be spelled out in any RCT report. These disclosures are of great assistance to readers, and often provide striking contrasts in credibility. Compare the following two examples:

- "The sponsors of the two trials had no role in study design, data collection, data analysis, data interpretation, or writing of the report" (124).
- "Employees and consultants of the sponsor developed the protocol, enrolled patients, and coordinated the trial. The study sponsor was responsible for data collection and analysis ... " (125).

No surprise, then, that the credibility of industry-controlled RCTs is falling in places like Canada, where internists find the results of industry-based trials 20 times as likely to be judged "not at all credible," of "only low credibility," or of "questionable credibility" as the results of trials carried out by independent investigators (126).

✓ Will your RCT be terminated for market considerations?

Once an RCT begins, trialists like us consider it unethical to stop it until there is clear evidence of:

- superiority (one treatment is clearly superior to the other, or to placebo),
- noninferiority (one treatment is clearly not inferior to the other active treatment),
- harm (one treatment is clearly inferior, or harmful side effects outweigh any benefit from it), or
- futility (not enough patients or events or effects to ever be able to answer the study question).

Stopping for other reasons treats study patients as objects, and places them at risk with no prospect of a valid answer to the study question. In our own RCTs, our sponsors have always agreed with this view.

Unfortunately, the funding of other RCTs has been cut off when sponsors decide that their money is better spent elsewhere. For example, the Steering Committee of an RCT of fluvastatin (to reduce cardiovascular risk and preserve cognitive function in the elderly) was told that their funding was being cut off "because it was feared that a similar trial of pravastatin ... would reach its conclusion before the fluvastatin trial" and that the sponsor said it was necessary "to reallocate resources from Lescol (fluvastatin) to the newer growth assets" (127). And in 2003, investigators in a a trial of verapamil (to reduce cardiovascular risk for hypertensive patients) reported that their funding was stopped 2 years early by its sponsors "with no written rationale or further details about the decision" given to the investigators (128). As this book was being written, Bruce Psaty and Drummond Rennie documented six cases of what they labeled "a broken pact with researchers and patients" (129).

Will Your Sponsors and Investigators Behave Ethically After the Trial is Over?

The final three items raise ethical issues following the completion of an RCT.

✓ Will you be free to report your RCT, regardless of its results?

RCTs with indeterminate (often mislabeled "negative") results are both slower (130) and less likely (131) to be published. Although both these behaviors are understandable, we believe that they (especially the latter) are unethical on the bases of both transparency and accountability. The failure to publish indeterminate trial results is all the more unethical with the advent of the systematic review, which can only meta-analyze what it can find. This latter conviction has been well put by Iain Chalmers: "All unbiased comparative studies should be published, so that the totality of the relevant evidence can be evaluated in the systematic reviews that are needed by those making choices and decisions in health care and about further research" (132).

Sometimes, RCT sponsors make this problem much worse by suppressing publications that threaten profits. Thomas Bodenheimer documented several examples in which funding companies stopped the publication of trial results (122). In others, they delayed publication while they prepared (sometimes in secret) competing papers on the same topic that were favorable to the company's viewpoint.

Before you even begin your trial, you need to have a written understanding with all your sponsors about the ownership and reporting of its results. For example, the agreement between the manufacturer and investigators in a trial I am presently monitoring is crystal clear:

- The manufacturer retains sole property rights to the drug's formula, method of manufacture, and related scientific data.
- The investigator reserves the right to publish the results as he sees fit.
- The investigator must give the manufacturer 15 working days to review and comment on (but not censor) the draft report.
- The investigator must give the manufacturer an additional 90 days if the sponsor needs to file a patent or otherwise protect its proprietary rights.
- These 15-day and 90-day rules are waived if there are concerns related to participant safety.

Finally, given the availability of Web-based entities for registering trials, posting protocols, and publishing results, the excuses for delayed and absent publication have vanished.

✓ Will your RCT publications be "ghost-written"?

Sometimes pharmaceutical firms hire "ghost writers" to convert trial results into manuscripts, and encourage investigators to substitute their names for that of the ghost. Annette Flanigin led a team at The Journal of the American Medical Association (JAMA), which surveyed 809 corresponding "authors" of articles published in major general medical journals in 1996 (133). They found that 11% of these articles had evidence of being ghostwritten, with the true author's name excluded from the paper. They also found that 19% of these articles had evidence of "honorary authorship" in which a person who didn't contribute of the writing of the paper was listed as an author. Two percent of papers had apparently committed both offenses.

Ghostwriters, paid by their industry employers, shouldn't surprise us if they follow the lyrics of the Johnny Mercer (134) standard: "accentuate the positive, eliminate the negative, and don't mess with Mr. In-Between." In commenting on ghostwriting, Drummond Rennie, an editor at JAMA, was quoted as saying: "The practice is well-known, scandalous, and outrageous. It is a perfect illustration of deceptive authorship practices for commercial reasons" (135). Trialists like me agree, and consider ghostwriting suitable for both censure and satire (136).

✓ Will your RCT's investigators declare their potential conflicts of interest in subsequent speeches, publications, and guideline committee participations?

Clinicians and patients must be able to trust the guidelines that are produced by governments and voluntary health agencies. The credibility, if not validity, of these therapeutic recommendations and guidelines is destroyed when their "expert" authors fail to declare potential conflicts of interest. For example, based on recommendations from a committee of experts, the American Heart Association (AHA) upgraded its recommendation for using alteplase (a patented thrombolytic) for stroke from "optional" to "definitely recommended." Afterward, Jeanne Lenzer, a medical investigative journalist, claimed that there were two potential conflicts of interest in this recommendation (137). First, on the 9-member "expert" AHA panel, she claimed that six of the eight "experts" who recommended the drug had financial ties to its manufacturer (as paid lecturers, consultants, and even grant holders). Second, she claimed that the drug's manufacturer had contributed $2.5 million to new AHA buildings. As this chapter was being written, the US National Institute of Neurological Disease and Blindness was assembling an independent committee to reanalyze the study's data.

This is not an isolated case. Niteesh Choudhry and colleagues quantified the extent and nature of interactions between the authors of guidelines and the pharmaceutical industry (138). Among those who responded to their survey, 87% had ties to industry (58% as grantees and 38% as consultants or employees), and over half had relationships with firms whose drugs were considered in their guideline. Furthermore, over half reported that their committees had no formal process for declaring financial ties. This team made three recommendations for the authors of clinical practice guidelines:

1. disclosure of potential conflicts of interest to other participants at the beginning of the guideline creation process
2. exclusion of authors with substantial financial conflicts
3. complete disclosure of each author's potential conflicts to readers of guidelines.

To close this section on a brighter note, the Steering Committee of the Global Utilization of Streptokinase and Tissue Plasminogen Activator for Occluded Coronary Arteries (GUSTO) trial, testing a thrombolytic drug with enormous potential sales, took this ethical concern one step further (139). As part of their trial planning, their Steering Committee "unanimously voted to prohibit any honoraria for speaking engagements, payment for consultancy or travel, or reimbursement of any kind from any of the five corporate sponsors until 1 year after the publication of the results."

✓ Will you make the results of your RCT available for updating all relevant systematic reviews?

We've come full circle. If the trialist who follows you conscientiously reviews the relevant systematic review before he or she designs his or her study, yours had better be there.

5.10 MONITORING FOR EFFICACY, SAFETY, AND FUTILITY

Consider the following four scenarios:

1. In the RRPCE, three of us at the Methods Centre at McMaster carried out the monitoring for safety, efficacy and futility: Mike Gent, the co-PI Biostatistician, Wayne Taylor, the Study Statistician, and I. None of the trial participants were my personal patients, and we kept the PI, Steering Committee, and participating neurologists blind to our analyses. Both study drugs had been in widespread use for years, but we nonetheless maintained a telephone "hotline" so that both anticipated (e.g., gastrointestinal) and unanticipated adverse drug reactions could be assessed at once. We continuously monitored for safety, but carried out a single analysis for efficacy at the scheduled end of the trial. It showed statistically significant efficacy for aspirin, and we then unblinded the PI, who discussed the findings with us and his Steering Group and started an "orderly termination" of the trial.

2. Fifteen years later, when we began the NASCET, our sponsor (the US National Institutes of Health) insisted on naming, and sitting on, our Data Safety and Monitoring Board. We were dissatisfied with its procedures and with some of its members, who, we thought, had conflicts of interest. We had developed statistical warning rules for efficacy and futility, and obtained the Data, Safety, and Monitoring Board (DSMB)'s grudging agreement to remain blind to our efficacy analyses until those warning rules were triggered. Subsequent DSMB meetings were positive and placid during discussions of accrual, surgical performance, follow-up, and data quality. They became stormy and confrontational when we refused to show them unblinded data and limited our efficacy report to a statement that the warning rules had not been triggered. Tempers would flare, we would threaten to quit, and some DSMB members appeared eager to accept our resignations. Then things would settle down and our report would be accepted. However, this cycle would recur at the next meeting. Our statistical warning rules (for patients with highgrade symptomatic stenosis) were triggered shortly before a regularly scheduled DSMB meeting. We presented the unblinded results to them, and they recommended stopping the trial. We showed the results to the PI and Steering Group that afternoon, and they decided to stop the trial. They announced the results to their clinical collaborators that same day, and a control patient underwent endarterectomy the next day.

3. In the interim, I had frequently provided a one-person, volunteer monitoring service for small (<100 patient) RCTs. I closely monitored their unblinded data for safety, and periodically examined their unblinded data for efficacy. Based on my assessments, I recommended either the continuation of these trials or the unblinding of their PIs.

4. Another 15 years later, as this edition was being written, I was asked to chair the TMC for an RCT of drugs that might delay or prevent the onset of diabetes. With agreement from the PI, I banned employees from any sponsor (government or industry) from the committee, and rejected any potential members who owned stock with the drugs' manufacturers. None of us will receive salaries or honoraria for serving on this TMC. Our committee will never be blind. The Data Center and I have established a system for alerting me within 24 hours of any unanticipated serious adverse event in any trial patient. Our TMC and the PIs have agreed upon and adopted statistical warning rules for efficacy and safety. It was understood from the outset that we are serving in an advisory (not executive) capacity to the PIs and their Steering Committee. That is, if we decide that the study treatment clearly works (or is clearly harmful), we will unblind the PIs, not stop the trial.

This section is about the external person(s) who serve the patients and investigators in RCTs by alerting them as soon as clear-cut evidence emerges about the safety or efficacy of the experimental treatment, or about the futility of continuing an indeterminate trial. These groups bear a wide array of names and acronyms, and Susan Ellenberg's collection (140) appears in Table 5–12. Some of the more common monikers are DSMB; Data Monitoring Committee (DMC); and TMC. In this section, I'll use the last term: TMC.

If this section whets your interest in TMCs, or it becomes clear that you need one for your RCT, there are two very good resources where you can learn more about them. The first is a book by Susan Ellenberg, Thomas Fleming, and David DeMets (141), and the second is a report from the UK DAMOCLES project (142) that carried out a systematic review and several interviews on issues in data monitoring and the interim analysis of RCTs.

TABLE 5–12 **Names Assigned to Monitoring Groups**

Subject	Function	Organization
Trial	Monitoring	Committee
Data	Review	Board
Safety	Advisory	Panel
Policy		
Efficacy		
Endpoint		
Ethics		

From Ellenberg SS. Independent data monitoring committees: rationale, operations and controversies. *Stat Med* 2001;20: 2573–2583. Copyright 2001. Copyright John Wiley & Sons Limited, with permission.

Monitoring checklist:

✓ Can you justify **not** monitoring your RCT for safety, efficacy, and futility?

If you decide to monitor your RCT

✓ Specify what's to be monitored.

✓ Specify your monitors' requirements in terms of expertise, experience, and freedom from conflicts of interest.

✓ Recruit your monitor(s).

✓ Get on with it.

✓ *Can you justify not monitoring your RCT for safety, efficacy, and futility?*

Current opinion among trialists is that virtually every RCT needs external monitoring for safety, efficacy and futility (e.g., the British MRC made monitoring of its trials mandatory in 1998). Current opinion also dictates that this monitoring be done by an individual or group who have no personal interest in its outcome. As shown in the third scenario above, this doesn't mean that every RCT needs a full-blown TMC. A single individual often can carry out these functions.

Exceptions to the need for monitoring are rare, but do occur. In some cases, monitoring is *not necessary* because no patients are at risk. An example here is an RCT that randomizes clinicians to receive the same efficacy information in relative or absolute terms, in order to determine whether these different formats lead to different conclusions about efficacy.

In other cases, monitoring is *not feasible* because all study patients have already been recruited and treated (and perhaps have experienced outcomes) before any monitoring function could be launched. One example here would be a single RCT of sufficient size to determine whether marathoners' performance is importantly improved or worsened by different rehydration regimens. A second example would be an RCT into whether different vaccines administered today lead to different outcomes 10 years from now (although even this RCT would need short-term monitoring for safety).

Finally, some trialists propose waiving monitoring in RCTs that test well-established treatments with minor hazards for their effects on trivial, reversible outcomes. I'd accept this view only if the criteria for "minor hazards" and "trivial, reversible outcomes" originated with the patients in these trials, and not from the investigators.

✓ *Specify what's to be monitored.*

Table 5–13 lists some possible functions that monitors could carry out. For a more detailed list, see the report of the DAMOCLES project (142).

TABLE 5-13 Some Monitoring Functions

Before the RCT	Review, discuss with, and advise the Principal Investigator/Steering Group about the protocol and the logistics of its execution
During the RCT	Immediately review every serious unanticipated adverse event, taking necessary steps to protect patients in the trial
	Periodically review accumulating safety data, taking necessary steps to protect patients in the trial
	Review any emerging external evidence that might influence a recommendation to stop or continue the trial
	Periodically review (and provide feedback and advice about) actual vs. projected patient accrual; patients' compliance with treatments; investigators' adherence to the study protocol; the completeness, timeliness and accuracy of study data; and other measures of the quality of the conduct of the trial
	Periodically review unblinded outcome data, applying previously established statistical warning rules for safety, efficacy, equivalence, and futility.
	Integrate this review with the totality of evidence about the target disorder and study regimens, and make a recommendation about continuing the study, enlarging it, or unblinding the PI so that a decision can be made about stopping it
	Based on any of the foregoing, make other recommendations about changes to the protocol or conduct of the study, or in the analysis of its results
After the RCT	Review and provide feedback on draft reports, presentations, and publications
	Assist the Principal Investigator and Writing Committee in responding to comments and criticisms of the trial
	Review the ongoing care of study patients

RCT, randomized control trial.

As in the third scenario above, a single monitor can provide all these functions for small studies (say, less than 100 patients) with early outcomes (say, within 3 months of entry). For bigger, longer studies I recommend that you create a monitoring committee.

✓ *Specify your monitors' requirements of expertise, experience, and freedom from conflicts of interest.*

To begin with, you want monitors who are experts in the functions you listed in the previous step. Their collective expertise should extend from the clinical presentation and care of patients with the target disorder to the latest developments in trial design and statistical analysis.

Paradoxically, we usually exclude the most knowledgeable clinician, the PI, from the monitoring process. In recognition of this paradox, Curt Meinert has challenged the notion that the PI must be kept blind to the emerging results (143). The fourth scenario describes a partial solution to this paradox in which the triggering of a statistical warning rule leads monitors to unblind the PI, not stop the trial.

Monitors' experience in the conduct and monitoring of RCTs must be sufficient for them to have previously confronted all the problems you envisage in your trial, especially in the consideration of early, unstable trends in efficacy and safety. Stopping an RCT early for an evanescent trend in efficacy or safety that subsequently would have disappeared is every trialist's nightmare.

Avoiding conflicts of interest (whether real or potential) among trial monitors is vital to both the validity and the credibility of your or anybody else's RCT. Some conflicts are obvious; others are subtle. Table 5–14 lists

TABLE 5-14   Real and Potential Conflicts of Interest for Monitors

Financial	Owns stock in the company that stands to gain from a positive trial of their product or process
	Owns stock in a competing company that stands to lose from a positive trial of the product or process
	Buys stock in the former company, or sells stock in the latter, based on unblinded data available only to monitors
	Is a paid consultant or honorarium-recipient of either company
	Receives research or educational grants, fellowship support, or free travel-accommodation from either company
	Receives payment beyond reimbursements for travel to, and accommodation at, monitoring meetings (Exception: income offsets required by some universities and governments, paid directly to them)
Professional	Career success is tied to applying the product or process
	Is (or will be) admitting patients to the RCT
	Is involved in running any part of the RCT
	Is a member of the regulatory agency that will approve/ disapprove the product or process
	Is a member of the funding agency whose prestige and budget will be affected by the outcome of the RCT
Academic	Already on record as certain about the efficacy and safety (good or bad) of the experimental treatment
	Would get credit for authorship of publications arising from the RCT

RCT, randomized control trial.

the ones the DAMOCLES gang and I could think of. Note that most of them apply as well to the authors of the letters, editorials, and guidelines that appear following the publication of the trial results.

The final entry in Table 5–14 stresses the "servant" role of monitors. They should seek neither fame nor publications for their efforts. They have to get all the satisfaction they need from working and learning behind the scenes, with nothing to show for it but an acknowledgement in small print at the end of a publication.

Even when monitors with conflicts of interest behave impeccably, their presence can detract from the credibility and acceptance of the trial result. Moreover, as described in the second scenario, their presence on a TMC can seriously impair its function. It was, in part, growing concern about these conflicts that has led to the organization and operation of TMCs like the one described in the fourth scenario.

✓ Recruit your monitor(s).

For small, short, simple trials (say, of the next advance in the short-term treatment of a common condition), you can recruit a single monitor who can carry out the functions you require. For larger, longer, more complex trials you can begin by recruiting a TMC chair, and then work together to select the other members. The chair must have prior experience in trials and trial monitoring, plus the interpersonal skills required to resolve differences of opinion within the committee. The TMCs I chair have six members, a number I find large enough both to provide the required range of expertise and to generate a quorum for our meetings and conference calls.

This recruitment process must include hammering out the policies and procedures for how the monitors will function and, crucially, how they will relate to you and your other investigators. The key issue here is whether they will act as advisors or executives. This distinction is best illustrated by how they behave when they conclude that the emerging results demonstrate efficacy, harm, or futility. An executive-style TMC would order the trial to stop. An advisory-style TMC would unblind the PI, show him or her the data, and collaborate with him or her and any others he or she chooses (such as the Steering Group) in deciding whether to stop or continue the trial.

By incorporating the PI's (and Steering Group's) greater clinical and biological expertise, the expanded, advisory-style TMC can intelligently examine the totality of evidence. The ultimate termination decision is left to the PI and Steering Group, and third party mediators are called in if the monitors disagree with them. Writing from experiences on both sides of the PI–monitor interface, I have found the advisory approach preferable from both perspectives. This advisory approach not only brings the most knowledgeable person (the PI) into the decision to stop the trial. It also renders the identification and solution of problems much more pleasant and productive when PIs and monitors work as collaborators, rather than as defendants and judges.

Another key policy decision to settle before the trial begins is how to monitor events that are both unanticipated and serious. In useful operational terms, events are designated "unanticipated" when they are not already specified in the trial protocol as determining the efficacy of the experimental treatment. These events are "serious" as well when their occurrence beyond chance would require unblinding the PI and changing the protocol or even stopping the trial.

It is vital that clinicians looking after trial patients identify and manage every "SUAE" as soon as it occurs. It is also vital that an unblinded monitor (who can combine this event with other, similar SUAEs) reviews this occurrence and determines whether it is happening at other centers with a combined frequency greater than chance. Thus, in the fourth scenario, the monitor is informed of any SUAE within 24 hours of its recognition.

✓ *Get on with it.*

Once the monitor(s) have been named, you should meet with them face-to-face for a detailed discussion of your protocol, how you will execute it, how they will protect study patients, and how they will help you achieve a result that is both valid and credible. This first meeting should also agree on the statistical warning rules and how everybody will act when they are triggered.

Subsequent monitors' meetings should be held when they can be most helpful to the trial. The second one could be held when patient recruitment is at a point where problems in accrual, eligibility, initial treatment, patient compliance, protocol adherence, data quality and timeliness, and the like can be identified and solutions suggested. Subsequent meetings might most sensibly be scheduled on the basis of study progression (such as when half the projected events have occurred, or when half of the projected follow-up has been reported) rather than on the passage of time (unless recruitment is lagging and the trial is bogging down).

Typical Agenda for a Monitoring Meeting

The agenda for the TMC meetings that follow the fourth scenario observe the following sequence:

1. A *"closed"* session among just the monitors, to identify concerns and other issues for discussion later in the meeting.
2. An *"open"* session with the blinded PI (perhaps accompanied by other members of the blinded Steering Group), the blinded Study Coordinator, and the unblinded Study Statistician(s). Patient accrual, data quality and timeliness, patient compliance and protocol adherence are usual topics, as well as any other issues raised by, and appropriate for discussion among blinded participants. Special attention is given to emerging results from external studies of the efficacy and safety of this or related treatments.
3. A *"semiclosed"* session between the monitors and the unblinded Study Statistician(s), to examine and discuss unblinded data on safety

and efficacy, and to determine the results of applying the statistical warning rules. This session often generates specific requests and recommendations that apply to just the Study Statisticians, and these are transmitted on the spot.

4. A *"closed"* session among just the monitors, to discuss all the foregoing and to generate appraisals and recommendations for the study statisticians, the PI, and the trial patients and staff.

5. A final *"open"* session with everyone, to present, explain, discuss and (if necessary) revise monitors' recommendations. The session closes with a decision on the timing and format (face-to-face or conference-call) for the next TMC meeting.

Following such a TMC meeting, its chair drafts two letters. The first is for general distribution to all the trial participants, makes comments on its (blinded) progress, offers praise where deserved, and concludes that it should continue as planned. The second is for the blinded PI and Steering Group, and includes recommendations about proposed protocol changes, recruitment, follow-up, and the quality and timing of field data. The PI decides whether to forward this second letter to the sponsors.

When the "semiclosed" session reveals that a statistical warning rule for safety, efficacy, or futility has been triggered, the "closed" session becomes a lengthy consideration of the totality of evidence for its completeness, consistency, sensibility, and coherence. If these criteria are met, the final "open" session unblinds the PI. At that point the PI assumes lead responsibility for deciding whether to stop the trial, involving Steering Group members and anyone else who could be helpful, and continuing to use the TMC as advisors.

If you have a question or comment about any of this chapter (or if you've caught us in a typo!) go to the book's Web site at *http://hiru. mcmaster.ca/CLEP3*. There you also will find comments from us and other readers, chapter updates, and examples of how the authors and others use the book in teaching.

REFERENCES

1. Antiplatelet Trialists' Collaboration. Secondary prevention of vascular disease by prolonged antiplatelet treatment. *BMJ* 1988;296:320–331.

2. Antithrombotic Trialists' Collaboration. Collaborative meta-analysis of randomised trials of antiplatelet therapy for prevention of death, myocardial infarction, and stroke in high risk patients. *BMJ* 2002;324:71–86.

3. Simon RN. An agenda for *Clinical Trials*: clinical trials in the genomic era. *Clin Trials* 2004;1:468–470.

4. Israel E, Chinchilli VM, Ford JG, et al., for the National Heart, Lung, and Blood Institute's Asthma Clinical Research Network. Use of regularly scheduled albuterol treatment in asthma: genotype-stratified, randomised, placebo-controlled cross-over trial. *Lancet* 2004;364:1505–1512.

5. Sackett DL, Gent M. Controversy in counting and attributing events in clinical trials.*N Engl J Med.* 1979;301:1410–1412.

6. Gent M, Blakely JA, Easton JD, et al. Canadian American Ticlopidine Study (CATS) in thromboembolic stroke. *Lancet* 1989;1:1215–1220.

7. Hass WK, Easton JD, Adams HP Jr, et al., Ticlopidine Aspirin Stroke Study Group. A randomized trial comparing ticlopidine hydrochloride with aspirin for the prevention of stroke in high-risk patients. *N Engl J Med* 1989;321:501–507.

8. Topol EJ. The GUSTO V Investigators. Reperfusion therapy for acute myocardial infarction with fibrinolytic therapy or combination reduced fibrinolytic therapy and platelet glycoprotein IIb/IIIa inhibition: the GUSTO V randomised trial. *Lancet* 2001; 357:1905–1914.

9. Altman DG. *Practical statistics for medical research*. London: Chapman & Hall, 1991:404–409.

10. Baigent C. The need for large-scale randomized evidence. *Br J Clin Pharmacol* 1997; 43:349–353.

11. Horton R. From star signs to trial guidelines. *Lancet* 2000;355:1033–1034.

12. Meinert CL. Data collection considerations; and data items and forms illustrations. *Clinical trials; design, conduct and analysis*. Oxford: Oxford University Press, 1986:119–137 and 379–416.

13. Pocock SJ. Forms and data management. *Clinical trials; a practical approach*. Chichester, UK: John Wiley & Sons, 1983:160–166.

14. Spilker B. Preparing data collection forms. *Guide to clinical trials*. Philadelphia, PA: J.B. Lippincott, 1991:262–271.

15. Kunz R, Vist G, Oxman AD. Randomisation to protect against selection bias in health care trials (Cochrane Review). *The Cochrane Library*, (Issue 3). Oxford: Update Software, 2002.

16. Braunholtz DA, Edwards SJL, Lilford RJ. Are randomized clinical trials good for us (in the short term)? Evidence for a "trial effect.". *J Clin Epidemiol* 2001;54:217–224.

17. Vist GE, Hagen KB, Devereaux PJ, et al. Outcomes of patients who participate in randomised controlled trials versus those of similar patients who do not participate (Protocol for a Cochrane Review). *The Cochrane Library*, (Issue 3). Oxford: Update Software, 2002.

18. Ferguson D, Aaron SD, Guyatt G, et al. Post-randomisation exclusions: the intention to treat principle and excluding patients from analysis. *BMJ* 2002;325:652–654.

19. Moher D, Schulz KF, Altman D, The CONSORT Group. The CONSORT statement: revised recommendations for improving the quality of reports of parallel-group randomized trials. *JAMA* 2001;285:1987–1991.

20. Schulz KF, Grimes DA. Allocation concealment in randomised trials: defending against deciphering. *Lancet* 2002;359:614–618.

21. Hallstrom AP, Paradis NA. Pre-randomization and de-randomization in emergency medical research: new names and rigorous criteria for old methods. *Resuscitation* Resuscitation. 2005;65:65–69.

22. Schulz KF, Chalmers I, Grimes DA, et al. Assessing the quality of randomization from reports of controlled trials published in obstetrics and gynecology journals. *JAMA* 1994;13:125–128.

23. The University Group Diabetes Program. A study of the effects of hypoglycemic agents on vascular complications in patients with adult-onset diabetes: II. Mortality results. *Diabetes* 1970;19:785–830.

24. Seltzer H. A summary of criticisms of the findings and conclusions of the University Group Diabetes Program. *Diabetes* 1972;21:976–979.

25. Cornfield J, The University Group Diabetes Program. A further statistical analysis of the mortality findings. *JAMA*. 1971;217:1676–1687.

26. Taves DR. Minimization: a new method of assigning patients to treatment and control groups. *Clin Pharmacol Ther* 1974;15:443–453.

27. Haynes RB, Sackett DL, Gibson ES, et al. Improvement of medication compliance in uncontrolled hypertension. *Lancet* 1976;1:1265–1268.

28. Schulz KF, Grimes DA. Generation of allocation sequences in randomized trials: chance, not choice. *Lancet* 2002;359:515–519.

29. Treasure T, MacRae KD. Minimization: the platinum standard for trials? *BMJ* 1998;317: 362–363.

30. Peto R. Clinical trial methodology. *Biomedicine* Special Issue 1978;28:24–36.

31. Devereaux PJ, Manns BJ, Ghali WA, et al. Physician interpretations and textbook definitions of blinding terminology in randomized controlled trials. *JAMA* 2001;285:2000–2003.

32. Moseley JB, O'Malley K, Petersen NJ, et al. A controlled trial of arthroscopic surgery for osteoarthritis of the knee. *N Engl J Med* 2002;347:81–88.

33. Horng S, Miller FG. Is placebo surgery unethical? *N Engl J Med* 2002;347:137–139.

34. Manandhar DS, Orsin D, Shrestha BP et al, MIRA Makwanpur trial team. Effect of a participatory intervention with women's groups on birth outcomes in Nepal: cluster-randomised controlled trial. *Lancet* 2004;364:970–979.

35. The Complications of Age-Related Macular Degeneration Prevention Trial Study Group. The Complications of Age-Related Macular Degeneration Prevention Trial (CAPT): rationale, design and methodology. *Clin Trials* 2004;1:91–107.

36. Meinert CL. Sequential versus fixed sample size designs. *Clinical trials; design, conduct and analysis.* Oxford: Oxford University Press, 1986:72–74.

37. Friedman LM, Furberg CD, DeMets DL. *Fundamentals of clinical trials*, 3rd ed. Berlin: Springer-Verlag, 1998:72–73.

38. Sackett DL. Why randomized controlled trials fail but needn't: 2. Failure to employ physiological statistics, or the only formula a clinical trialist is ever likely to need (or understand!). *CMAJ* 2001;165:1226–1237.

39. Kahn KS, Daya S, Colins JA, et al. Empirical evidence of bias in infertility research: overestimation of treatment effect in crossover trials using pregnancy as the outcome measure. *Fertil Steril* 1996;65:939–945.

40. Pocock SJ. *Clinical trials; a practical approach.* Chichester, UK: John Wiley & Sons, 1983:110–122.

41. Zelen M. A new design for randomized clinical trials. *N Engl J Med* 1979;300:1242–1245.

42. Ellenberg SS. Randomization designs in comparative clinical trials. *N Engl J Med* 1984; 310:1404–1408.

43. The EC/IC Bypass Study Group. Failure of extracranial-intracranial arterial bypass to reduce the risk of ischemic stroke: results of a randomized trial. *N Engl J Med* 1985;313: 1191–1200.

44. Moseley JB, O'Malley K, Petersen NJ, et al. A controlled trial of arthroscopic surgery for osteoarthritis of the knee. *N Engl J Med* 2002;347:81–88.

45. Goldstein AJ, de Beurs E, Chambless DL, et al. EMDR for panic disorder with agoraphobia: comparison with waiting list and credible attention-placebo control conditions. *J Consult Clin Psychol* 2000;68:947–956.

46. Hull RD, Raskob GE, Hirsh J, et al. Continuous intravenous heparin compared with intermittent subcutaneous heparin in the initial treatment of proximal-vein thrombosis. *N Engl J Med* 1986;315:1109–1114.

47. Sackett DL. Turning a blind eye: Why we don't test for blindness at the end of our trials. *BMJ* 2004;328:1136–113a. May

48. Veterans Administration Cooperative Study Group on Antihypertensive Agents. I. Results in patients with diastolic blood pressures averaging 115 through 129 mm Hg. *JAMA* 1967;202:1028–1034.

49. Haynes RB, Taylor DW, Sackett DL, eds. *Compliance in health care.* Baltimore, MD: The Johns Hopkins University Press, 1979.

50. Haynes RB, McDonald H, Garg AX, et al. Interventions for helping patients to follow prescriptions for medications (Cochrane Review). In: *The Cochrane Library*, (Issue 3). Oxford: Update Software; 2002.

51. Thomson O'Brien MA, Oxman AD, Davis DA, et al. Audit and feedback versus alternative strategies: effects on professional practice and health care outcomes (Cochrane Review). In: *The Cochrane Library*, (Issue 3). Oxford: Update Software; 2002.

52. Thomson O'Brien MA, Freemantle N, Oxman AD, et al. Continuing education meetings and workshops: effects on professional practice and health care outcomes (Cochrane Review). In: *The Cochrane Library*, (Issue 3). Oxford: Update Software; 2002.

53. Thomson O'Brien MA, Oxman AD, Davis DA, et al. Educational outreach visits: effects on professional practice and health care outcomes (Cochrane Review). In: *The Cochrane Library*, (Issue 3). Oxford: Update Software; 2002.

54. Hayden GF. Alliteration in medicine: a puzzling profusion of p's. *BMJ* 1999;319:1605–1608.

55. Yusuf S, Sleight P, Pogue J et al., The Heart Outcomes Prevention Evaluation Study Investigators. Effects of an angiotensin-converting-enzyme inhibitor, ramipril, on cardiovascular events in high-risk patients. *N Engl J Med* 2000;342:145–153.

56. Freemantle N, Calvert M, Wood J, et al. Composite outcomes in randomized trials: greater precision but with greater uncertainty? *JAMA* 2003;289:2554–2559.

57. Hughes MD, Society for Clinical Trials. Experience with the validation of surrogate endpoints in HIV. New Orleans, LA, May 2004.

58. Currie GP, Lee DK, Haggart K, et al. Effects of montelukast on surrogate inflammatory markers in corticosteroid-treated patients with asthma. *Am J Respir Crit Care Med* 2003;167:1232–1238

59. Guyatt GH, Cranney A, Griffith L, et al. Summary of meta-analyses of therapies for postmenopausal osteoporosis and the relationship between bone density and fractures. *Endocrinol Metab Clin North Am.* 2002;31:659–680.

60. D'Agostino RB. Debate: The slippery slope of surrogate outcomes. *Curr Control Trials Cardiovasc Med* 2000;1:76–78.

61. DeGruttola VG, Clax PC, DeMets DL, et al. Considerations in the evaluation of surrogate endpoints in clinical trials: summary of a National Institutes of Health workshop. *Control Clin Trials* 2001;22:485–502.

62. Bucher H, Guyatt G, Cook D, et al. Therapy and applying the results. Surrogate outcomes. In: Guyatt G, Rennie D, eds. *Users' guides to the medical literature.* Chicago, IL: AMA Press, 2002.

63. Lasser KE, Allen PD, Woolhandler SJ, et al. Timing of new black box warnings and withdrawals for prescription medications. *JAMA* 2002;287:2215–2220.

64. Sackett DL, Haynes RB, Gent M. Compliance. In: Inman WHW, ed. *Monitoring for drug safety*, Lancaster, CA: MTP Press, 1980.

65. Hull RD, Raskob GE, Hirsh J, et al. Continuous intravenous heparin compared with intermittent subcutaneous heparin in the initial treatment of proximal-vein thrombosis. *N Engl J Med* 1986;315:1109–1114.

66. The Heart Outcomes Prevention Evaluation Study Investigators. Effects of an angiotensin-converting-enzyme inhibitor, ramipril, on cardiovascular events in high-risk patients. *N Engl J Med* 2000;342:145–153.

67. Myers MG, Cairns JA, Singer J. The consent form as a possible cause of side effects. *Clin Pharmacol Ther* 1987;42:250–253.

68. Cairns JA, Gent M, Singer J, et al. Aspirin, sulfinpyrazone, or both in unstable angina. Results of a Canadian multicenter trial. *N Engl J Med.* 1985;313:1369–1375.

69. Peto R, Pike MC, Armitage P, et al. Design and analysis of randomized clinical trials requiring prolonged observation of each patient. *Br J Cancer* 1976;34:585–612, and 1977;35:1–39.

70. Altman DG. *Practical statistics for medical research.* London: Chapman & Hall, 1991:461.

71. Pocock SJ, Assmann SE, Enos LE, et al. Subgroup analysis, covariate adjustment and baseline comparisons in clinical trial reporting: current practice and problems. *Stat Med* 2002;21:2917–2930.

72. Haynes RB, Taylor DW, Sackett DL, et al. North American Symptomatic Carotid Endarterectomy Trial Collaborators. Prevention of functional impairment by endarterectomy for symptomatic high-grade carotid stenosis. *JAMA* 1994;271:1256–1259.

73. O'Brien JR, Etherington MD. How much aspirin? *Thromb Haemost* 1990;64:486.

74. Taylor DW, Barnett HJM, Haynes RB et al, ASA and Carotid Endarterectomy (ACE) Trial Collaborators. Low-dose and high-dose acetylsalicylic acid for patients undergoing carotid endarterectomy: a randomised controlled trial. *Lancet* 1999;353:2179–2184.

75. Sackett DL, Haynes RB, Guyatt GH, et al. *Clinical epidemiology*, 2nd ed. Boston, MA: Little, Brown and Company, 1991:13.

76. Altman DG. *Practical statistics for medical research*. London: Chapman & Hall, 1991.

77. Kaplan EL, Meier P. Nonparametric estimation from incomplete observations. *JASA* 1958;53:457–481.

78. Donner A, Klar N. *Design and analysis of cluster randomized trials in health research*. London: Arnold, 2000.

79. Bailar L. Hormone-replacement therapy and cardiovascular diseases. *N Engl J Med* 2003;349:521–522.

80. James W. *What pragmatism means. Pragmatism: a new name for some old ways of thinking*. New York: Longman Green and Company 1907:17–32.

81. Schmid CH, Lau J, McIntosh MW, et al. An empirical study of the effect of the control rate as a predictor of treatment efficacy in meta-analysis of clinical trials. *Stat Med* 1998;17:1923–1942.

82. Furukawa TA, Guyatt GH, Griffith LE. Can we individualize the 'number needed to treat'? An empirical study of summary effect measures in meta-analyses. *Int J Epidemiol* 2002;31:72–76.

83. McAlister FA, Straus SE, Guyatt GH, et al. Evidence-Based Medicine Working Group. Users' guides to the medical literature: XX. Integrating research evidence with the care of the individual patient. *JAMA* 2000;283:2829–2836.

84. Cook RJ, Sackett DL. The number needed to treat: a clinically useful measure of treatment effect. *BMJ* 1995;310:452–454.

85. Haybittle JL. Repeated assessment of results in clinical trials of cancer treatment. *Br J Radiol* 1971;44:793–797.

86. Meinert CL. *Clinical trials, design, conduct, and analysis*. New York: Oxford University Press, 1986:215–216.

87. Bosch J, Yusuf S, Pogue J, et al. On behalf of the HOPE Investigators. Use of ramipril in preventing stroke: double blind randomised trial. *BMJ* 2002;324:1–5.

88. P Badrinath, AP Wakeman, JG Wakeman Preventing stroke with ramipril (Letter). *BMJ* 2002;325:439.

89. Yusuf S, Bosch J, Sleight P. Responding to issues raised (Electronic letter). *BMJ* 2003;326:52

90. Bucher HC, Weinbacher M, Gyr K. Influence of method of reporting study results on decision of physicians to prescribe drugs to lower cholesterol concentration. *BMJ* 1994; 309:761–764.

91. Fahey T, Griffiths S, Peters TJ. Evidence based purchasing: understanding results of clinical trials and systematic reviews. *BMJ* 1995;311:1056–1059.

92. Pocock SJ, Hughes MD, Lee RJ. Statistical problems in the reporting of clinical trials. A survey of three medical journals. *N Engl J Med* 1987;317:426–432.

93. Oxman AD, Guyatt GH. A consumer's guide to subgroup analyses. *Ann Intern Med* 1992;116:78–84.

94. Freiman JA, Chalmers TC, Smith H Jr, et al. The importance of beta, the type II error and sample size in the design and interpretation of the randomized control trial. Survey of 71 "negative" trials. *N Engl J Med* 1978;299:690–694.

95. Moher D, Dulberg CS, Wells GA. Statistical power, sample size, and their reporting in randomized controlled trials. *JAMA* 1994;272:122–124.

96. Detsky AS, Sackett DL. When was a "negative" clinical trial big enough? How many patients you needed depends on what you found. *Arch Intern Med* 1985;145:709–712.

97. Chalmers I. Proposal to outlaw the term 'negative trial.' *BMJ* 1985;290:1002.

98. Chan AW, Krleza-Jeric K, Schmid I, et al. Outcome reporting bias in randomized trials funded by the Canadian Institutes of Health Research. *CMAJ* 2004;171:735–740.

99. Roberts R, Hoey J. An amnesty for unpublished trials. CMAJ 1997;157:1548. Medical Editors Trial Amnesty. Fax: 0171-383-6418. *BMJ*, BMA House, Tavistock Square, London WC1H 9JR., UK or send by e-mail to: *Meta@ucl.ac.uk*

100. Clarke M, Alderson P, Chalmers I. Dis sections in reports of controlled trials published in general medical journals. *JAMA* 2002;287:2799–2801.

101. McAlister FA, Straus SE, Sackett DL, et al. Analysis and reporting of factorial trials: a systematic review. *JAMA* 2003;289(19):2545–2553.

102. Guyatt GH, Juniper EF, Walter SD, et al. Interpreting treatment effects in randomised trials. *BMJ* 1998;316:690–693.

103. Friedman LM, Furberg CD, DeMets DL. *Fundamentals of clinical trials*, 3rd ed. New York: Springer-Verlag, 1998:120 ff.

104. Klar N, Donner A. Current and future challenges in the design and analysis of cluster randomization trials. *Stat Med* 2001;20:3729–3740.

105. Friedman LM, Furberg CD, DeMets DL. *Fundamentals of clinical trials*, 3rd ed. New York: Springer-Verlag, 1998:112 ff.

106. Ross S, Grant A, Counsell C, et al. Barriers to participation in randomised controlled trials: a systematic review. *J Clin Epidemiol* 1999;52:1143–1156.

107. Mapstone J, Elbourne D, Roberts I. Strategies to improve recruitment to research studies (Cochrane Review). In: *The Cochrane Library*, (Issue 1). Chichester, UK: John Wiley & Sons, 2004.

108. Sackett DL. Why randomized controlled trials fail but needn't: 1. Failure to gain "coalface" commitment and to use the uncertainty principle. *CMAJ* 2000;162:1311–1314.

109. The EC/IC Bypass Study Group. The international cooperative study of extracranial/intracranial arterial anastomosis (EC/IC Bypass Study): methodology and entry characteristics. *Stroke* 1985;16:397–406.

110. Wootton R, Bloomer SE, Corbett R, et al. Multicentre randomised control trial comparing real time teledermatology with conventional outpatient dermatological care: societal cost-benefit analysis. *BMJ* 2000;320:1252–1256.

111. Thomson O'Brien MA, Oxman AD, Haynes RB, et al. Local opinion leaders: effects on professional practice and health care outcomes (Cochrane Review). In: *The Cochrane Library*, (Issue 1). Oxford: Update Software, 2001.

112. Warlow C. Clinical research under the cosh again. This time it is ethics committees *BMJ* 2004;329:241–242.

113. Rothman KJ. The continuing unethical use of placebo controls. *N Engl J Med* 1994; 331:394–398. (plus the subsequent correspondence and rebuttals)

114. Angell M. Investigators' responsibilities for human subjects in developing countries. *N Engl J Med* 2000;342:967–969. (plus the subsequent correspondence and rebuttals)

115. Lo B, Bayer R, The Ethics Working Group of the HIV Prevention Trials Network. Establishing ethical trials for treatment and prevention of AIDS in developing countries. *BMJ* 2003;327:337–339.

116. Bhutta Z. Standards of care in research: should reflect local conditions and not the best western standards. *BMJ* 2004;329:1114–1115.

117. Braunholtz DA, Edwards SJL, Lilford RJ. Are randomized clinical trials good for us (in the short term)? Evidence for a "trial effect.". *J Clin Epid* 2001;54:217–224.

118. Vist GE, Hagen KB, Devereaux PJ, et al. Outcomes of patients who participate in randomised controlled trials versus those of similar patients who do not participate (Protocol for a Cochrane Review). In: *The Cochrane Library*, (Issue 2). Oxford: Update Software, 2003.

119. Di Blasi Z, Kaptchuk TJ, Weinman J, et al. Informing participants of allocation to placebo at trial closure: postal survey. *BMJ* 2002;325:1329–1331.

120. Marnocha RM. Clinical research: business opportunities for pharmacy-based investigational drug services. *Am J Health Syst Pharm* 1999;56:249–252.

121. Canadian Medical Association Policy. Physicians and the pharmaceutical industry (Update 2001). *CMAJ* 2001;164:1339–1341.

122. Bodenheimer T. Uneasy alliance—clinical investigators and the pharmaceutical industry. *N Engl J Med* 2000;342:1539–1544.

123. Davidoff F, DeAngelis C, Drazen JM, et al. Sponsorship, authorship, and accountability. *Lancet* 2001;358:854–856.

124. Angelini G, Taylor FC, Reeves BC, et al. Early and midterm outcome after off-pump and on-pump surgery in beating heart against cardioplegic arrest studies (BHACAS 1 and 2): a pooled analysis of two randomised controlled trials. *Lancet* 2002;359:1194–1199.

125. Waksman R, Raizner AE, Yeung AC, et al. The INHIBIT investigators. Use of localized intracoronary ß radiation in treatment of in-stent restenosis: the INHIBIT randomised controlled trial. *Lancet* 2002;359:551–557.

126. Sackett D, Sackett B. A survey of the credibility of identical trial results when generated by independent investigators or by drug manufacturers. *Society for clinical trials annual meeting* 2004.

127. Lievre M, Menard J, Brucket E, et al. Premature discontinuation of clinical trial for reasons not related to efficacy, safety, or feasibility. *BMJ* 2001;322:603–606.

128. Black HR, Elliott WJ, Grandits G et al, The CONVINCE Research Group. Principal results of the controlled onset verapamil investigation of cardiovascular end points (CONVINCE) trial. *JAMA* 2003;289:2073–2082.

129. Psaty BM, Rennie D. Stopping medical research to save money. A broken pact with researchers and patients. *JAMA* 2003;289:2128–2131.

130. Hopewell S, Clarke M, Stewart L, et al. Time to publication for results of clinical trials (Cochrane Review). In: *The Cochrane Library*, (Issue 2). Oxford: Update Software, 2003.

131. Scherer RW, Langenberg P. Full publication of results initially presented in abstracts (Cochrane Review). In: *The Cochrane Library*, (Issue 2). Oxford: Update Software; 2003.

132. Chalmers I. All unbiased comparative studies should be published. *BMJ* 2002;324:483.

133. Flanigin A, Carey LA, Fontanarosa PB, et al. Prevalence of articles with honorary authors and ghost authors in peer-reviewed medical journals. *JAMA* 1998;280:222–224.

134. Arlen H, Mercer J. "Ac-Cent-Tchu-Ate the Positive." Circa 1945. *http://www.leoslyrics.com/listlyrics.php?id=8492*

135. Larkin M. Whose article is it anyway? *Lancet* 1999;354:136.

136. Sackett DL, Oxman AD. HARLOT plc: an amalgamation of the world's two oldest professions. *BMJ* 2003;327:1442–1445.

137. Lenzer J. Alteplase for stroke: money and optimistic claims buttress the "brain attack" campaign. *BMJ* 2002;324:723–729. (The rapid electronic responses make for lively reading!)

138. Choudhry NK, Stelfox HT, Detsky AS. Relationships between authors of clinical practice guidelines and the pharmaceutical industry. *JAMA* 2002;287:612–617.

139. Topol EJ, Armstrong P, Van de Werf F et al, Global Utilization of Streptokinase and Tissue Plasminogen Activator for Occluded Coronary Arteries (GUSTO) Steering Committee. Confronting the issues of patient safety and investigator conflict of interest in an international clinical trial of myocardial reperfusion. *J Am Coll Cardiol* 1992;19:1123–1128.

140. Ellenberg SS. Independent data monitoring committees: rationale, operations and controversies. *Stat Med* 2001;20:2573–2583.

141. Ellenberg SS, Fleming TR, DeMets DL. *Data monitoring committees in clinical trials: A practical perspective*. Chichester, UK: John Wiley & Sons, 2003.

142. Grant AM, Altman DG, Babiker AB, Campbell MK, Clemens FJ, Darbyshire JH, Elbourne DR, McLeer SK, Parmar MK, Pocock SJ, Spiegelhalter DJ, Sydes MR, Walker AE, Wallace SA; and the DAMOCLES study group. Issues in data monitoring and interim analysis of trials. Health Technol Assess. 2005;9:1–238.

143. Meinert CL. Masked monitoring in clinical trials – blind stupidity? *N Engl J Med* 1998; 338:1381–1382.

THE PRINCIPLES BEHIND THE TACTICS OF PERFORMING THERAPEUTIC TRIALS

Dave Sackett

Chapter Outline

6.1 CONFOUNDING, AND HOW TO BREAK IT

Show Me the Money!

One day I made a site-visit to a group of clinicians who had applied for funds to start a post–myocardial infarction (post-MI) exercise program. I asked them to justify their request. They described a cohort study in which they had enrolled and followed two cohorts of MI survivors. One cohort had engaged in regular exercise after their myocardial infarctions, and the other cohort had remained sedentary. Their outcomes were as shown in Table 6–1.

What do you think? Did these clinicians have a convincing case for getting the money?

I asked them whether they had included patients with hypertension or effort-induced angina in their study. Pause for a moment, and see if you can figure out why this question was important.

TABLE 6–1 Exercise and Mortality After a Heart Attack

	Dead within 5 Y
Exercised after their MI	4%
Sedentary (did not exercise) after their MI	12%

MI, myocardial infarction.
Fisher exact probability for this (or an even greater) difference in death rates <0.05.

I thought it was important because of three attributes of hypertension and angina in MI survivors:

- These patient attributes were *extraneous to the question posed* (which was: "Among patients who have survived an MI, does exercise reduce mortality over the next 2 years?")
- They were *determinants of the outcome* (death).
- They were almost certainly *unequally distributed between the comparison groups.* Patients with effort-induced angina couldn't exercise for long, and clinicians caring for patients with hypertension often advised them against vigorous exercise. As a result, the nonexercising cohort would have lots of patients with these potentially lethal complications, and the exercising cohort would have just a few of them. Their hypothetical distribution is shown in Table 6–2.

Even if exercise were worthless for post-MI patients, the imbalance in these extraneous determinants of death would make it look beneficial. The shorthand term for attributes with these three properties is *confounder.* The trouble with confounders is that they can lead to *biased* conclusions that an intervention is beneficial when it is not. Thus, confounders prevent us from executing a "fair test" of the effects of an intervention.

You Can Carry Out "Fair Tests" of Benefit by "Breaking" Confounding

As it happens, there are eight strategies for overcoming confounding of this sort. I'll come back to several of them in detail later in this chapter. Thinking your way through them now will give you a nice review of the shortcomings of observational research as a means of determining treatment benefit. It also will make the later bits of this chapter easier to understand. All of these

TABLE 6–2   Potentially Lethal Post–myocardial Infarction Complications in the Two Cohorts

	Types of Patients	
Exercised after their MI (label them E)	Lots at normal risk	E-1
	Very few at high risk	E-2
Sedentary after their MI (label them S)	Some at normal risk	S-1
	Very many at high risk	S-2

MI, myocardial infarction.

strategies tackle the "unequal distribution" property of confounders. In brief, these strategies are:

1. *Exclusion:* We can exclude patients with hypertension or effort-induced angina from both groups (setting their frequency at zero in both groups).

2. *Stratified sampling:* As we pick patients for our study, we can restrict or reduce the number of sedentary patients with confounders (S-2) until their number is equal to the number of exercising patients with these same confounders (E-2).

3. *Pair-wise matching:* We can enter patients in pairs, one exercising, and one sedentary, making sure they are similar ("matched") for the presence or absence of the confounders.

4. *Stratified analysis:* We can permit the unequal distribution shown in Table 6–2 to occur, but then perform two analyses, stratified for the confounder. That is, we can compare death rates between E-1 and S-1 separately from our comparison of death rates between E-2 and S-2.

5. *Standardization or Adjustment:* We can apply the death rates we generated in each of our four strata (E-1, E-2, S-1, and S-2) to the same "standard" theoretical population. This standard population is created so that the frequency of the confounder is identical between exercising and sedentary patients. Applying the rates for exercising and sedentary patients to this standard population will generate a single pair of "adjusted" death rates.

6. *Multivariate Modeling:* We can extend our adjustment for hypertension and angina to any other real or potential confounders we desire. In our example, these could include unstable ventricular rhythms, heart failure, social class, and so on. Once again, we generate a single set of rates. The most popular current method for doing this is the Cox "proportional hazards model" (1). (Don't try it at home; this is why I told you to get yourself a statistician co-principal investigator back in Table 4–2.)

7. *Randomization:* We can take all the patients who are capable of exercising and assign each of them to either an exercise or sedentary program by the "casting of lots" (2). We could cast lots in the time-honored versions of a coin-toss or a roll of the dice, or we could employ their modern-day equivalent, a formal "random allocation system." This casting of lots has an advantage overall the other methods of breaking confounding: randomization renders the exercising and sedentary groups equivalent, on average, for unknown as well as known confounders. Indeed, as described in Section 5.4 ("Allocation of Patients to Treatments"), we could even start by stratifying for the presence or absence of known confounders and then randomize separately from each stratum.

8. *Minimization:* This more recently introduced method identifies all potential confounders and assigns them 1 point each. Thus, a patient with neither hypertension nor angina has a score of 0, a patient with only hypertension has a score of 1, and a patient with both hypertension and angina has a score of 2. A minimization strategy randomizes the first patient. It then assigns each subsequent patient to whichever group will minimize the difference in the total scores between the groups (randomizing again only when the running totals are equal). Randomization and minimization are described in detail in Section 5.4 ("Allocation of Patients to Treatments").

What Happened to the Exercise Program?

To finish my story, I recommended that this group receive a large amount of money, not for an exercise program but for a randomized controlled trial (RCT) to see whether it was effective. They got the money and started the trial. Alas, half of their patients dropped out and their result was indeterminate.

Reprise: Can't We Use the First Six Confounding-breaking Strategies to Avoid the Effort Required for a Randomized Controlled Trial?

If we apply the foregoing strategies 1 to 6, mightn't a high-quality cohort study be as good as, or even better than, an RCT for determining treatment benefit? Some methodologists have vigorously adopted this view (3). I disagree with them, for two reasons. First, there are abundant examples of the harm done when clinicians treat patients on the basis of cohort studies. Two recent examples of cohort-based treatment recommendations that failed in RCTs are postmenopausal estrogen plus progestin for healthy women (4) and vitamin E for coronary heart disease (5). (Note: my argument here does not apply to determining treatment harm, where observational studies are often the only way to detect a treatment's rare but awful adverse effects.)

My second justification is an unprovable act of faith. It professes that the gold standard for determining the effectiveness of any health intervention is a high-quality systematic review of all relevant, high-quality RCTs. When the other study architectures are measured against this gold standard, they have generated less reliable estimates of effectiveness. For example, Regina Kunz and her colleagues performed a Cochrane Review of randomization as a protection against selection bias in health care trials (6). They frequently found a worse prognosis at entry among control patients in nonrandomized studies. Moreover, they documented the overestimation of treatment effects when the randomization schedule was not concealed from the clinicians who were inviting patients to join RCTs, converting these "RCTs" into cohort studies.

Surprise!

Now for a surprise (for some of you at least). Why do you suppose Bradford Hill used randomization to assign tuberculosis patients to receive either bed rest plus streptomycin or bed rest alone in the trial that opened the modern era of RCTs (7)? As it happens, the ability of randomization to balance potential confounders between the streptomycin and control groups was of only secondary importance (8)! Bradford Hill randomized these patients in order to *conceal* the treatment allocation of the next eligible patient from the clinician who was determining that patient's eligibility for the trial. As you saw in the preceding paragraphs on confounding, there are lots of other, sometimes better, ways than randomization to equalize (and thereby eliminate bias from) known confounders.

If this surprise makes you want to know a tiny bit more of the history of RCTs, continue on to the next section.

6.2 A TINY BIT OF HISTORY

This tiny bit of history is not intended to bore you with irrelevant tales from the past. Rather, I want to show you that yesteryear's "experts," just like today's, had a powerful tool at hand for finding out whether their expert opinions were correct. Accordingly, they deserve as much criticism as today's "experts" for failing to use a tool that could have shown everyone whether their therapeutic pronouncements were worthy, worthless, or harmful (9).

Casting Lots to Achieve Fair Tests of Treatment Effects Has Been Around for Centuries

In the description of randomization, you learned that the simple "casting lots" by a coin-toss or roll of the dice creates comparable groups of patients for therapeutic trials. If you go to the Web site for the James Lind Library (*http://www.jameslindlibrary.org/*), you'll discover that this strategy for avoiding confounding has been in use for centuries.

Venesection

In 1662, about a hundred years *before* the famous American physician (and signer of the Declaration of Independence) Benjamin Rush was pontificating on the benefits of venesection, Jean-Baptiste van Helmont issued a challenge to "experts" like him: "Let us take out of the Hospitals ... 200 or 500 poor People, that have Fevers, Pleurisies. Let us divide them into Halfes, let us *cast lots*, that one half of them may fall to my share, and the other to yours; I will cure them without bloodletting and sensible evacuation; but you do, as ye know ... We shall see how many Funerals both of us shall have" (10).

All that Benjamin Rush lost by not carrying out a fair test of the effects of venesection was a small portion of his posthumous reputation. But generations of patients paid with their lives for his expert advice. It was, after all, one of Benjamin Rush's disciples who, when asked to consult on George Washington's epiglottitis, killed him by completing the venesection of 5.5 pints of his blood in less than 12 hours (11).

In 1816, after centuries of its use, but only 17 years after it killed George Washington, venesection was finally subjected to a fair test of its effectiveness (12). Alexander Lesassier Hamilton and two of his army surgical colleagues admitted 366 sick soldiers to each of them in turn ("by lot"). One surgeon employed routine venesection, but the other two never applied "the lancet." The patients treated with venesection were *ten times* more likely to die following treatment. The fact that so harmful a treatment was applied by so many generations of intelligent, observant physicians is breathtaking. But I hope it also warns you how uncontrolled observations of treatment effects can mislead even you, even today.

Belladonna

Shortly after George Washington's death-by-venesection, another "expert" pontificated that belladonna (atropine) could prevent scarlet fever. This time it was Dr. Samuel Hahnemann, the father of homeopathy. Such was his prestige that his "divine remedy as a preservative" had been adopted subsequently by allopaths as well as homeopaths.

In 1854, about 50 years after Dr. Hahnemann delivered his belladonna "guideline," a scarlet fever epidemic broke out in an orphan's home at

Chelsea, United Kingdom. Thomas Graham Balfour (then a surgeon at the orphan's home but later the President of the Royal Statistical Society) carried out a fair test of belladonna as a preventive by "casting lots" (13). He withheld or gave belladonna to alternate orphans in order, as he later reported, "to prevent the imputation of selection." Belladonna failed to protect against scarlet fever. Brilliantly, Thomas Balfour went on to state "but the observation is good, because it shows how apt we are to be misled by imperfect observation. Had I given the remedy to all the boys, I should probably have attributed to *it* the cessation of the epidemic."

Are Today's Experts Any Smarter?

At this point I'll bet that some of you are sighing with relief that the "foolish" experts of yesteryear have been replaced by "real" experts today. If so, you'd better find out what today's experts were saying before and even during the Women's Health Initiative (WHI) trial of estrogen plus progestin for healthy postmenopausal women and the Corticosteroid Randomisation after Significant Head Injury (CRASH) trial of steroids for head injury. As long as even our most brilliant clinicians fail to apply some remarkably simple ways for finding the truth, they will continue to say some breathtakingly dumb things. Worse, patients will continue to pay with their lives for expert pronouncements on untested treatments.

For a Cornucopia of Historic Trials

I hope this brief side-trip into medical history has whetted your appetite for more of it. If so, visit the brilliant contents of The James Lind Library at *http://www.jameslindlibrary.org/*.

6.3 PHASE I–IV TRIALS

In case you've forgotten the scenario that opened Chapter 4, here is a thumbnail of it again:

> In 1969, two methodologists met with a senior neurologist and a basic scientist ...
> We met because we shared the idea that drugs that affect platelet function in the laboratory (aspirin and sulfinpyrazone) might be beneficial to patients with transient ischemic attacks. Could we design and execute a study that would determine whether the drugs that worked so well at the bench, on blood platelets, did more good than harm in the clinic, to patients with transient ischemic attacks?

As you probably already know, a new drug never jumps directly from its first synthesis in a test tube to a definitive RCT in sick patients. Drug developers and trialists have created a nomenclature to describe the orderly series of studies that intervene. If you consider it useful to understand the nature and names of these intervening phases, read on.

Pre-phase I

A compound with interesting molecular structure not only might reap billions of dollars for its creator, but also might kill or otherwise seriously harm the humans who take it and bankrupt its manufacturer. Similarly, a new operation might make its inventor famous, but might also do terrible damage to patients. Most humans prefer to learn this bad news from studies on somebody else. Accordingly, we begin the evaluation of therapeutic innovations with extensive testing in laboratory animals.

For new drugs, these *animal studies* look at four things. First, we quantify the time course of the candidate drug's distribution in various tissues and organs (pharmacokinetics). Second, we determine its effects on the structure and function of cells, tissues, organs, and organ systems (pharmacodynamics). Third, we find out the substances into which it is metabolized, their effects, and their mechanisms of excretion. Fourth, we give it in ever-increasing doses until it kills half the animals that receive it (the so-called lethal dose for 50% of the experimental animals or LD_{50}). We examine the half that die at once. The survivors are killed at various intervals thereafter and examined. If the compound's ultimate human targets include pregnant or nursing mothers, we administer it to their counterparts in other species, and both these recipients and their offspring are studied for birth defects and infant growth and development.

If the drug's LD_{50} is comfortably above the dose required for the desired pharmacodynamic effect, if its other attributes are favorable, and if it looks affordable and/or profitable, we might select it for further study, this time in humans.

Phase I Trials

First, we give tiny doses of the compound to a handful (perhaps a dozen) "volunteers" (usually paid) to see if humans display the same pharmacokinetics, metabolic fate, and freedom from toxicity as their animal cousins. If so, we then give it in increasing amounts to "appropriate" persons until the pharmacodynamic effects found among laboratory animals are replicated in humans. Healthy volunteers may still be appropriate, but we usually test drugs with serious side effects on seriously ill patients who have failed to respond to currently established therapy. We closely monitor these participants for intended and unintended effects through frequent clinical examinations, large batteries of lab tests, and so on. The name we give to this sort of investigation is "Phase I Trial." I hope you noted that it is not randomized.

Phase II Trials

If the compound still looks promising after Phase I testing, we administer it to two or three dozen patients who have the target disorder that the compound is designed to benefit. Our objectives here are four: first, to set and confirm the dose necessary for the desired pharmacodynamic effect; second, to estimate the proportion of patients who do (responders) and

don't (nonresponders) display this desired effect: third, to confirm the results of the previous pharmacokinetic and metabolic studies: and fourth,
to continue our look for toxicity. The shorthand term for this sort of investigation is "Phase II Trial." We can employ several different designs in
Phase II, ranging from case-series to parallel or crossover RCTs.

Phase II trials are extremely unlikely to provide convincing evidence
for efficacy (unless the compound saves lives in a previously universally
fatal condition). Even if the compound looks good in a Phase II trial, the
confidence interval around its effect will usually be huge and will include
harm and uselessness, as well as benefit.

Phase II "Futility" Trials

The real and opportunity costs of taking a promising Phase II drug into a
full-scale Phase III efficacy or effectiveness trial are huge. Moreover, the
chances of success in a Phase III trial can be very low. For example, by
the year 2000, there had been 173 Phase III trials of neuroprotective
and/or rheologic/antithrombotic agents for acute stroke, but only three of
them yielded positive results (14). Might these 170 futile Phase III trials
have been prevented?

Yuko Palesch and Barbara Tilley led a group of us who explored this
question among the treatment arms of six of the 173 Phase III trials, only
one of which was "positive." (15) We analyzed the emerging results in
their Phase III active treatment arms as if they were happening in hypothetical single-arm Phase II "futility" studies in which all patients received
the active treatment. These hypothetical success rates were compared
with the success rates specified by the investigators in justifying their sample size calculations for the Phase III trials. Finally, we created a "futility" stopping rule for each Phase II futility trial that would be triggered if
the accumulating rate of successful outcomes observed in it was too low
to be compatible with the success rates predicted for the corresponding
Phase III trial.

Our results were striking. We would have correctly declared three of
these trials futile in Phase II, and none of them demonstrated efficacy in
Phase III. In one case, we would have concluded that the treatment was
futile after just 19 patients, only 4% of the number actually enrolled in the
corresponding Phase III trial before it was abandoned. The single positive
Phase III trial would have "passed" our futility criterion. This "Phase II futility trial" approach is receiving further study.

Phase III Trials

If the compound still looks promising through Phase II and if no competing compound is ahead of it in the race to approval and marketing, we
may carry out a full-scale Phase III RCT, with sufficient sample size and
power to establish or refute the compound's predicted benefit. The design,
execution, analysis, interpretation, and presentation of such Phase III trials constitute the prime focus of this chapter.

Phase IV Studies (Monitoring, or Postmarketing Surveillance)

Finally, even if a Phase III RCT is positive and its compound goes on the market, we must not stop its critical appraisal. First, and most important, we must carry out some sort of surveillance for its rare but awful side effects. Of course, we already began this search for adverse outcomes in the initial animal studies. However, some simple arithmetic will show why Phase I, II, and III trials are far too small to detect rare but awful side effects.

The simple truth, described as the "inverse rule of 3," is that to be 95% sure of observing at least one adverse event that occurs once per x-many patients, we have to observe $3x$ patients (16). For example, acute muscle damage (rhabdomyolysis) that is severe enough to cause hospitalization occurs only about once per 23,000 patients who take a statin drug for a year. The inverse rule of 3 tells us we'd have to follow $23,000 \times 3 = 69,000$ statin takers for a year before we could be 95% confident that we'd observe even one episode of rhabdomyolysis. Moreover, we'd have to follow several times that many to be confident that this rare but serious unexpected adverse event is more common among statin takers (the study that documented this risk followed over 250,000 patients taking statins) (17).

We call such "postmarketing" surveillance *Phase IV Monitoring*. It can serve other purposes besides determining a drug's safety. These studies can address the drug's interactions with other drugs or dietary components, the distribution and determinants of its use (pharmacoepidemiology), and the measurement of its cost-effectiveness (pharmacoeconomics). Finally, it is these postmarketing studies that may provide our first opportunity to assess benefits and harms among the very young, the very old, and those with comorbidity.

What About Nondrug Trials?

Are there parallels to these phases for nondrug innovations? I think so. Surely, we should carry out a similar sequence of investigations before we introduce a new operation, behavioral intervention, or complementary therapy. For example, we can perfect the new operation and identify its serious complications on nonhumans. Then, we can carry out a few Phase I operations in humans with the target disorder (there are no volunteers here, unless the procedure is innocuous). We could then invite several surgeons to perfect their skills in carrying out the operation in a longer Phase II case-series, and could use promising results to design a full-scale Phase III RCT. In Phase IV, we could analyze routine hospital discharge information for the immediate effects of the operation. We also could carry out formal follow-up studies, tracking both the patients who undergo the operation and the surgeons who carry it out. This combination of Phase IV monitoring will reveal long-term outcomes for patients and will document whether surgeons (and institutions) with more frequent operations have fewer complications.

Compared with drug treatments, fewer surgical, complementary, or nonprescription treatments are subjected to this rigorous testing series. Unfortunately, the same must be said for several forms of devices (e.g., heart valves and stents), radiations (e.g., lithotripsy), procedures (e.g., shaving before delivery), and ways of looking after patients (e.g., multidisciplinary care). We can neither justify nor excuse these disparities in testing non-drug interventions by invoking less valid rules of evidence or less rigorous methods for testing their efficacy. I believe we can validate or reject every one of them through RCTs, and I have devoted Section 6.9 of this chapter ("Special Issues in Nondrug Trials") to nondrug trials.

6.4 EXPLANATORY VERSUS MANAGEMENT TRIALS

Consider the following two (of several) versions of the question we might pose about aspirin, sulfinpyrazone, and the prevention of stroke or death in patients with transient ischaemic attacks (TIAs):

1. *Among highly compliant patients who are under the care of expert neurologists for TIAs (or minor completed strokes), can exposure to the pharmacodynamic effects of aspirin or sulfinpyrazone, singly or in combination, reduce their risk of subsequent ipsilateral (same-sided) stroke (at an acceptably low rate of adverse drug effects)?*

   I call this an "explanatory" or "efficacy" question (18,19) because its biologically oriented answer will tell us whether these drugs, when prescribed by experts and taken faithfully by patients, exhibiting their full pharmacodynamic effects, and causing an acceptably low risk of adverse drug effects, do more good than harm to the cerebral circulation downstream from the presumed source of their TIA.

2. *Among all-comers who are under the care of any licensed physician for TIAs (or minor completed strokes), does offering aspirin or sulfinpyrazone, singly or in combination, reduce their risk of subsequent stroke or death from any cause (also at an acceptably low rate of adverse drug effects)?*

   I call this a "pragmatic" or "management" or "effectiveness" question because its clinical- and community-oriented answer will tell us whether these drugs, when offered by a wide range of clinicians to patients who might or might not take them, causing an acceptably low risk of adverse drug effects, will reduce the risk of all subsequent strokes and death.

These two questions share a few attributes, such as the necessity for high ethics and total follow-up. However, the appropriate tactics for answering them differ in at least ten important ways, as shown in Table 6–3.

To answer an explanatory question (*can* the treatment produce more good than harm under *ideal* circumstances?), we could go to great pains to:

- enroll only those patients who meet the eligibility criteria of high-risk and high-response.
- enroll only those patients who prove to us that they'll take their medicine.
- throw out any patients subsequently discovered not to have met the foregoing criteria (as long as this exclusion was bias-free).
- show that they can tolerate the experimental treatment before they are randomized.

TABLE 6–3   The Differing Attributes of Explanatory and Management Trials

Attribute	Explanatory Trial (Efficacy)	Management Trial (Effectiveness, Pragmatic)
Nature of the question posed	Can the Rx work under ideal circumstances (of risk, responsiveness, compliance, and follow-up)?	Does the Rx work under usual circumstances?
Patient eligibility criteria	Very strict, limited to high-risk, highly responsive, highly compliant patients	All-comers with the target disorder
Patients subsequently found to be ineligible at entry	Excluded from the analysis whenever it is valid to do so	Usually included in the analysis
Treatment	Given by the best hands and closely monitored for dose and side effects	As in routine clinical care
Intensity of follow-up	High, with frequent visits	No greater frequency than in routine practice
Patient compliance	Closely monitored, with compliance-maintaining/ improving strategies for all patients	Monitored unobtrusively if possible, but no enhancing interventions
Clinician adherence to the study protocol	Closely monitored, with feedback for incomplete performance	Little or no monitoring
Events of interest	Restricted to just those that answer the biologic question (or constitute adverse effects of treatment)	All harmful events, regardless of their causes
Duration of follow-up for individual participants	Stops ("censored") as soon as they have the event of interest	Continues to the death or the end of the trial, whichever comes first
Eligibility of events for analyses for "good"	Restricted set of outcomes, excluding those occurring before the Rx "takes hold" and after Rx has been abandoned or contaminated	All outcomes, from the instant of allocation, through treatment, to the close of the trial

- place them under the care of experts.
- closely monitor their drugs, compliance, and health status.
- intervene if their compliance falls (20).
- intervene if their clinicians falter in following the study protocol.
- restrict the patient outcome events—we collect and analyze just those that answer our precise study question.
- stop our follow-up as soon as an outcome event occurs (or a worse event prevents us from observing them).
- exclude events occurring before and after a drug's maximum pharmacodynamic effect (risky).
- "censor" (exclude from any further analyses) patients as soon as they stop complying (very risky).

Interpretations Differ for Positive and Negative Conclusions from Explanatory and Management Trials

The final two tactics in the preceding paragraph are labeled "risky" and "very risky" because they can lead to "false-positive" trials, and are avoided by most trialists. Even without them, however, we can carry out small, tight RCTs that generate explanatory answers, as shown in the upper row of Table 6-4.

TABLE 6-4   The Conclusions that Can Be Drawn from Explanatory and Management Trials

	Conclusion from this trial	
	Benefit clearly greater than harm ("positive result")	Benefit clearly no greater than harm ("minimally important improvement" ruled out)
Explanatory trial	*Ambiguous*; it "works" but will patients and clinicians jump through the hoops necessary for its success? a	*Clearly sensible to abandon* this treatment for this condition b
Management trial	c *Clearly worthwhile* to adopt this treatment	d *Ambiguous*; did it fail because it was worthless or because too few patients and clinicians followed directions and took their medicine?

When the confidence interval around the treatment effect excludes any minimally important difference (MID) in the form of a treatment benefit (especially from the patient's perspective), we have definitive evidence (in cell b) that the treatment is useless for this condition (a "true-negative" trial). However, when an explanatory trial reaches the positive conclusion that the treatment exceeds this MID and is efficacious in this set of patients (cell a), ambiguity remains about what we should advise clinicians and patients. Would the ordinary run of clinicians, prescribing the treatment to the ordinary run of patients, get enough (but not too much) of the drug on board enough patients that they would, on average, benefit from it? Alas, a positive explanatory trial can't answer that question.

But, as shown in the lower row of Table 6–4, the management trial can. To answer a management question (*does* the treatment do more good than harm under *usual* circumstances?), we could practice good science by:

- setting our eligibility criteria very loose (perhaps even based on the mutual conclusion of a patient and his or her clinician that both are *uncertain* about what treatment should be administered).
- taking all eligible comers, regardless of risk, likely responsiveness, compliance record, or site of care.
- retaining every admitted patient in the analysis.
- leaving the clinician and patient alone to get on with treatment, free of any monitoring of (or intervention into) the precise treatment process or patient compliance (unless the former can be done unobtrusively).
- ascertaining a broad range of events and including them in the analysis.
- counting every event from the moment of randomization and charging it against the randomized treatment.

The result can be a large, simple trial with a very pragmatic answer.

When a pragmatic trial reaches the positive conclusion that the treatment does more good than harm to this broad array of patients (cell c), a case can be made for its immediate adoption in everyday clinical practice. On the other hand, when a pragmatic trial rules out an MID by generating a confidence interval around the treatment effect that excludes any important benefit or harm (cell d), ambiguity remains. We shouldn't jump to the conclusion that the treatment lacks efficacy. Might it simply be that the ordinary run of clinicians, prescribing an efficacious treatment to the ordinary run of patients, fail to get enough of it on board enough patients for them to display its underlying efficacy?

Equivocal, "nonstatistically significant," or "indeterminate" results haunt both explanatory and management trials, and some of the tactics described in this chapter are designed to avoid this sad situation.

Explanatory and Management Trials Constitute a Continuum, Not a Dichotomy

Before you get carried away with this "polar" discussion, I want to emphasize that this explanatory-management construct comprises a continuous spectrum, not an either–or dichotomy. Moreover, I reckon it's impossible ever to perform a "pure" explanatory or "pure" management trial. For example, no patient is perpetually compliant, and the hand of the most skilled surgeon occasionally slips, so you'll never perform a "pure" explanatory trial. Similarly, a "pure" management trial bites the dust as soon as its first eligible patient refuses to be randomized.

Several conclusions can be drawn from the foregoing discussion of explanatory and management trials. The most important ones for you are three:

1. Neither the explanatory nor the management trial is the "right" (or "wrong") one to perform. Each of them follows directly from the nature of the question being posed. On the one hand, our trial of endarterectomy for symptomatic carotid artery stenosis set our question nearer the explanatory pole (21): "Among patients with high-grade symptomatic carotid artery stenosis who agree to surgery, can the addition of endarterectomy, performed by highly skilled surgeons, to best medical therapy (compared with best medical therapy alone), reduce their risk of severe stroke or death, at an acceptable rate of surgical complications?" On the other hand, the Adjuvant Tamoxifen—Longer Against Shorter (ATLAS) trial (*http://www.ctsu.ox.ac.uk/~atlas/1st_page.htm*) set its question nearer the management pole: "Among women currently taking tamoxifen for breast cancer (irrespective of their original type of surgery, histology, nodal status, estrogen receptor status, or adjuvant therapy) who are apparently free of disease, and who share their physician's uncertainty as to whether they should continue taking tamoxifen, would at least 5 additional years of tamoxifen (compared with stopping this drug), improve their 10-year survival?"

2. The right way to design, conduct, analyze, and interpret any individual RCT is determined by the question it poses. Thus, North American Symptomatic Carotid Endarterectomy Trial (NASCET), based on the explanatory nature of its question, screened prospective surgical collaborators for their expertise, intensely followed its study patients, and intervened when their hypertension wasn't well controlled, and its principal clinical investigator frequently visited every participating center to be sure that they were adhering to the letter of the protocol. By contrast, the Web site for the pragmatic ATLAS trial reads: "To encourage wide participation, the ATLAS study involves virtually no extra work for collaborators, so that even the busiest clinicians can take part. The entry procedure is quick and easy [a 1-page entry form], no examinations are required beyond those given as part of routine care, and minimal, annual follow-up information is requested." (*http://www.ctsu.ox.ac.uk/~atlas/1st_page.htm*)

3. Given the consequences of the conclusions of positive and negative explanatory and management trials displayed in Table 6–4, a strong case can be made for initially testing a novel treatment in a small, quick, tight explanatory trial. Only if that were positive would it be retested in a large pragmatic trial. Alas, that second, pragmatic trial often isn't done, sometimes because of the conviction that it's

unethical to withhold a treatment once it is shown to be efficacious in an explanatory trial. On the other hand, despite the high utility of large, simple trials, they rarely constitute the first test of novel treatments.

A Strategy Exists for Performing Simultaneous Explanatory and Management Trials

Before leaving this pragmatic/management versus explanatory trial discussion, I want to show you a novel design suggested by Sikhar Banerjee when he was a graduate student working with me. The "Banerjee Simultaneous Explanatory-Management Design" (22) brilliantly converts an explanatory *versus* pragmatic dilemma into an explanatory *plus* management trial. This is illustrated in Figure 6–1.

In the Simultaneous Explanatory-Management Design, all eligible patients undergo a preliminary test of compliance or of their ability to tolerate the treatment. Those who pass are randomized and studied in the usual fashion. Their analysis answers the explanatory question.

Sikhar Banerjee's great contribution is to *not* discard study patients who flunk this preliminary test. Instead, they become a second stratum and are randomized and followed just like those who passed. The explanatory (efficacy) analysis is restricted, as usual, to those patients who passed the pretrial test. However, it is now possible to combine the patients who passed the test with those who flunked it, thereby generating a management (effectiveness) analysis as well.

Even in a "simultaneous" trial, however, the "explanatory versus management" ways in which we carry out the other steps of this compound trial (frequent versus less frequent follow-up visits, whether we apply compliance-improving strategies, and the like) will determine how confident we will be about its explanatory and management conclusions.

6.5 SUPERIORITY, EQUIVALENCE, AND NONINFERIORITY TRIALS

Don't Blame Me for These Terms

In this section I hope to explain (or at least demystify) what trialists mean by "superiority" trials, "noninferiority" trials, and maybe even "equivalence trials" (sorry for the awful jargon, but it wasn't my doing).

Let's start from a clinical perspective and then tiptoe through the accompanying statistical minefield. To make the latter presentation easier to follow, let's assume that our measure of patient outcomes combines both benefit and harm, as in a global measure of function or quality of life. In addition, because these ideas can be difficult to grasp the first time you encounter them, I'll describe them in both words and pictures.

Clinicians Ask One-sided Questions

When busy clinicians bump into a new treatment, they ask themselves two questions (23). First, is it *better* than ("superior to") what they are using

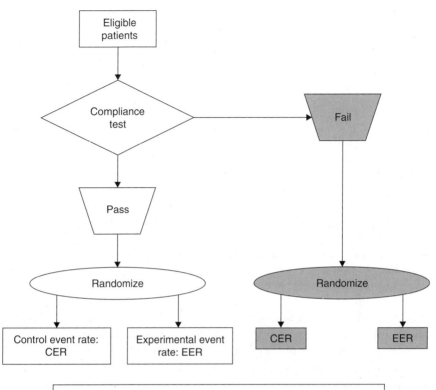

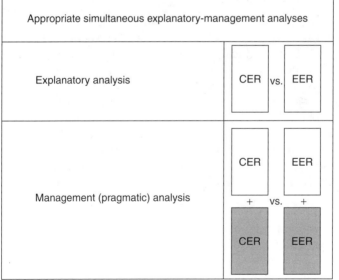

FIGURE 6–1 Execution and analysis of the simultaneous explanatory-management design. CER, control event rate (the rate of events among patients assigned to the control treatment); EER, experimental event rate (the rate of events among patients assigned to the experimental treatment).

now? Second, if it's not superior, is it *as good as* what they are using now ("noninferior") and preferable for some other reason (e.g., fewer side effects or more affordable)? Moreover, they want answers to these questions right away. *ACP Journal Club* and its related evidence-based journals do their best to answer these questions in their "more informative titles."

But Traditional Statistics is Two-sided

Progress toward this "more informative" goal has been slow because we have been prisoners of traditional statistical concepts that call for two-sided tests of statistical significance and require rejection of the null hypothesis. We have further imprisoned ourselves by misinterpreting "statistically nonsignificant" results of these two-tailed tests. Rather than recognizing such results as "indeterminate" (uncertain), we conclude that they are "negative" (certain, providing proof of no difference between treatments).

At the root of our problem is the "null hypothesis," which decrees that the difference between a new and standard treatment ought to be zero. Two-sided P values tell us the probability that the results are compatible with that null hypothesis. When the probability is small (say, $<5\%$), we "reject" the null hypothesis and "accept" the "alternative hypothesis" that the difference we've observed is not zero. In doing so, however, we make no distinction between the new treatment being better, on the one hand, or worse, on the other, than the standard treatment.

The Consequences of Two-sided Answers to One-sided Questions

There are three consequences of this faulty reasoning. First, by performing "two-sided" tests of statistical significance, investigators turn their backs on the "one-sided" clinical questions of superiority and noninferiority. Second, they often fail to recognize that the results of these two-sided tests, especially in small trials, can be "statistically nonsignificant" even when their confidence intervals include important benefit or harm. Third, investigators (abetted by editors) frequently misinterpret this failure to reject the null hypothesis (based on two-sided P values $>5\%$, or 95% confidence intervals that include zero). Rather than recognizing their results as uncertain ("indeterminate"), they report them as "negative" and conclude that there is "no difference" between the treatments.

The Fallacy of the "Negative" Trial

Not only authors, but also editors and especially readers regularly fall into the trap of concluding that the "absence of proof of a difference" between two treatments constitutes "proof of an absence of a difference" between them. This mistake was forcefully pointed out by Phil Alderson and Iain Chalmers: "It is never correct to claim that treatments have no effect or that there is no difference in the effects of treatments. It is impossible to prove … that two treatments have the same effect. There will always be some uncertainty surrounding estimates of treatment effects, and a small difference can never be excluded" (24).

The Solution Lies in Employing One-sided Statistics

A solution to both this incompatibility (between one-sided clinical reasoning and two-sided statistical testing) and confusion (about the clinical interpretation of statistically nonsignificant results) has been around for decades but is just now gaining widespread recognition and application. I assign most of the credit to a pair of biostatisticians, Charles Dunnett and Michael Gent (25) (others have also contributed to its development (26), although they sometimes refer to "noninferiority" as "equivalence," a term whose common usage fails to distinguish one-sided from two-sided thinking). I'll illustrate Charlie Dunnett's and Mike Gent's contribution with a pair of trials in which their thinking helped me and my colleagues escape from the prison of two-sided null hypothesis testing and, by doing so, prevented the misinterpretation of statistically nonsignificant results.

Examples of Employing One-sided Statistics

Thirty years ago, a group of us performed an RCT of nurse practitioners as providers of primary care (27). We wanted to know if patients fared as well under their care as under the care of general practitioners. Guided by Mike Gent, we came to realize that a two-sided analysis that produced an "indeterminate," statistically nonsignificant difference in patient outcomes could confuse rather than clarify matters. We therefore abandoned our initial two-sided null hypothesis and decided that we'd ask a noninferiority question: Were the outcomes of patients cared for by nurse practitioners noninferior to those of patients cared for by general practitioners? Mike then helped us recognize the need to specify our limit of acceptable "inferiority" in terms of these outcomes. With his prodding, we decided that we would tolerate no worse than 5% lower physical, social, or emotional function at the end of the trial among patients randomized to our nurse practitioners as we observed among patients randomized to our general practitioners. As it happened, our one-sided analysis revealed that the probability that our nurse practitioners' patients were worse off (by $\geq 5\%$) than our general practitioners' patients was as small as 0.008. We had established that nurse practitioners were not inferior to general practitioners as providers of primary care.

Twenty years ago, a group of us performed an RCT of superficial temporal artery–middle cerebral artery anastomosis ["extracranial–intracranial (EC/IC) bypass"] for patients with threatened stroke (28). To the disappointment of many, we failed to show a statistically significant superiority of surgery for preventing subsequent fatal and nonfatal stroke. It immediately became important to overcome the ambiguity of this "indeterminate" result. We therefore asked the one-sided question: What degree of surgical benefit could we rule out? That one-sided analysis, which calculated the upper end of a 90% (rather than a 95%) confidence interval, excluded a surgical benefit as small as 3%. When news of this one-sided result got around, use of this operation rapidly declined.

Thanks to statisticians like Charlie Dunnett and Mike Gent, we now know how to translate rational, one-sided clinical reasoning into sensible, one-sided statistical analysis. Moreover, this modern strategy of asking one-sided noninferiority and superiority questions in RCTs is gathering momentum. The Consolidated Standards of Reporting Trials (CONSORT) statement on recommendations for reporting RCTs omits any requirement for two-sided significance testing. By the time this chapter was being written in 2004, even some mainline journal editors were getting the message, and one-sided noninferiority and superiority trials had started to appear in the *New England Journal of Medicine, The Lancet, JAMA*, and quite regularly in the *ACP Journal Club*.

One-sided Statistical Analyses Need to be Specified Ahead of Time

An essential prerequisite to doing one-sided testing is the specification of the exact noninferiority and superiority questions before the RCT begins. As with unannounced subgroup analyses, readers can and should be suspicious of authors who apply one-sided analyses without previous planning and notice. Have they been slipped in only after a peek at the data revealed that conventional two-sided tests generated indeterminate results? This need for prior specification of one-sided analyses provides yet another argument for registering RCTs in their design stages and for publishing their protocols in open-access journals such as Biomed Central (*www.biomedcentral.com*).

A Graphic Demonstration of Superiority and Noninferiority

Because these ideas of superiority and noninferiority can be tough to master, I'll now go over that verbal ground again, this time with pictures. Along the way, I'll use these pictures to illustrate other important issues, such as how we should test a new treatment when an effective one already exists. As before, I'll employ a single outcome measure that incorporates both the benefits and the risks of the experimental treatment. And, for your statistical comfort, I'll start by thinking in terms of two-sided tests of statistical significance and double-pointed 95% confidence intervals. Have a look at Figure 6–2.

This figure (and the two that follow it) uses "forest" plots to illustrate different sorts of trial results and their interpretation. In each of the figures, the *horizontal arrows* present the two-sided 95% confidence intervals for the differences in outcomes between experimental and control treatments. For purposes of this discussion, think of these *horizontal arrows* as expressing a composite of both good and harm, such as a quality-of-life measure. When there is no difference in outcomes between experimental and control treatments, the confidence interval would be centered on the heavy vertical line at **0**. When the average patient fares better on experimental therapy than on control therapy, the confidence interval is centered to the left of **0**. But when the average patient fares worse on experimental therapy than on control therapy, the confidence interval is centered to the right of **0**. Okay so far?

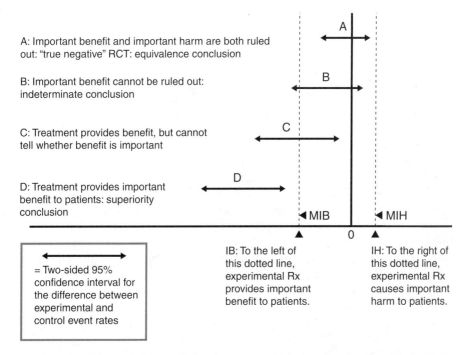

A: Important benefit and important harm are both ruled out: "true negative" RCT: equivalence conclusion

B: Important benefit cannot be ruled out: indeterminate conclusion

C: Treatment provides benefit, but cannot tell whether benefit is important

D: Treatment provides important benefit to patients: superiority conclusion

= Two-sided 95% confidence interval for the difference between experimental and control event rates

IB: To the left of this dotted line, experimental Rx provides important benefit to patients.

IH: To the right of this dotted line, experimental Rx causes important harm to patients.

FIGURE 6–2 Randomized controlled trials (RCTs) in which the control Rx is a placebo or no treatment at all.

How to Think About and Incorporate Minimally Important Differences (MIDs)

Now notice that there are dashed vertical lines on either side of **0**. These lines show the points where patients (and, we hope, their clinicians) reckon that these differences in outcomes on experimental versus control treatment exceed some MIDs in benefit and harm. As a consequence, patients would want, and their clinicians should offer, treatments that meet or exceed a positive MID in good outcomes. Similarly, patients would refuse, and their clinicians would not even offer, treatments that meet or exceed a negative MID in bad outcomes.

I've illustrated these MIDs in Figure 6–2. On the left, you can see the dotted line for minimally important benefits (MIB), and on the right, the dashed line for minimally important harm (MIH) to patients. Patients and clinicians usually place the MIH line closer to **0** than they do the MIB line, consistent with most people's greater concern about avoiding harm.

The locations of the MIB and MIH lines ought to be based on what patients consider important benefit and harm. As it happens, patient considerations are rarely determined in any formal way but are informally incorporated by the investigators as they set these lines. Their location depends on the question posed by the trial. For an awful disease with no known cure (say, a rapidly fatal untreatable cancer), any benefit would be welcomed by patients and their clinicians, and the MIB line might be placed very close to the **0** line. For a trivial self-limited disease like the common cold, the MIB line might be placed far to the left of **0**, but its MIH line might be only slightly to the right of **0**.

Incorporating Confidence Intervals for Treatment Effects

When a treatment's confidence interval is centered to the left of the MIB line, we are encouraged. If its entire confidence interval lies to the left of the MIB line, we can be confident that experimental treatment provides important benefits (IB) to patients (if you are looking ahead, the double-tipped confidence interval arrow labeled **D** describes this happy case). In a similar fashion, any confidence interval centered to the right of the MIH line is discouraging, and if the entire confidence interval lies to the right of the MIH line, we can be confident that experimental treatment causes important harm to patients.

To give you a comfortable starting point, Figure 6–2 illustrates four of several results we might obtain in RCTs performed with a promising new drug on a disorder for which "no effective treatment" exists. (By "no effective treatment," I mean that no prior RCT has found any treatment whose confidence interval lies entirely to the left of the **0** line.) These initial trials typically employ placebos, and seek a treatment that is superior to that placebo.

Trial Result **A** is highly informative, isn't it? Its entire confidence interval lies to the right of the **IB** line, so we have ruled out any MIB to patients. By contrast, Trial Result **B** isn't very helpful, is it? Its confidence interval stretches all the way from being slightly (but not importantly) harmful at its right tip to being importantly beneficial at its left tip.

Why We Should Never Label an "Indeterminate" Trial Result as "Negative" or as Showing "No Effect"

Trial Results **A** and **B** nicely illustrate the confusion that arises from stating that a treatment "has no effect" or that an RCT was "negative" just because its confidence interval crosses the **0** line. These "negative" and "no effect" labels imply that we should throw the experimental treatment into the dustbin. And I agree that's what we should do with Treatment **A**, where you've ruled out any important patient benefit.

But should we throw Treatment **B** into the bin along with Treatment **A**? After all, its confidence interval also crosses the **0** line. Of course, we shouldn't. The confidence interval for Treatment **B** also crosses the important benefit line, so it might, in fact, produce important benefit to patients. We simply don't know whether Treatment **B** is worthwhile. A useful word that most of us use to describe such a trial result is "indeterminate."

Because of this confusion in labeling, some leading trialists have called for banning the terms "negative" and "no effect" from health care journals. Remember that earlier quote from Phil Alderson and Iain Chalmers that:

"It is never correct to claim that treatments have no effect or that there is no difference in the effects of treatments"? For my part, I reserve the term "true negative" for only those A-type RCTs that rule out any important treatment benefit for patients. For example, in our previously noted trial of superficial temporal–middle cerebral artery anastomosis ("EC/IC bypass"), we ruled out a surgical benefit as small as 3% in the relative risk of fatal and nonfatal stroke (29). One way to distinguish A-type results from merely indeterminate ones is to label the A-types "true-negative" trials.

How Does a Treatment Become "Established Effective Therapy?"

Trial Result **C** shows a definite benefit (the right tip of the arrow lies to the left of the **0** line). The treatment in **C** lies entirely to the good side of **0**, so it works better than nothing. However, because it straddles the MIB line, we can't tell whether its benefit is great enough to be important to patients. Result **D** is what you'd hope to find in most trials. The *right arrow tip* lies to the left of the MIB line, and we can be confident that Treatment **D** provides IB to patients. Treatment **D**, especially when it is confirmed in a meta-analysis of several independent trials, now deserves the title of "established effective therapy (EET)" and you'd urge your clinical colleagues to offer it to all patients who could get their hands on it and tolerate it (alas, economic, geographic, political, and cultural barriers deny EET to millions of patients on every continent).

Most Trials are Too Small to Declare a Treatment "Established Effective Therapy"

As you'll learn elsewhere in Chapters 4 through 6, the sample sizes enrolled in most trials are only large enough to generate Result **C** (treatment is better than nothing). Although its point estimate of efficacy (the midpoint of its two-tipped arrow) lies to the left of the IB line, the lower bound of its confidence interval extends to the right of that IB line. It requires lots more patients for that same treatment to shrink its confidence interval enough to drag its right tip to the left of that IB line. This degree of shrinkage may not be achieved until several trials of this treatment have been combined in a meta-analysis.

How Do We Achieve a D-type of Result?

Most commonly, a **D**-type result, with the entire confidence interval beyond the MIB line, is achieved only in meta-analyses of several comparable trials. Otherwise, I have seen it in trials that met two conditions. First, the experimental treatment turned out to be so much better than expected that the number of enrolled patients was far greater than necessary for generating Result **C**. Second, the trial was short-term, and virtually all its patients had been admitted and treated before any interim analysis could have detected its favorable result.

What Do We Do When Established Effective Therapy Already Exists?

So far, I have described how we might think about placebo-controlled trials. Where do we go from here? What should we do when we already have an EET such as **D**, but a new, promising (but untested) treatment comes along? How would we find out whether the new treatment was "superior" to **D** and ought to replace it as EET? Alternatively, how should we try to find out whether this new promising treatment is just as good as ("noninferior" to) the current EET but safer or less expensive?

Trialists like me believe that we should *not* test such promising new treatments against a placebo when EET already exists. Our reasons for this strong stand are both ethical and clinical. The ethical reason is that it's simply wrong to replace EET (something we know *does* work among patients who can and will take it) with a placebo (something we know does *not* work). It's tough enough to justify withholding EET from the promising new treatment arm that only might work. Surely, it is wrong in this situation to assign half the study patients to a treatment we *know* doesn't work.

The clinical reason for our position is that, when we already have an EET, it's stupid to test the next promising treatment against a placebo. Who cares if the promising new treatment is better than a placebo? That won't tell clinicians whether they should offer it, rather than the EET, to future patients. Surely, what we all want to know is the answer to one of two questions. First, is the promising new treatment better than the EET (a "superiority" question)? Second, if it's not better, is the promising new treatment "as good as" ("noninferior" to) EET but preferable on other grounds (such as safety or cost)? The best way to answer these questions depends on whether the new treatment, if effective, would replace EET or simply be added to it.

Disputes over the Use of Placebos When Established Effective Therapy Already Exists

A strong case can and has been made [e.g., by Kenneth Rothman and K. Michels in 1994 (30)] that it is always unethical to substitute placebos for EET. However, the US Food and Drug Administration (FDA) regularly proposes arguments about the need for "assay sensitivity" (too esoteric for me, but often rejected by my statistical betters) and continue not only to permit but also to require promising new drugs to be tested against placebo even when EET already exists (31). And trialists such as I recognize two exceptions to the rule that it is always unethical to substitute placebos for EET.

Exception no. 1: When Patients Can't or Won't Take Established Effective Therapy

What sort of trial should we carry out if the EET is contraindicated for, or refused by, a subset of patients? In this case, I'd argue that no EET exists for them, and that a placebo controlled trial is both clinically sensible and ethical.

Or, what should we do if another subset of patients can't get at the EET because of geography, politics, local tradition, or economics? Shouldn't they be invited to join an RCT of the promising untested (PU) treatment versus placebo? I think they should. My reasoning isn't an exception to the rule, but a strict application of the definition of EET (in patients who can tolerate *and afford* it). For these subsets of patients, there *is no* EET, and inviting them to join an RCT of the promising treatment versus placebo is, I think, both good science and good ethics.

Exception no. 2: When a Promising New Treatment Might Replace Established Effective Therapy

In this situation, the only comparison that makes clinical (and ethical) sense to trialists like me is a "head-to-head" comparison of the EET and the promising new therapy. If the promising but untested treatment would *replace* EET, the head-to-head comparison would be similar to the "placebo-controlled" trials I've already described, but with EET in place of the placebo.

When a Promising New Treatment Might Be Added to Established Effective Therapy

What if the promising but untested treatment is touted as a beneficial *addition to* EET? By the same ethical and clinical reasoning presented in the preceding paragraphs, the appropriate RCT compares the combination of EET *plus* the new treatment versus EET *alone*. Peter Tugwell led the first trial to successfully challenge the FDA's position that such "add-on" treatments had to be tested against placebos (32). Peter and his coinvestigators insisted on testing a promising new therapy, cyclosporine, by adding it or a placebo to methotrexate, the EET for rheumatoid arthritis. We call this sort of trial an "add-on" RCT.

Using Placebos in a Trial Needn't Mean the Absence of Treatment

A brief reminder: don't equate the use of placebos with the absence of any treatment. They might be used in both sorts of the RCTs that test the promising new treatment. Let's label the established effective therapy "EE" and the promising untested treatment "PU." In a head-to-head trial of EE versus PU (and unless the two drugs are identical in appearance), the treatment groups would be:

(active EE + placebo PU) versus (placebo EE + active PU).

Similarly, the "add-on" RCT to test PU would have treatment groups of:

(active EE + active PU) versus (active EE + placebo PU).

Demonstrating Trials of Promising New Treatments Against (or in Addition to) Established Effective Therapy

To repeat these latest ideas in picture form, take a look at Figure 6–3.

The first thing you should notice in Figure 6–3 is that the "goalpost has been moved" to the left. The vertical 0 line that was used when there

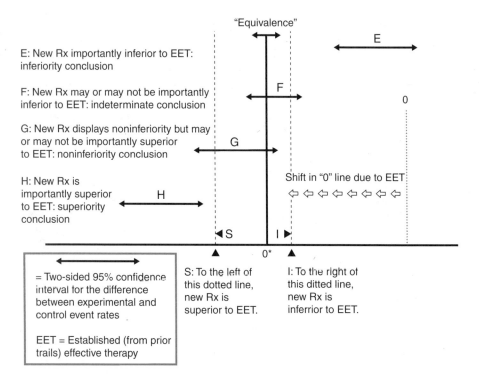

E: New Rx importantly inferior to EET: inferiority conclusion

F: New Rx may or may not be importantly inferior to EET: indeterminate conclusion

G: New Rx displays noninferiority but may or may not be importantly superior to EET: noninferiority conclusion

H: New Rx is importantly superior to EET: superiority conclusion

= Two-sided 95% confidence interval for the difference between experimental and control event rates

EET = Established (from prior trails) effective therapy

S: To the left of this dotted line, new Rx is superior to EET.

I: To the right of this ditted line, new Rx is inferrior to EET.

FIGURE 6–3 Randomized controlled trials (RCTs) in which the control Rx is established effective therapy (EET) [conventional two-sided 95% confidence interval (CI)].

was no EET has been replaced with the 0^* line that sets the new standard by which benefit and harm is to be judged. I hope that these "shifting goal posts" reinforce my argument that, when a promising but untested treatment joins a clinical arena with an EET, the sensible questions require testing the promising treatment against (or in addition to) EET, not against placebo.

The second thing I want you to notice is that the MIB line has been replaced by the superiority line (**S** line) that identifies the boundary, to the left of which the new treatment is minimally importantly superior to EET. In a similar fashion, the MIH line has been replaced by the inferiority line (**I** line) that identifies the boundary, to the right of which the new treatment is minimally importantly inferior to EET. As before, the locations of these superiority and inferiority lines should be based on what's important to patients.

Why We Almost Never Find, and Rarely Seek, True "Equivalence"

Here is where the convoluted terminology comes in. Although it would be nice to prove that the efficacy of the promising new treatment was "equivalent" to EET (but safer or cheaper), the number of patients required for that proof is huge; in fact, the determination of identical efficacy (a confidence interval of zero) requires a sample size of infinity. Even the "equivalence" result shown at the top of Figure 6–3, where the entire confidence interval lies between the superiority and inferiority lines, requires massive numbers of patients (as you'll discover in the following section, to halve a 95% confidence interval you'll need to quadruple your sample size). Unfortunately, some authors use "equivalence" to denote "noninferiority," a usage that should further increase your suspicion when you see the word "equivalence."

The Graphical Demonstration of "Superiority" and "Noninferiority"

As is already (I hope) burned into your brain, head-to-head trials of promising new versus EET usually ask two questions. A stroll though Figure 6–3 will illustrate this noninferiority and superiority business. Trial Result **E** shows that the new treatment is importantly inferior to EET (and should be abandoned). At the other extreme, Result **H** shows that it is importantly superior to EET (and, if it is safe and affordable, should replace it).

Results for treatments **F** and **G** are the troublesome ones. Result **F** is indeterminate for noninferiority because it crosses the inferiority line **I**, and the new treatment might or might not be inferior to EET. Similarly, result **G** is indeterminate for superiority because it crosses the superiority line **S**, and the new treatment might or might not be superior.

However, I hope you noticed both ends of these 95% confidence intervals. If you did, you discovered that the upper (left) bound of the confidence interval for Treatment **F** lies to the right of the superiority line **S**. Thus, you can confidently conclude that Treatment **F** is *not superior* to EET. You also may have noticed that the lower (right) bound of the confidence interval for **G** lies to the left of the inferiority line **I**. Thus, treatment G is *not inferior* to EET.

Converting One-sided Clinical Thinking into One-sided Statistical Analysis

Is there some way to avoid the indeterminate noninferiority conclusion about Treatment **F** and the indeterminate superiority conclusion about **G** without having to greatly increase the numbers of patients in these trials? The solution is illustrated in Figure 6–4, where some key results from the previous two-tailed figure are presented in their one-tailed forms.

As I hope you recall from my earlier verbal description of this dilemma, Charlie Dunnett and Mike Gent (25) have argued persuasively that the first question usually posed in an RCT (Is treatment X superior to placebo or EET?) is a "one-sided" (not a "two-sided") question. That is, it asks only about superiority. As investigators, we wouldn't care if the answer was "no" due to equivalence or inferiority; both would lead us to abandon the new treatment.

What does that mean in graphic terms? It means that only the right-hand tip of the confidence interval arrow for treatment **G** is relevant and

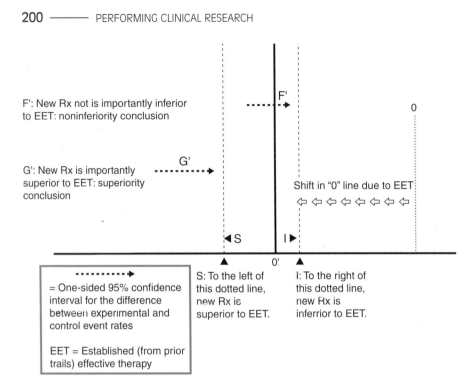

F': New Rx not is importantly inferior to EET: noninferiority conclusion

G': New Rx is importantly superior to EET: superiority conclusion

Shift in "0" line due to EET

= One-sided 95% confidence interval for the difference between experimental and control event rates

EET = Established (from prior trails) effective therapy

S: To the left of this dotted line, new Rx is superior to EET.

I: To the right of this dotted line, new Rx is inferrior to EET.

FIGURE 6–4 Randomized controlled trials (RCTs) in which the control Rx is the established effective therapy (EET) [using one-sided 95% confidence interval (CI)].

that it should extend rightward only to its 5% boundary, not to its 2.5% boundary. Now, with the less stringent one-sided 95% confidence interval, indeterminate study Result **G** in the previous figure becomes the definitive superiority Result **G′** in this one.

As I hope you'll also recall, Charlie Dunnett and Mike Gent then maintained that, if both a superiority and a noninferiority question were posed in the design phase of the trial, the answers to both can be sought in the analysis. Thus, even if their one-sided "superiority" question is answered "no," they can still go on to ask the other one-sided "noninferiority" question: Is the new treatment not importantly inferior to EET? This would be a highly relevant question if the promising new treatment might be safer, or easier to take, or produce fewer or milder side effects, or less expensive.

What does that mean in graphic terms? It means that only the right-hand tip of the confidence interval arrow for treatment **F** is relevant, and that it should extend rightward only to its 5% boundary, not to its 2.5% boundary. Now, with the less stringent one-sided 95% confidence interval, indeterminate study Result **F** in the previous figure becomes the definitive noninferiority Result **F′** in this one.

Once again, the projection of one-tailed clinical reasoning into one-tailed statistical analysis has provided very useful results for patients.

"Me-too" Drugs

Often, the promising new treatment is a "me-too" drug from the same class as EET, and was developed by a competing drug company to gain a share of the market already created by the EET. In this case, they aren't interested in whether the new drug is superior to the standard drug, but only in whether it is *not* inferior to it. As before, this question is best answered in a "head-to-head" RCT.

This strategy is viewed with suspicion by some (especially some licensing authorities). They fear that the noninferiority trial may be a tool used by ambitious trialists and profit-oriented drug companies to promote treatments of little value. What's to keep them from "shifting the goal posts" by moving either or both the superiority line **S** and the inferiority line **I** to the right? There are two safeguards against this abuse. First, patients' values should determine the location of the superiority and inferiority lines. Second, through the registration of trials and protocols, the precise noninferiority questions can be made public before the trial begins.

I hope that these verbal and pictorial discussions have made the concepts of superiority and noninferiority (if not their technical jargon) understandable and reasonable.

6.6 PHYSIOLOGICAL STATISTICS (33)

"Because statistics has too often been presented as a bag of specialized computational tools with morbid emphasis on calculation it is no wonder that survivors of such courses regard their statistical tools as instruments of torture [rather] than as diagnostic aids in the art and science of data analysis."

–George W. Cobb (34)

The myriad statistical formulae that appear in textbooks and articles about how to do Phase III RCTs are frightening to behold. They are tough to remember, and exist in isolation without relation to each other. In addition, they require an understanding of mathematics and statistics far beyond most would-be trialists' background knowledge and expertise. Finally, they take so much time to master that clinicians who do so risk losing their clinical competence, social life, positive self-image, and sense of humor.

All the foregoing is true until we realize that the importance of these statistical formulae lies not in their individual application but in their thoughtful combination. Although it's possible (and in statistical circles, mandatory) to describe this combination in mathematical terms, clinicians might understand them far better by thinking of them in physiological terms, analogous to combining the determinants of systemic arterial blood pressure.

A patient's blood pressure represents the net effects of multiple cardiac, central nervous, endocrinal, renal, and vascular factors (that can interact both synergistically and antagonistically). By wonderful analogy, the confidence we have in an RCT's results (i.e., the narrowness of the confidence interval around the effect of the experimental treatment) is the net result of the interaction of patients, treatments, and study factors that, as you'll see, also can behave synergistically and antagonistically.

The Only Formula You'll Ever Need

The "only formula" of physiological statistics is ridiculously simple, and looks like this:

$$confidence = \frac{signal}{noise} \times \sqrt{sample\ size}$$

Expressed in words, the *confidence* we have in the conclusion of an RCT is the ratio of the size of the *signal* generated by our treatment to the size of the background *noise*, times the square root of the *sample size*. Let's define these terms so that they are clear.

Confidence describes *how narrow the confidence interval is* (the narrower the better) around the effect of treatment, whether expressed as an absolute or relative risk reduction (RRR) or as some other measure of efficacy. For readers still imprisoned by *P* values, this sort of "confidence" becomes greater as the *P* value becomes smaller.

The *signal* describes the differences between the effects of the experimental and control treatments. In the RCTs in which I've taken part, the most useful signal in understanding their design, execution, analysis, and interpretation has been the (absolute) arithmetic difference between the rate (or average severity) of events in experimental and control patients. When, as in most RCTs, these outcomes are "discrete" clinical events such as strokes, bleeds, or death, we'll call this arithmetic difference (the control event rate, or CER, minus the experimental event rate, or EER) the *absolute risk reduction* (ARR).

Why don't we prefer the more frequently reported RRR (which is the ARR divided by the CER)? This is because the RRR doesn't distinguish important treatment effects from trivial ones [slashing deaths from 80% down to 40% generates the same RRR (0.5) as teasing them from 0.008% down to 0.004%].

Finally, in some RCTs the outcomes are "continuous" measures such as blood pressure, time elapsed on a treadmill before chest pain occurs, or location on a 0 to 100 scale of disease activity or functional status. In the latter cases, the signal is best represented for me by the *absolute difference* (AD) in this continuous measure.

The *Noise* (or uncertainty) in an RCT is the sum of all the factors ("sources of variation") that can affect the ARR or AD. Why might patients' responses to treatment, or our measurements of them, vary? Some of these sources are obvious but others aren't, so I'll use plenty of examples along the way.

Finally, *sample size* is the number of patients in the trial. Note that its influence on confidence occurs as its square root. Accordingly, if we want to cut the confidence interval around a study's ARR in half by adding more patients to it, we need to *quadruple* their number. Alternatively, an

RCT designed to detect a 0.10 ARR (from 0.50 to 0.40) needs to quadruple its size in order to confidently detect a 0.05 ARR (from 0.50 to 0.45).

A Simple Way to Demonstrate the Formula at Work or Play

For a quick appreciation of the "physiology" described by this formula, I suggest that you perform a simple experiment. Place a CD player alongside a radio. Ask a friend to insert one of your favorite melodies (the signal) into the former but not to tell you which one it is. Next, tune the radio to a spot between stations where you hear only static (the noise) and turn up the volume. Then start the CD at low volume. Note the "confidence" with which you can identify the melody within, say, 2 seconds. Then vary the volume of the CD (signal), the radio static (noise) and note the amount of time (analogous to sample size) it takes you to discern the former amidst the latter.

Large, Simple Trials

In order to generate extremely small and highly convincing confidence intervals around moderate but important benefit signals, a very strong case can be, and has been, made for really large, really simple RCTs (35) and systematic reviews (36). Their success in revolutionizing the treatment and improving the outcomes of patients with heart disease, cancer, and stroke attests to their success. When study patients number in the tens of thousands they can overcome, by the brute force of numbers, the negative influences of small but highly important ARRs (e.g., the polio vaccine trials that required hundreds of thousands of study individuals) in the presence of considerable noise (as long as the latter does not result from bias). They are described and discussed in Section 6.11 ("Large, Simple Trials").

However, most trials, even when carried out in multiple centers, are of small to moderate size, and they must confront and solve the challenges of small (but useful) signals in the face of lots of noise and a shortage of eligible patients.

Effects of Signal, Noise, and Sample Size on the Confidence or Our Conclusions

Table 6–5 summarizes the independent effects of changes in each of these three elements on the confidence interval around a trial's ARR or RRR

TABLE 6–5 Effects of Changes in a Single Element on Confidence

Element that is Changed	Effect on Our Confidence in the RCT Result	
	When This Element *Increases*	When This Element *Decreases*
Signal (ARR)	Confidence rises	Confidence falls
Noise	Confidence falls	Confidence rises
Sample size	Confidence rises	Confidence falls

RCT, randomized controlled trial; ARR, absolute risk reduction.

Confidence increases as the confidence interval around the absolute risk reduction (ARR) signal narrows.

when the other two elements are held constant. If any of its entries are confusing, I suggest that you repeat the CD/radio experiment until they all make sense.

You are now ready to understand how each of these elements can raise or lower the confidence in any RCT result. But first a cautionary note. Because this pursuit of confidence may involve restricting the entry of certain sorts of patients into our RCT, it may shift it away from a "pragmatic" orientation ("Does offering the treatment to all patients do more good than harm under usual circumstances?") toward an "explanatory" one ("Can rigorously applying the treatment to just some subgroup of patients do more good than harm under ideal circumstances?"). I'll discuss the implications of this shift as they arise.

Determinants of the Signal, and How They Can Be Manipulated to Maximize It

Four determinants affect the magnitude of the signal generated in an RCT (as you will see later, they can also affect noise). They are the "baseline" or control group's risk of an outcome event, the potency of our experimental treatment, the responsiveness of experimental patients to it, and the completeness with which we detect outcome events. Our understanding of how these determinants operate begins and ends with our realization that the important number in an RCT is *not* the *number of patients* in it, but the *number of outcome events* among those patients.

All four determinants operate in every group of individuals we consider for, or later invite to join, a Phase III RCT. Sometimes they are already at optimum levels: our patients are at high risk, our experimental treatment is powerful, all our patients can respond to it, and we can capture every outcome event. In that case, we won't need to apply any restrictive eligibility criteria on their account.

More often, however, these determinants are optimum only in certain subgroups of potential study patients. Accordingly, you'll need to decide whether to selectively enroll just these optimum subgroups. As I'll show you in a moment, changing the eligibility criteria to achieve this selective enrollment can result in large, indeed definitive, increases in the signal we produce in our trial. On the other hand, the opportunity costs of examining, lab testing, and imaging all patients in order to find that optimum subgroup can be prohibitive. Moreover, as noted earlier, restricting patient eligibility criteria might shift our RCT away from its intended "pragmatic" orientation toward an "explanatory" one. With this *caveat* in mind, I'll now demonstrate each of these four determinants and how they can be manipulated to maximize a treatment signal.

Maximizing the Signal by Selectively Enrolling "High-risk" Patients

Restricting eligibility to patients who are at higher than average "baseline" risks of outcome events leads to higher CERs on control (and experimental) therapy. The ARR signal is the product of this CER and the RRR from therapy. In terms of simple maths, ARR = CER × RRR (37). If the RRR is constant over different CERs, the experimental treatment will generate a larger ARR signal when the CER is high than when it is low. This is illustrated in Table 6–6. If the RRR is one fourth for all patients in the RCT (regardless of their CERs), notice the different impacts on the ARR signal and the corresponding confidence in the trial result when we enroll all patients and when we restrict enrollment to just the subgroups at high and low baseline risk. Recruiting and randomizing just the subgroup of 120 high-risk patients in Panel B generated both a higher ARR (up from 0.125 to 0.20) and a 20% narrower confidence interval around it (from ±100% to ±80%) than randomizing all 240 patients in Panel A. An examination of the low-risk patients in Panel C shows how they inflate the confidence interval around the ARR signal. In fact, every low-risk patient admitted to this trial makes the need for additional patients go up, not down!

Remember that this strategy works only when the RRR is either constant or increasing as CERs increase. Although there isn't much documentation about this, and there are some exceptions, I've concluded that RRR is pretty constant over different CERs when the treatment is designed to slow the progression of disease and prevent its complications. This has been observed, for example, in meta-analyses of aspirin and the secondary prevention of cardiovascular disease (38), and of both angiotensin-converting enzyme (ACE) inhibitors (39) and β blockers (40) in heart failure. Moreover, in an examination of 115 meta-analyses covering a wide range of medical treatments, the CER was twice as likely to be related to the ARR as to a surrogate for the RRR (the odds ratio), and in only 13% of the analyses did the RRR significantly vary over different CERs (41). When the treatment is designed to reverse the underlying disease, I've concluded that RRR should increase as CERs increase, exemplified by carotid endarterectomy for symptomatic carotid artery stenosis where the greatest RRRs are seen in patients with the most severe stenosis (and greatest stroke risks) (42).

When outcomes are "continuous" we can look for evidence on whether the experimental treatment will cause the same relative change in a continuous outcome (say, treadmill time) for patients with severe starting values (e.g., awful exercise tolerance, analogous to high-risk patients for discrete events) and good starting values (e.g., good but not wonderful exercise tolerance, analogous to low-risk patients for discrete events). If this evidence suggests a consistent relative effect over the range of the continuous measure, I hope it's clear why the AD signal generated by experimental treatment is greater (and its confidence interval narrower) among the initially severe patients than among the less severe ones (if this isn't clear, consider how much "room for improvement" there is in a patient who already is doing pretty well versus one who is doing poorly).

The Harsh Truth

Harsh as it may sound, we need people in our RCT who are the most likely to have the events we hope to prevent with our experimental treatment

TABLE 6–6 Effect of Enrolling only "High-risk" Patients with Higher Control Event Rates

	Panel A		Panel B		Panel C	
	All Eligible Patients ($n = 240$)		Just High-risk Patients ($n = 120$)		Just Low-risk Patients ($n = 120$)	
	Control	Exper.	Control	Exper.	Control	Exper.

E
v
e
n
t
s

Panel A Control	Panel A Exper.	Panel B Control	Panel B Exper.	Panel C Control	Panel C Exper.
	45			12	9
	75			48	51
60			36		
60			24		
		48			
		12			

	Panel A	Panel B	Panel C
Control event rate	0.50	0.80	0.20
Relative risk reduction	1/4	1/4	1/4
Experimental event rate	0.375	0.60	0.15
Absolute risk reduction	0.125	0.20	0.05
Size of the 95% confidence interval around that absolute risk reduction	±100%	±80%	±270%
P value	0.07	0.03	0.63

In Panel A we have randomized 240 patients into equal-sized control and experimental groups (and have lost none of them to follow-up). Although their overall risk of an event if left on conventional therapy is 50% (control event rate = 0.50), they are a heterogeneous lot and half of them (Panel B) are at high risk if left untreated (control event rate = 0.80) and half (Panel C) are at low risk (control event rate = 0.20). The relative risk reduction (1/4) is the same in all groups. Confidence intervals shown here are calculated as CI for a difference in absolute risk reductions, as described by Douglas Altman in: Sackett DL, Straus SE, Richardson WS, Rosenberg W, Haynes RB. *Evidence-based medicine*, 2nd ed. Edinburgh: Churchill Livingstone, 2000, p. 235.

(e.g., myocardial infarctions, relapses of a dreadful disease, or death). And, as long as the RRR from treatment is constant or rises with increasing CERs, these high-risk patients also have the most to gain from being in the trial. Finally, to be practical this "high-risk" strategy requires not only solid prior evidence that high- and low-risk patients exist, but also that their identification is easy and cheap enough to make their inclusion and exclusion cost-effective in conducting the trial.

The foregoing should cause second thoughts among trialists who are considering arbitrary upper age limits for their trials; they may be excluding precisely the high-risk patients who will benefit the most, raise the ARR, and make the largest contribution to the confidence in a positive result. On the other hand, if high-risk (or severe) patients are too far gone to be able to respond to the experimental therapy, or if competing events (e.g., all-cause mortality) swamp those of primary interest in the trial, the ARR's confidence interval will expand and its signal might decrease. This discussion introduces a second element, responsiveness.

Maximizing the Signal by Selectively Enrolling "Highly Responsive" Patients

The second way that we can increase the ARR signal and the confidence in a positive trial result is by *selectively enrolling highly responsive patients* who are more likely (than average) to respond to the experimental therapy. Their greater-than average RRRs translate to increased ARRs and higher confidence in positive trial results. This increased responsiveness can arise from two different sources. The first and most easily determined cause is patients' compliance with an efficacious experimental therapy. Those who take their medicine might respond to it, but those who don't take their medicine can't respond to it. No wonder, then, that so much attention is paid to promoting and maintaining high compliance during RCTs, and why some RCTs put patients through a prerandomization "faintness-of-heart" task, rejecting those who are unwilling or unable to comply with it. This is because once patients are randomized all of them must be included in subsequent analyses, even if they don't comply with their assigned treatment. The second cause for increased responsiveness is the result of real biologic differences in the way that subgroups of patients respond to experimental treatment. This biologic difference may be much more difficult (and expensive) to determine among otherwise eligible patients. Table 6–7 illustrates how either cause works among another 240 patients, this time with subgroups at the same baseline risk but with differing degrees of compliance (or other aspect of responsiveness).

Panel A of Table 6–7 is identical to Panel A of Table 6–6. If, as in Panel B of Table 6–7, just the highly compliant subgroup is recruited, the resulting confidence intervals around the ARR are narrower than those observed among all 240 patients. However, every patient with low compliance (Panel C) admitted to this trial made the need for additional patients go up, not down! Note that this high-response strategy works best when CERs are either constant or increasing among subgroups with progressively

TABLE 6–7 **Effect of Enrolling only Highly Responsive Patients**

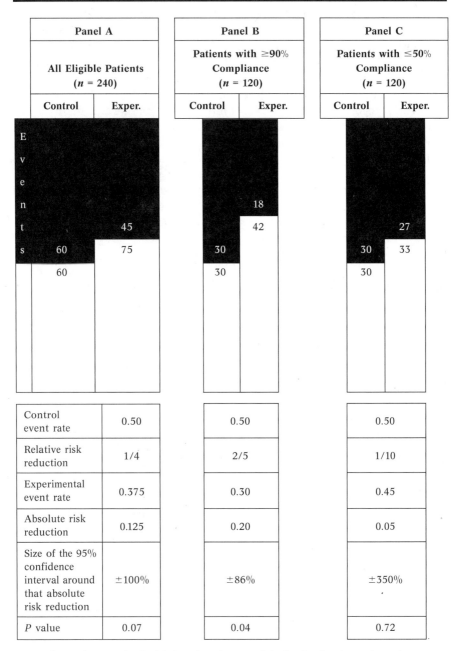

	Panel A		Panel B		Panel C	
	All Eligible Patients (*n* = 240)		**Patients with ≥90% Compliance** (*n* = 120)		**Patients with ≤50% Compliance** (*n* = 120)	
	Control	**Exper.**	**Control**	**Exper.**	**Control**	**Exper.**
Events	60	45	30	18 42	30	27 33
		60 75		30		30
Control event rate	0.50		0.50		0.50	
Relative risk reduction	1/4		2/5		1/10	
Experimental event rate	0.375		0.30		0.45	
Absolute risk reduction	0.125		0.20		0.05	
Size of the 95% confidence interval around that absolute risk reduction	±100%		±86%		±350%	
P value	0.07		0.04		0.72	

In Panel A we have randomized 240 patients into equal-sized control and experimental groups (and have lost none of them to follow-up). Although their overall compliance rate is great enough to achieve a relative risk reduction of 1/4, they are a heterogeneous lot and half of them (Panel B) take 90% or more of their study medication and achieve a relative risk reduction of 2/5, whereas the other half (Panel C) take 50% or less of it and achieve a relative risk reduction of only 1/10. The control event rate (0.50) is the same in all groups.

higher RRRs. Once again, although there isn't much documentation of CERs among subgroups with different responsiveness, patients in our carotid endarterectomy trials with higher CERs also enjoyed greater RRRs with surgery (19). As in the case of high-risk patients, the identification of high-response patients has to be both accurate and inexpensive if it is to decrease the total effort necessary for achieving a definitive trial result.

Maximizing the Signal by Combining Risk and Responsiveness

The foregoing elements of risk and responsiveness can usefully be combined as shown in Table 6–8, where I have summarized the "attractiveness" (in terms of maximizing the ARR signal and the confidence of a positive trial result) of different sorts of patients whom we might consider entering into our RCT. This will come home to haunt us if, toward the end of our recruitment phase, we are short of "ideal" patients (cell a) and decide to relax our inclusion criteria and start admitting patients who are at lower risk (cell c), less compliant (cell b) or both (cell d). As predicted in Tables 6–6 and 6–7, admitting low-risk, low-response patients may increase, rather than decrease, the remaining sample size requirement (and administrative burdens) that must be satisfied to achieve a sufficiently large ARR and sufficiently narrow confidence intervals around it.

There are 11 strategies that we can employ to either increase our sample size or make the most of whatever sample size we do recruit. These are presented in Section 5.8 ("Sample Size").

Once again, maximizing the signal by restricting admission to a trial forces it toward the explanatory pole and limits its extrapolation to all patients with the target disorder. We can have our cake and eat it too by admitting all-comers, but stratifying for risk and responsiveness before

TABLE 6–8 The Attractiveness of Different Sorts of Potential Randomized Controlled Trial Patients

		Responsiveness to (compliance with) the experimental Rx (relative risk reduction)	
		High	Low
Risk (control event rate)	High	Ideal! a	Are they too sick to benefit? Admit with caution b
	Low	c Are they too well to need any treatment? Admit with caution	d Keep out!

randomizing them, and prespecifying the subgroup analysis of the high-risk, highly responsive patients in cell a.

Maximizing the Signal by Giving Enough Treatment over Enough Time

The third way that we can tend to raise an ARR signal and the confidence in a positive trial result is to *employ a potent experimental treatment and to give it a chance to exert its effect.* We shouldn't expect patients to experience better outcomes when we don't give them sufficient doses of the experimental treatment for a sufficiently long time. Thus, an RCT to see whether drastic reductions in blood pressure reduce the risk of stroke must employ a drug that, in Phase 2 trials, really does reduce blood pressure to the desired level. This "be-sure-your-experimental-treatment-is-potent" strategy is dramatically demonstrated in surgical trials, where the principal investigators may restrict their clinical collaborators to just those surgeons with excellent skills and low perioperative complication rates. In a similar fashion, we should be sure that the experimental treatment is applied long enough to be able to achieve its favorable effects, if they are to occur.

If you digested the foregoing, you'll quickly grasp the incremental price of therapeutic progress that trialists must pay as they search for marginal improvements over treatments they already have shown, in previous RCTs, to do more good than harm. When today's standard treatment is already known (through prior RCTs) to do more good than harm, clinicians, and ethics committees should and will insist that this EET (rather than a placebo) be provided to the control patients in any subsequent RCT of the next generation of potentially more effective treatments. As a result, the CERs are progressively reduced in subsequent trials (they behave like the low-risk patients described above), and even if an RRR is maintained at its former level, its confidence interval will widen. It is not a surprise, then, that RCTs in acute myocardial infarction have become huge and hugely expensive, not (only) because cardiologists are an entrepreneurial lot, but (also) because they already are reducing CERs with the thrombolytics, β blockers, aspirin, and ACE inhibitors that they validated in previous positive trials.

As forecast in the introduction, the foregoing strategies for increasing the ARR and narrowing its confidence interval by restricting trial participants to just the high-risk, high-response group, by maximizing compliance, by employing just the best surgeons, and so forth moves the resultant trial away from a "pragmatic" study question ("does offering the treatment do more good than harm under usual circumstances?") toward an "explanatory" study question ("can rigorously applying the treatment do more good than harm under ideal circumstances?") (19). If the original question was highly pragmatic and was intended to compare treatment policies rather than rigorous regimens, the strategies described above may be unwise and it becomes more appropriate to conduct a really large, simple trial. Similarly, these restrictive strategies may raise concerns (and not a few hackles) about the "generalizability" of the trial result. As I've argued elsewhere (43), it is my contention that front-line clinicians do not want to "generalize" an RCT's results to all patients but only want to "particularize" its results to their individual patients and already routinely adapt the trial result (expressed, say, as a number needed to treat or NNT, which is the inverse of the ARR) to fit the unique risk and responsiveness of their individual patient, the skill of their local surgeon, the patient's preferences and expectations, and the like (44). Moreover, cautionary pronouncements about generalizability have credibility only if the failure to achieve it leads to qualitative differences in the kind of responses patients display such that, for example, experimental therapy is, on average, unambiguously helpful for patients inside the trial but equally unambiguously harmful or powerfully useless, on average, to similar patients outside it. This issue is discussed in Section 6.11 ("Large, Simple Trials").

Maximizing the Signal by Ascertaining Every Event

The fourth way that we can maximize an ARR signal and the confidence in a positive trial result is to make sure that we identify and record (that is, ascertain) every event suffered by every patient in the trial. Up to this point, I have assumed that all events have been ascertained in both control and experimental patients and that the resulting ARR signal, regardless of whether it is large or small, is true. In other words, although the ARRs displayed in Tables 6–6 and 6–7 are affected by the risk-responsiveness composition of the study patients, they nonetheless provide unbiased estimates of the effects of treatment. What happens in the real world of RCTs, where the ascertainment of events is virtually always incomplete? As you will see, this leads to systematic distortion of the ARR signal away from the truth; that is, this estimate of the signal becomes biased. Suppose that the RCT's follow-up procedures were loose, and many patients were lost. Or, suppose that the outcome criteria were so vague and subjective that lots of events were missed. If experimental and control patients are equally affected by this incomplete ascertainment, the situation depicted in Table 6–9 would occur, with a loss in the strength of the ARR signal even though the RRR is preserved. Accordingly, the fourth way that we can increase the ARR signal and the confidence in a positive trial result is by *improving the ascertainment of events during the RCT.* This is shown in Table 6–9.

The Price of Unequal Ascertainment Among Control and Experimental Patients

But what if the accuracy of ascertainment differed between control and experimental patients, such as might occur in nonblinded trials when experimental patients are more closely followed (e.g., for dose-management and the detection of toxicity) than control patients? What if that greater scrutiny of experimental patients led to missing only 5% of events in the experimental group while continuing to miss 25% of control events? This situation is shown in Table 6–10. Missing more events among control than experimental patients not only decreases the ARR signal but also widens its confidence interval. In this case, the bias leads to a "conservative" type

TABLE 6–9   **What Happens with Equally Incomplete Ascertainment of Events in Both Control and Experimental Patients**

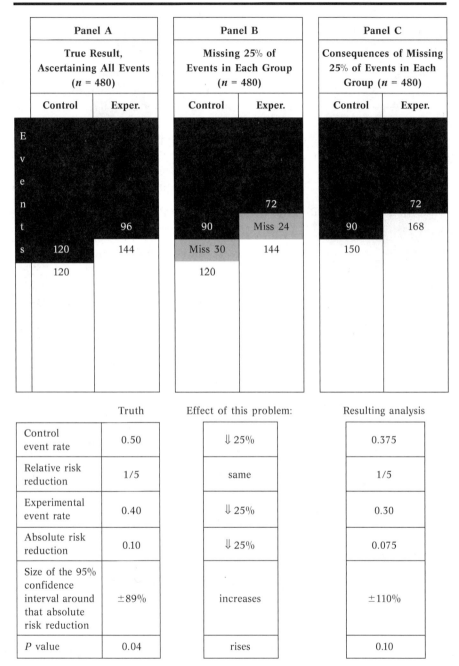

	Panel A		Panel B		Panel C	
	True Result, Ascertaining All Events (*n* = 480)		Missing 25% of Events in Each Group (*n* = 480)		Consequences of Missing 25% of Events in Each Group (*n* = 480)	
	Control	Exper.	Control	Exper.	Control	Exper.
E v e n t s		96	90	72 Miss 24	90	72 168
	120	144	Miss 30	144	150	
	120		120			

	Truth	Effect of this problem:	Resulting analysis
Control event rate	0.50	⇓ 25%	0.375
Relative risk reduction	1/5	same	1/5
Experimental event rate	0.40	⇓ 25%	0.30
Absolute risk reduction	0.10	⇓ 25%	0.075
Size of the 95% confidence interval around that absolute risk reduction	±89%	increases	±110%
P value	0.04	rises	0.10

Panel A of Table 6–9 displays the true effect of the experimental treatment: a relative risk reduction of 1/5, generating an absolute risk reduction signal of 0.10 whose confidence intervals exclude zero. If experimental and control patients are equally affected by this incomplete ascertainment (missing, say, 25% of events in both groups) the misclassification of events depicted in Panel B would occur. As a consequence, shown in Panel C, although the relative risk reduction is preserved, the absolute risk reduction signal declines from 0.10 to 0.075, its confidence interval now crosses zero, and the trial result becomes indeterminate.

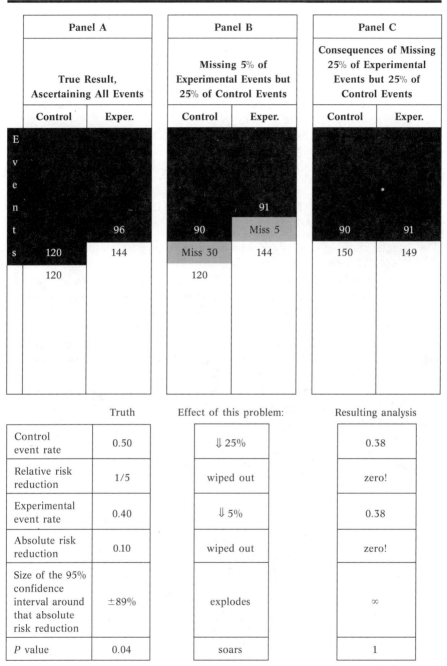

	Panel A		Panel B		Panel C	
	True Result, Ascertaining All Events		Missing 5% of Experimental Events but 25% of Control Events		Consequences of Missing 25% of Experimental Events but 25% of Control Events	
	Control	Exper.	Control	Exper.	Control	Exper.
Events				91		
		96	90	Miss 5	90	91
	120	144	Miss 30	144	150	149
	120		120			

	Truth	Effect of this problem:	Resulting analysis
Control event rate	0.50	⇓ 25%	0.38
Relative risk reduction	1/5	wiped out	zero!
Experimental event rate	0.40	⇓ 5%	0.38
Absolute risk reduction	0.10	wiped out	zero!
Size of the 95% confidence interval around that absolute risk reduction	±89%	explodes	∞
P value	0.04	soars	1

Panel A of Table 6–10 displays the true effect of the experimental treatment: as in Table 6–9, there is a relative risk reduction of 1/5, generating an absolute risk reduction signal of 0.10 whose confidence intervals exclude zero. If experimental and control patients are unequally affected by this incomplete ascertainment (missing 25% of events in the control group but only 5% of events in the experimental group) the misclassification of events depicted in Panel B of Table 6–10 would occur. As a consequence, shown in Panel C, both the relative and absolute risk reductions are falsely reduced and the trial draws a false-negative conclusion.

213

II error (concluding that the treatment may be useless when, in truth, it is efficacious) and presents a powerful additional argument for blind RCTs (because they maintain equal scrutiny of experimental and control patients and equal ascertainment of their outcome events).

A parallel lesson here is the need to achieve complete follow-up of patients in both explanatory and pragmatic trials. Remember, the important number in an RCT is *not* the *number of patients* in it, but the *number of outcome events* among those patients.

Having defined the determinants of the signal generated in an RCT and demonstrated how they can be manipulated to maximize that signal, it is time to consider how noise affects our confidence in the trial result, and how that noise can be reduced.

Determinants of the Noise, and How They Can Be Manipulated to Minimize It

The effects of noise and its reduction are perhaps best understood by considering RCTs whose outcomes are continuous measures (blood pressure, functional capacity, quality of life, and the like) rather than discrete events (major stroke, brain metastasis, death, and the like). The key to understanding noise is to think of *all sorts of factors* ("sources of variation" or, better yet, "sources of uncertainty") *that might affect the end-of-study result* for this continuous measure, not just in the individual study patient but especially in the groups of patients that comprise the experimental and control groups in the RCT.

Consider blood pressure. We know from prior experience that we won't get the same blood pressure result for every patient in an RCT. Indeed, we know that repeat measurements of blood pressure in the same patient at the same visit will generate different results (depending on whether it's the first or the fourth measurement at that visit, on whether she is inhaling or exhaling, on whether she is talking, on whether we are supporting her arm and back, and so forth). At the group level we must add the variation in blood pressure that exists between study patients (based not only on differences in their individual endocrine, cardiovascular, and nervous systems and responses to therapy but also on how well they know their examiner and the timing of their last cigarette, their last meal, their last conversation, their last void, and by which of several types of sphygmomanometers is being applied to them by which examiners with what hearing acuity and which preferences for the terminal digits 0, 2, 4, 6, and 8). These sources of variation in recorded blood pressure may, in combination, create so much noise that it becomes impossible to detect the signal (e.g., a small but important reduction in blood pressure) being generated by the experimental treatment.

Strategies for Minimizing Noise

How might we minimize this noise, recalling from the first section of this chapter that decreases in noise are rewarded by decreases in confidence intervals around signals and, therefore, by increases in our confidence about the results of the trial? In this case, the link between statistics and

TABLE 6–11 **Strategies for Reducing Noise in a Randomized Controlled Trial**

Strategy	Tactics
Validate eligibility	Make sure study patients have the target condition..
Crossover trial	Give both treatments to every patient, in random order.
Homogenize	Restrict participants to a single risk-response subgroup.
Minimize	Render experimental and control patients as identical as possible in their risk and responsiveness.
Maintain high compliance	Monitor compliance with study regimens, and apply compliance-improving strategies when needed.
Ascertain all events	Achieve complete follow-up of all study patients and ascertain outcomes in every one of them.

physiology is just about perfect. As summarized in Table 6–11, we reduce the noise element in our trial by eliminating or minimizing sources of uncertainty. I'll illustrate this with the blood pressure example.

1. We can *make sure that every study patient actually has the target condition* whose natural history we are attempting to change. Misdiagnoses at patient entry create subgroups of patients with the wrong conditions who may be incapable of responding to our experimental treatment, thus adding noise to the trial.

2. We can remove the uncertainty that arises from studying the two different treatments in separate, "parallel" groups of different patients (with their different baseline blood pressures and responses to treatment) by *applying both treatments to every patient.* This is accomplished by randomizing, for each patient, the order in which they receive the experimental and control regimens, separated by an intervening period of sufficient length to "wash-out" any effects of the previous regimen. This *"within-patient"* or *"crossover"* design, if feasible, removes the effect of any variation between study patients and usually produces big reductions in noise that are reflected in big reductions in confidence intervals (ambitious readers can verify this by contrasting the results of paired and unpaired *t* tests on a data set obtained from a crossover trial). Although theoretically attractive, crossover trials are not suited for disorders subject to irreversible events or total cures, and patients who withdraw or drop-out before completing both treatment periods are tough to analyze. Moreover, it is impossible to tell whether there is a "carry-over" of the effects of the first treatment into the second treatment period until the trial is over. When these carry-over effects are large, the data for the second period may have to be thrown away, the trial's noise continues unabated, and we are no better off than if the trial had been of a more usual "parallel" design in the first place.

3. We can reduce variations in the outcomes of study patients by making them more homogeneous through the same strategies that we employed in the previous section: *assembling study patients with similar risks* (e.g., just those with the highest blood pressures) and similar *responsiveness* to the experimental treatment. This can be done either by "restricting" admission to the trial to just those patients with similar risk and responsiveness or by stratifying study patients for these features and then randomizing from each stratum. The result is a narrower band of blood pressures and blood pressure changes with therapy (smaller standard deviations for these measures) and reduced noise. As previously mentioned, in explanatory surgical trials we routinely reduce uncertainty in responsiveness by drafting only those surgical collaborators who can document their high success and low complication rates.

4. We can reduce noise by *making experimental and control patients as similar as possible in their risk and responsiveness*. Although random allocation tends to create similar groups (and is our only hope for balance in unknown determinants of responsiveness), we can ensure similarity for known determinants by stratification prior to randomization or even by *minimization* (allocation of the next patient to whichever treatment group will minimize any differences between the groups) (45). Minimization is described with an example in Section 5.4 ("Allocation of Patients to Treatments").

5. In a similar fashion, we can reduce noise by achieving similar (and *high*) *compliance* among all study patients.

6. We can minimize sloppiness and inconsistency in the *ascertainment* of outcomes. Not only should our outcome criteria be objective and unambiguous, they should also be applied (or at least adjudicated) by two or more observers who are "blind" to which treatment a study patient has received. In trials whose outcomes are measured in ADs (e.g., in hemoglobin levels), noise is reduced by analyzing the averages of duplicate or triplicate determinations of the outcome.

Increasing Sample Size: the Last Resort

Reducing confidence intervals by increasing the size of an RCT should be a last resort. There are two major reasons for this admonition. First, as I stated at the start of this section, in order to halve the width of the confidence interval around the ARR achieved by our experimental treatment, we need to quadruple the number of patients in our trial. For example, in Panel A of Table 6–6, to halve the confidence interval for an ARR from ±100% to ±50% demands a quadrupling in sample size from 240 to 960 patients. Only after exhausting the foregoing strategies for increasing the signal and reducing the noise should we take on the daunting task of increasing our sample size. The second reason why it may be dangerous to attempt to rescue an RCT that is too small is that scouring recruitment sites with relaxed inclusion/exclusion criteria leads to the recruitment of low-risk, low-response patients. Tables 6–6 to 6–8 reveal that adding patients of these sorts can paradoxically lower ARRs and increase the confidence interval around them. Of course, sample size requirements can be revisited during a trial (with care not to destroy blindness), and methods are available for determining the risk of drawing false-negative conclusions after a trial is completed (46).

Gaining First-hand Experience with (and the "Feel" of) Physiological Statistics

Just as the understanding of human physiology benefits from dynamic laboratory and bedside (real-life) observations of the effects of altering a single determinant (say, peripheral resistance) on a "final common pathway" (say, arterial blood pressure), aspiring trialists can increase their understanding of physiological statistics by creating the tables in this chapter from their own protocols and data sets and by examining the effects of altering these determinants, singly and in combination, on a final common pathway such as the confidence interval around an ARR.

The simple experiment with the CD player and radio that opened this chapter provided primitive insights. Better still, and analogous to what can be learned from interactive computer models of human physiology, aspiring trialists can study the combined effects of different signal strengths, different amounts of noise, and different sample sizes in computer models of randomized trials. For example, a Clinical Trials Simulator has been developed by an international consortium that is promoting and aiding the performance of pragmatic trials in low-income countries. Its current version can be accessed via the Web site maintained by its principal creator, Eduardo Bergel (The Web site for the Controlled Trial Simulator is: http://www.randomization.org, and the discussion group for comments and questions is: http://groups.yahoo.com/group/trial-simulator/).

Users of these simulators can input whatever risks, responsiveness, compliance, loss to follow-up, ascertainment of outcomes, drop-outs, cross-overs, and so on, as they desire. The simulator then carries out a few hundred simulations in a few seconds and displays the effects of these inputs on both the validity of the hypothetical trials and the confidence intervals around their signals.

I reckon the more that trialists use such CD and radio, pencil-and-paper, or computer simulations to "massage" their assumptions before they start a trial, the less they'll have to "massage" their inconclusive data after the trial is over.

6.7 THE UNCERTAINTY PRINCIPLE AND EQUIPOISE

Under what circumstances should we conduct a trial to determine whether one treatment is better than another? How should we decide whether to offer trial enrollment and allocation to our patient? When should our patient accept our offer? The literature on these core questions is pretty dense, but we think it can be boiled down to two contrasting notions.

"No Preference" Between Treatments: Theoretical Equipoise

The first notion finds an RCT appropriate and ethical only when there is a "state of balance or equilibrium between two alternative therapies (47)" such that "there is no preference between treatments (i.e., it is thought equally likely that treatment A or B will turn out to be superior). At this point we may be said to be 'agnostic' ... we would take odds of 1:1 on a bet (48)." This "no preference" or "indifferent" point of view is sometimes referred to as "theoretical equipoise." (49).

Theoretical equipoise has never been present in any planning stage of trials in which I've taken part. Why (on earth!) would any trialist subject himself or his patients to an RCT if he didn't think that one of the treatments was probably better than the other?

Uncertainty

On the contrary, we undertake trials because we have a hunch that a particular (often new) treatment is probably better than the current standard therapy (in terms of efficacy, safety, affordability, etc.), but we're uncertain whether our hunch is correct. Our intellectual state is one of *uncertainty, not indifference.* We think the new treatment is probably better, but our "zone" of uncertainty includes the possibility that it is no better, or even worse, than current standard therapy.

Community Uncertainty, or Clinical Equipoise

We initiate a trial protocol when there is a "genuine uncertainty on the part of the expert clinical community about the comparative merits of two or more treatments for a defined group of patients or population" (50). When this uncertainty is claimed in a high-quality research grant application, and accepted by the appropriate ethics committees and funding sponsors, the trial proceeds. This uncertainty at the level of the professional community was usefully described by Benjamin Freedman, who labeled it "clinical equipoise."

Three Levels of Uncertainty

We recognize, deal with, and sometimes incorporate into our protocols three levels of uncertainty:

1. *Uncertainty in the community (clinical equipoise).* As above, this denotes "genuine uncertainty on the part of the expert clinical community about the comparative merits of two or more treatments." When sufficient numbers of clinicians, methodologists, and ethics committees are sufficiently uncertain whether an intervention is beneficial, an RCT is judged to be both necessary and appropriate.

   However, we will find, and must deal with, second, and third levels of uncertainty in designing and executing our RCT.

2. *Uncertainty in the individual clinician.* The second level of uncertainty concerns individual clinicians who are invited to recruit patients into a trial. Simply put, they may disagree with the prevailing

community uncertainty. On the contrary, they may feel certain that one of the trial treatments is clearly better than the other. As a result of their certainty, they wouldn't want to subject their patients to the risk of being allocated to the inferior treatment.

For example, in the early 1990s, several of my senior medical residents were certain that magnesium was beneficial in acute myocardial infarction. Their certainty was based on a meta-analysis of seven small RCTs that concluded that magnesium reduced mortality in such patients (51). Their certainty was put to the test when our hospital joined the Fourth International Study of Infarct Survival (ISIS-4) mega trial that randomized such patients to magnesium or placebo. Most other, uncertain, residents offered the trial to their patients. But a few of the equally bright, equally well-read, equally conscientious young clinicians working with me decided it was unethical for them to offer the trial to any of their patients. Their certainty that magnesium saved lives made it impossible for them to justify risking any of their patients to the chance of receiving placebo in the trial.

This example of uncertainty at the level of the individual clinician has a second lesson in store. In fact, ISIS-4 convincingly showed that magnesium was not beneficial to patients with heart attacks (52). Thus, individual clinicians' certainty about efficacy needn't be correct for it to determine their behavior.

Some caution about assigning preeminence to the individual clinician's views rather than to the community's views (53). In certain circumstances, they consider it "important for the individual physician to set aside his or her opinion, bias or 'certainty' in deference to the reasoned uncertainty that exists within the larger community of experts." I've yet to meet a clinician who agrees that this view is compatible with his or her responsibility to provide what he or she considers the optimal care to individual patients.

3. *Uncertainty within the patient–clinician partnership.* The third level of uncertainty arises when an individual patient and his or her clinician are deciding whether that patient should join a trial. It begins with the "informed consent" notion that protects the patient's freedom to refuse an invitation to enter, or remain in, an RCT. If the patient thinks that one of the treatments on offer (or even some treatment outside the trial) is better or safer than the other, then he or she is free to stay out of the trial and seek the preferred treatment.

To the patient's judgment, we add that of the clinician's: although he or she might offer the trial to most of his or her patients, does this particular patient have some special features that strongly suggest that one of the treatments on offer is clearly better or safer than the other? If this is so, the clinician feels honor bound to tell the patient so and to help them seek the preferred treatment. It is *only when both the patient and their clinician are uncertain which treatment is preferable that the patient is offered the opportunity to join the trial.*

This third level of uncertainty has been labelled the "uncertainty principle" by the Clinical Trial Service Unit at Oxford (36). Briefly, it states that when *either* the patient *or* the clinician think that one of the treatments on offer is better, the patient should be offered that treatment openly at once and should not be entered into the RCT. The patient enters the trial only when *both* the patient *and* the clinician are uncertain which treatment arm of the trial is better. As you already learned in the section on trial participants, adopting this third-level "uncertainty principle" can markedly simplify the eligibility criteria for a trial.

We can usefully conclude this discussion by bringing it full-circle back to its roots in community uncertainty. One way to think about the job of trial monitors (Data Safety and Monitoring Boards, or whatever) is as guardians of uncertainty at the community level. One of their vital tasks is to help the investigators determine whether and when the emerging outcome data are convincing enough to resolve community uncertainty about the therapy being tested. This function is described in detail in Section 5.9 ("Ethics of RCTs"), and in Section 5.10 ("Monitoring of Trials").

6.8 PLACEBOS, PLACEBO EFFECTS, AND PLACEBO ETHICS

What Is a Placebo?

In this discussion I'll define *placebo* as an inert pill, mock procedure, or non-therapeutic patient–clinician interaction introduced into an RCT in order to:

- blind both patients and the clinicians who are following their progress as to whether they are receiving the experimental or control treatment;
- isolate the "active" portion of the experimental treatment that distinguishes it from routine care.

The first objective, blinding, is essential if we are to avoid four sources of bias in determining efficacy:

1. When clinicians or patients know that the latter are receiving a placebo, they may give and take the active treatment outside the trial ("contamination-bias").
2. When clinicians or patients know that the latter are receiving a placebo, they may slip in other, additional treatments that might improve outcomes ("cointervention-bias").
3. When clinicians know which treatment the patient is receiving, they may be more or less likely to search out and report mild events, improvements or deteriorations, symptoms, and side effects ("ascertainment-bias").
4. When patients know which treatment they are receiving they may be more or less likely to report mild events, improvements or deteriorations, symptoms, and side effects (an "information-bias").

The second objective of using placebos is to isolate the unique effects of the active treatment over and above the "laying on of hands," paying and receiving attention, and the other elements of routine care.

To accomplish these objectives in drug trials, the placebo is a pill that appears identical to the active treatment by the senses of sight, smell, touch, and taste. In surgical trials, the placebo can be a sham operation involving nothing more than an incision. In trials of education or psychologic interventions, the placebo can consist of interactions of equal duration but devoid of the experimental maneuver (an "attention placebo").

What is the "Placebo Effect?"

A lot has been written about "placebo effects" (54,55). Most of it is confusing and some of it, in the view of trialists like us, is simply wrong.

We think the placebo effect can only be understood if we begin by recognizing that there are seven reasons why the health states of patients who participate in a randomized trial tend to improve during the course of the trial. Moreover, these improvements occur in trial patients *regardless of whether they are receiving the active treatment or a placebo:*

1. *The natural history of any illness.* Patients can spontaneously recover, or their symptoms may decrease or disappear, as a result of the natural course of their disease *in the absence of any treatment whatsoever.* This regularly occurs even in serious conditions such as multiple sclerosis, severe depression, unstable angina pectoris or threatened stroke.

2. *Regression to the mean (56).* We often recruit patients into trials because they are displaying an extremely high (say, blood pressure) or low (say, hemoglobin) value for some measure of their health or of their risk for disease. When we repeat these measurements a few weeks or months later, they will have returned to or toward normal values *in the absence of any treatment whatsoever.*

3. *Extraneous treatment.* Patients or the clinicians who care for them (both inside and outside the trial) can use other treatments that will relieve symptoms, prevent complications, or cure the target disorder.

4. *Investigator-expectation bias.* When investigators think (rightly or wrongly) that they know which treatment a trial patient is receiving, their "hunch" about the efficacy of that treatment can, consciously or unconsciously, bias them to over- or under-report that patient's events, symptoms, and side-effects.

5. *Patient-expectation bias.* When patients think (right or wrong) that they know which treatment they are receiving, their "hunch" about the efficacy of that treatment can, consciously or unconsciously, bias them to over- or under-report their own events, symptoms, and side-effects.

6. *Patient-appreciation bias.* When patients appreciate the attention and care they receive in an RCT, they can, consciously or unconsciously, show that they are "good" ("socially desirable") patients by

reporting spurious improvements in their symptoms and function in the absence of any real improvement.

7. *The effect of the active or placebo treatment that they received.* Finally, patient outcomes may be affected by the experimental or control (including placebo) treatments they receive in an RCT.

The first six improvements occur in *both* active treatment and placebo patients, and occur even when patients receive *neither active nor placebo treatment.*

It necessarily follows that the "placebo effect" (or "placebo response") during a trial can only be determined by correcting for these other six causes. Thus, the valid determination of the placebo effect is *not* a comparison of placebo patients at the start and end of a trial (for this "observed response in the placebo arm" is confounded with all the other causes for improvement). Alas, some investigators, especially in psychiatry, fail to make these corrections and incorrectly apply the term "placebo response (57)" to what is really the very much larger "observed response in the placebo arm."

The only valid determination of the "placebo effect" is a comparison of improvements among blinded placebo patients with those of patients who have received no treatment (active or placebo) at all during the trial. Fortunately, there have been more than 100 such "3-arm" trials in which patients agreed to be randomized to active treatment, to placebos, or to no treatment at all. A recent systematic review of these trials concluded that it had found no important placebo effects on objective or binary outcomes (58). Moreover, the placebo effect they observed in continuous or subjective outcomes was small, producing only 6.5% reductions in pain and shortening the time it took to fall asleep by about 10 minutes.

These conclusions are hotly debated, but if they are even half-right it becomes vital, in any discussion about placebos, that we carefully distinguish between the "placebo response/effect" and the very much larger "observed response in the placebo arm."

What are the Ethics of Using Placebos in Randomized Controlled Trials?

In our view, this boils down to whether an "EET" already exists for patients who are eligible for the RCT in question. By "EET" we mean a treatment that does more good than harm based on an examination of the totality of evidence derived from:

- systematic reviews of randomized trials (even though there may be just one trial), coupled with all available data about late or rare adverse effects of the treatment.
- "all or none" evidence (when, in a universally fatal condition, the therapy is followed by survival; or when a less frequent adverse outcome is totally eliminated following therapy).

The rules Penny Brasher (a cancer trialist–statistician), Stan Shapiro (a biostatistician–ethicist) and Dave Sackett suggested to a Canadian National Placebo Working Committee in 2002 for trials inside Canada were the following:

When there is NO established effective therapy. First, when there is NO "EET" for patients eligible for the trial (including patients who have previously refused EET, experienced severe adverse reactions to it, or are from subgroups known to be nonresponsive to it), we maintained that the methodologically sound and ethical trial is one in which experimental patients receive *general supportive care plus the new treatment*, and control patients receive *general supportive care plus placebo or no treatment*.

Indeed, in the absence of solid evidence regarding "EET" for patients with the target disorder, we held that it was unethical NOT to do a randomized trial of promising but untested therapy.

When there IS established effective therapy. Second, when there IS solid evidence for "EET" for patients with the target disorder and a promising new drug may provide *additional* benefit, we maintained that the scientifically sound and ethical trial is either:

1. When the promising new treatment, if effective, would be added to the EET: an "add-on" placebo trial in which experimental patients receive the EET *plus the new treatment* and control patients receive the EET *plus placebo or no treatment*.

2. When the promising new treatment, if effective, would be given in place of EET: a "head-to-head" trial in which experimental patients receive *the new treatment*, and control patients receive the EET (employing complementary placebos as necessary for blindness).

Our third recommendation stated that when there IS solid evidence for EET for patients with the target disorder, it is neither sensible (from a methodologic or clinical perspective) nor ethical to withhold that EET from control patients.

The recommendations we developed didn't address RCTs in places, inside as well as outside Canada, where the only EET was validated in RCTs conducted in high-income, urban situations. What if it can't be brought to geographically isolated patients (e.g., coronary angioplasty for the acute phase of myocardial infarction in the high Arctic)? What if it is too expensive to provide to low-income patients (e.g., costly retroviral drugs for patients with HIV–AIDS in sub-Saharan Africa)? When a low-income country or remote area seeks to determine the efficacy of affordable or accessible treatments, many trialists consider it ethical to withhold the "established effective *but unaffordable/inaccessible* therapy," and to test the promising, affordable/accessible treatment against placebo.

6.9 SPECIAL ISSUES IN NONDRUG TRIALS

Most RCTs test new drugs. They possess three advantages over trials of new operations, behavioral interventions, and organizational innovations. First, it is relatively easy to obtain support for them, especially from the drug industry. Second, they usually test patented compounds, so that their sponsors (and sometimes their investigators as well) can control and profit from their future use following positive trials. Third, their investigators pay only a small price when their experimental arms are shown to be useless or even harmful: reputations are rarely at stake, clinical earnings are rarely diminished, and no additional clinical training is required before moving on to test a different drug.

None of these conditions applies to surgical trials. Financial support for most surgical trials is abysmal (save for the occasional trial of an implantable device). The surgeon who "invented" the carotid endarterectomy didn't patent it nor did he receive commissions from all the surgeons who took it up subsequently. Moreover, when surgeons put "their" operation to the RCT test, the price for discovering that it is useless or harmful may not only tarnish their reputations; they may lose income if it is their "bread and butter" operation, and they may have to retrain in another procedure. For these reasons, trialists like me view surgical trialists as far more courageous than their medical colleagues.

These disadvantages also apply to behavioral interventions such as cognitive therapy or care giver support for postpartum depression. Funding for such nondrug trials is simply inadequate.

A relatively recent use of the RCT has been to test health care organizational interventions, and Cochrane Reviews of the RCTs have generated important conclusions (59). These trials have tested different sorts of clinicians, different educational and electronic ways of trying to improve their effectiveness and efficiency, different ways of organizing and paying them, and different ways of providing care to special populations in both high- and low-income countries.

Nonetheless, the fundamental scientific principles and requirements are identical for all trials, regardless of who is applying what experimental treatment to whom, and the rules of evidence can never be waived through "special pleading" by any group of health care providers or investigators. That being said, nondrug trials face special challenges to their ability to generate valid answers, and this section of the chapter will briefly consider them.

Surgical Trials

Trials of surgical procedures face eight methodologic challenges that are usually avoided by drug trials (60). Each of them must be identified and solved, or at least acknowledged, during the design phase. I think Robin McLeod has written the most useful paper on managing these challenges (61). They can be summarized as follows:

1. *Surgeons learn how to do things better; drugs don't need to.* A new drug has an identical effect on the cells, tissues, and organs of

the first and the millionth patient who takes it; not so for surgeons. There is a "learning curve" for a new operation, and individual surgeons' complication rates typically fall, sometimes dramatically, as they carry out the operation on more and more patients. For example, a study of 55 surgeons who performed 8,839 laparoscopic cholecystectomies calculated that the risk of bile duct injury was 10 times higher during their first attempt than during their fiftieth (62).

The surgical learning curve raises an interesting dilemma for the timing of surgical trials. Tom Chalmers, a famous trialist (and non-surgeon), suggested that his surgical colleagues should begin to randomize with the very first patient who is a candidate for their new operation. When they strenuously objected to his proposal, citing the learning curve for an operation that made it much safer and more effective on later patients, Tom's eyes would twinkle as he said: "Then shouldn't those first patients have a 50:50 chance that you'd learn how to do it right on somebody else?"

2. *Drugs work the same, regardless of the clinical competence of their prescribers; not so for operations.* Besides the learning curve, some surgeons are just plain better, safer operators than other surgeons. How surgical trialists handle this challenge depends on the question they are trying to answer. Suppose they are asking the explanatory or efficacy question that usually launches the first trial of an operation: "Among patients with disease X, can operation Y, carried out by the best of hands, do more good than harm?" In this case, it makes sense for the trialists to require potential surgical participants to have their case-records and track records scrutinized, letting only the best of them (who have completed their learning curves) join the trial. For example, in NASCET we appointed a panel of expert surgeons who scrutinized the last 50 carotid endarterectomies performed by potential collaborators, and invited only those with the fewest surgical complications to join the trial. However, suppose they are asking a pragmatic question: "Among patients with disease X, does a policy of referring them for operation Y, as carried out by the usually available surgeons, do more good than harm?" In this case, they would not screen out the less experienced or less competent surgeons.

A team of us led by PJ Devereaux has been exploring the implications of surgeon-to-surgeon differences in their preferences for, and expertise in, performing different operations (say, A and B) for the same clinical indication (63). If community uncertainty (clinical equipoise) exists over which operation is better, the operations warrant head-to-head comparisons in an RCT. But what should we do when, as is usually the case, some surgeons prefer, and are better at performing, operation A, and other surgeons, operation B. We believe a strong case can be made for "expertise-based" trials in which consenting patients are allocated to expert surgeons (who carry out just the operation they prefer and are expert in performing), rather than allocating patients to different operations, both performed by the same surgeon (who prefers, and is better at, just one of them).

3. *It is difficult or impossible to standardize a surgical intervention.* Most surgeons develop their own, idiosyncratic modifications of "standard" ways for dissecting and isolating target organs and tumors, removing organs, stopping bleeding, handling intra-operative emergencies and managing post-operative complications. A surgical aphorism I learned from David Grimes says it well: "The magic is in the magician, not in the wand." As a result, it is often impossible to define the experimental surgical intervention with precision. One solution is to attempt to standardize the procedure for all the important details. For example, the Dutch ColoRectal Cancer Group preceded its RCT of total mesorectal excision with a series of conferences and videos. Once the trial began, a senior surgeon directly supervised the first five operations at each participating hospital (64). A surrogate standardization can be inferred from a pre-trial requirement for equally favorable "outcomes" of the surgery. As previously mentioned, in the NASCET study of carotid endarterectomy surgeons had a free hand in selecting from a variety of approaches they used, but all had to have a perioperative complication rate less than 6% before they could join the trial (65).

4. *Surgeons are never "blind," and their patients are rarely "blind," to their operation.* "Blindness" to whether the experimental or control surgical maneuver has been carried out is never possible for the surgeon and often impossible for the patient. This becomes a major problem any time the psychological consequences of knowing one's treatment can affect the occurrence or reporting of key outcomes. Prime examples here are symptoms like pain, functional measures like exercise tolerance, and global measures like quality of life. Ingenious surgeons have sometimes devised, and enlightened ethics committees have sometimes allowed, the performance of "sham" operations on control patients. Sham procedures have proven crucial in "debunking" trials where the investigators' hunches are that the procedure is worthless. Back in the late 1950s, a group of surgeons made skin incisions and isolated the internal mammary arteries of patients with angina pectoris (a simple procedure done under local anesthetic). Only then were patients randomized to have their arteries tied off or simply to get closed up (66). Although these trials were far too small to generate powerful "no effect" analyses, the similarly rosy outcomes in both experimental and control patients was enough to convince clinicians that the emperors of internal mammary ligation might have no clothes.

About five decades later, another group of surgeons randomized patients with osteoarthritis of the knee to undergo arthroscopic debridement, arthroscopic lavage, or a sham ("placebo") procedure that involved just the skin incision and simulated debridement without insertion of the arthroscope (67). As they reported, "the 95% confidence intervals for the differences between the placebo group and the intervention groups (for pain and function) exclude any minimally important difference."

However, unblinded surgical trials are the rule. In such trials, surgical trialists do their best to develop "hard" outcome measures (such as tumor recurrence or death) that are relatively immune to the knowledge of one's treatment and have these measures applied by assessors who are blind to treatments.

5. *A surgical trial patient's ineligibility may not become known until after randomization.* A patient in a surgical trial may appear to be eligible until they are opened up and found to have the wrong disease, too extensive a disease (e.g., multiple metastases), or co-morbid conditions that violate the trial's eligibility criteria. Although ever more sensitive diagnostic imaging has improved the determination of ineligibility prior to surgery, this remains a problem, especially in explanatory trials, and sample size estimates need to be raised enough to overcome the need to retain unoperated patients in its surgical arm.

6. *Experimental drugs can be started within minutes of randomization; operations cannot.* Patients who die between randomization and operation are extreme examples of ineligibility. Trialists can minimize the number of such patients by requiring an operating room booking before randomization. For example, the median interval between randomization and carotid endarterectomy in the NASCET trial was 2 days.

7. *Cointervention is the rule in surgical trials.* Preop consultants, anesthesiologists, and recovery room staff add all sorts of treatments to patients in the surgical arms of surgical trials. Sometimes it is possible to standardize these cointerventions and apply them to control patients as well, but, many times, it is impossible, nonsensical, or unethical to do so. Often the best that can be done is to record and report cointerventions.

8. *Surgical trials may face special problems in recruitment.* Often, patients can obtain a new drug only within an RCT. This is not so for new operations, where the patient who wants it usually can get it outside the trial. This can hamper the recruitment of the required numbers of trial patients. Recruitment of surgeons can be difficult as well. Some surgeons fear a loss of their "referral base" if they offer the latest operation only within a trial. Others don't like the need to put trial patients through a much more rigorous consent process than would apply outside the trial. Although multicenter surgical trials can overcome these problems, they are difficult to fund and run.

Finally, surgical trials share other methodological challenges with drug trials. For example, one survey of 90 "negative" surgical trials found that only 24% had sufficient power to detect RRRs of 50% (68). Moreover, only 29% of them reported a formal sample size calculation. A set of users' guides for interpreting surgical trials has been developed, and it includes several pointers for their methodological improvement (69). Finally, a discussion of these problems in the BMJ in 2002 (70) suggested that training surgeons in clinical epidemiology, or at least employing epidemiologists in academic departments of surgery, could improve the quality of surgical trials.

On the other hand, surgical trials have some distinct advantages. One bright spot in surgical trials that include "no-surgery" control groups is their ability to debunk "operative complication" rates (that typically include all the bad things that happen at surgery or within 30 days afterward). We can correct this rate by subtracting from it what happened in the "no-operation" control patients over a similar period of time. For example, as described previously, NASCET patients randomized to carotid endarterectomy had their surgery an average of 2 days after randomization. Their rate of disabling stroke or death over the next 30 days was 2.0%. However, patients randomized to the medical arm of the trial had a 32-day rate of disabling stroke or death of 0.7%, demonstrating just how risky symptomatic high-grade carotid stenosis is. The corrected surgical complication rate (2.0% − 0.7% = 1.3%) was about one third lower than it appeared from case-series of carotid endarterectomies.

Moreover, surgical trials have a "compliance-advantage" over most drug trials. Once the operation is finished, patient compliance with their surgical treatment is no longer an issue.

Behavioral and Educational Trials

Trials of educational and behavioral maneuvers designed to improve the compliance of patients and the practices of clinicians have had to cope with most of the same problems as surgical trials. These include the learning curve, standardization, the lack of "blindness," and cointervention. Moreover, "contamination" becomes a problem whenever study patients receiving different treatments describe and discuss them with each other. In addition, trials of behavioral interventions among prisoners or the emotionally ill can raise special ethical issues, especially around coercion and informed consent. As with surgical trials, these challenges have been met by waiting for the completion of the learning curve, standardizing interventions and cointerventions wherever possible, and providing "attention placebos." Moreover, early and frequent interaction and mutual education between investigators and ethics committees have avoided mistakes on both sides.

Health Care Organization Trials

Trialists have only recently applied RCT methodology to matters of the organization and delivery of health care. However, the growth, scope, and ingenuity of these health care trials are impressive. The impetus for their execution may have more to do with improving the efficiency of health care than its effectiveness. Nonetheless, the opportunity costs of not doing health care trials include wasting the health care budget on useless activity at the expense of effective health care, even when the latter is cheap.

Contamination is a major problem in health care trials. For example, it is unreasonable to expect a clinician to respond to feedback about the costs of lab tests for just one half of her patients, but not for the other half. To reduce this sort of contamination, health care trialists often employ "cluster randomization." In cluster randomization, the same intervention is applied to, or withheld from, all members of a family (in a trial of care by nurse practitioners versus family physicians), or of an entire clinical team or setting (in a trial of lab cost feedback versus no feedback), or of an entire village (in a trial of a public health maneuver). The price for reducing contamination by cluster randomization is the need for an increase in total sample size. This increase is proportional to the tendency of the members within the cluster to respond to the experimental maneuver in the same way (71).

I think that Duncan Neuhauser, Victoria Cargill, and David Cohen in Cleveland, and Kurt Kroenke at Fort Sam Houston in Texas, initiated the most innovative approach for conducting RCTs in clinical settings (72). They randomized not only patients but also housestaff (from the start of their training) to the clinical "firms" who operated their own outpatient and inpatient services at their hospitals. They then carried out a series of cluster-randomized trials of health care maneuvers such as giving feedback about the costs of diagnostic tests, giving seminars and checklists for offering preventive interventions, and providing intravenous therapy teams. They not only achieved very high comparability between both patients and clinicians in their control and experimental firms but also kept contamination low.

Cluster health care organization trials can be carried out at a fraction of the cost of drug, surgical, or behavioral trials. First, in the "firms trials" it cost about the same to randomize patients and housestaff into comparable firms as to assign them by the former system. Moreover, the investigators often could ascertain outcomes from routinely collected data. These strategies made the firms trials so cheap that their investigators didn't even apply for outside funding for the first two of them (and a later investigator claimed he could fund his <US $500 trial by selling brownies and tee shirts and have money left over). A special supplement to the July 1991 issue of *Medical Care* is devoted to firms trials.

Their cluster trial of intravenous (i.v.) teams applied a useful allocation strategy and generated a supremely useful result. First, all firms eventually received the services of an i.v. team; what was randomized was the *order* in which they received them. This allocation strategy is worth considering when any new program can't be started in all practices, villages, or provinces at the same time.

Second, when the hospital administration later tried to eliminate the i.v. teams to save money, the firms had RCT evidence to back their request that it be maintained. When they submitted evidence that the teams had reduced the frequency (and cost) of intravenous catheter-related complications, the administration backed down.

6.10 THE CONSOLIDATED STANDARDS OF REPORTING TRIALS (CONSORT) STATEMENT

In the mid-1990s a group of trialists (including me), statisticians, epidemiologists, and biomedical journal editors met in Ottawa to discuss our concerns over the deficiencies in the way that RCTs were being reported. Each of us had encountered too many instances in which trials were called "randomized" when they were not, participating clinicians were revealed to have had advance notice of the treatment to which their next patient would be allocated, definitions of primary events (outcome measures) appeared to have been changed after the investigators "peeked" at them during the progress of a trial, and trial patients unaccountably disappeared or were inappropriately declared "ineligible" for final analyses.

At about that same time, some participants had begun to carry out systematic reviews of trials that had committed and avoided these errors (73), and found that nonrandomized trials generated both over- and underestimates of efficacy, that the failure to conceal a randomization list led to the overestimation of efficacy, and that the return of "ineligible" patients to the final analysis often erased a treatment's apparent benefit.

We decided that both clinicians and patients would benefit if an RCT's strengths and weaknesses were made clear in its report and set about devising a "checklist" and "patient flow-diagram" that we thought authors ought to employ in writing up their trials. We also considered whether each recommendation was supported by solid evidence that it contributed to the validity of an RCT (see the note accompanying Table 6–12). Where possible, the inclusion of an item on the checklist was justified from empirical research (e.g., a systematic review of trials that met and failed that item), but other items were included based only on our "expert" opinions (and we acknowledged the deficiencies (9) of that approach). The eventual result was the CONSORT statement (74).

The CONSORT statement received a huge boost when it was endorsed by editors of the leading clinical journals, culminating with its support by the "Vancouver Group" (The International Committee of Medical Journal Editors). Its use expanded rapidly, and it probably made a difference. Some studies comparing the reporting of RCTs before and after the adoption of CONSORT suggested that it made trial reports more transparent. For example, clear statements about whether the destined allocation of the next patient was concealed from their clinician in one set of journals rose from 39% of trial reports in 1994 to 61% by 1998 (75). However, other studies documented how far we still have to go. For example, a team led by PJ Devereaux reported in 2002 that 6 of 11 methodological items in the CONSORT checklist were reported in less than 50% of the papers published in 29 medical journals (76).

On the other hand, "bad" reporting does not necessarily mean "bad" methods. For example, Heloisa Soares led a team who compared the protocols of 56 radiation oncology trials with their subsequent publications (77). Although all trials concealed their randomization, only 42% reported doing so. Alpha and beta errors were specified in 74% of the

TABLE 6–12 **Consolidated Standards of Reporting Trials (CONSORT) Checklist of Items to Include when Reporting a Randomized Trial**

PAPER SECTION And Topic	Item	Description
TITLE and ABSTRACT	1	How participants were allocated to interventions (e.g., "random allocation," "randomized," or "randomly assigned")
INTRODUCTION		
Background	2	Scientific background and explanation of rationale
METHODS		
Participants	3	Eligibility criteria for participants and the settings and locations where the data were collected
Interventions	4	Precise details of the interventions intended for each group and how and when they were actually administered
Objectives	5	Specific objectives and hypotheses
Outcomes	6	Clearly defined primary and secondary outcome measures and, when applicable, any methods used to enhance the quality of measurements (e.g., multiple observations, training of assessors)
Sample size	7	How sample size was determined and, when applicable, explanation of any interim analyses and stopping rules
Randomization– sequence generation	8	Method used to generate the random allocation sequence, including details of any restrictions (e.g., blocking and stratification)
Randomization– allocation concealment	9	Method used to implement the random allocation sequence (e.g., numbered containers or central telephone), clarifying whether the sequence was concealed until interventions were assigned
Randomization– implementation	10	Who generated the allocation sequence, who enrolled participants, and who assigned participants to their groups
Blinding (masking)	11	Whether the participants, those administering the interventions, and those assessing the outcomes were blinded to group assignment. When relevant, how the success of blinding was evaluated
Statistical methods	12	Statistical methods used to compare groups for primary outcome(s); methods for additional analyses, such as subgroup analyses and adjusted analyses

(continued)

TABLE 6–12 (Continued)

PAPER SECTION And Topic	Item	Description
RESULTS		
Participant flow	13	Flow of participants through each stage (a diagram is strongly recommended). Specifically, for each group, report the numbers of participants randomly assigned, receiving intended treatment, completing the study protocol, and being analyzed for the primary outcome. Describe protocol deviations from study as planned, together with reasons
Recruitment	14	Dates defining the periods of recruitment and follow-up
Baseline data	15	Baseline demographic and clinical characteristics of each group
Numbers analyzed	16	Number of participants (denominator) in each group included in each analysis and whether the analysis was by "intention-to-treat." State the results in absolute numbers when feasible (e.g., 10/20, not 50%)
Outcomes and estimation	17	For each primary and secondary outcome, a summary of results for each group, and the estimated effect size and its precision (e.g., 95% confidence interval)
Ancillary analyses	18	Address multiplicity by reporting any other analyses performed, including subgroup analyses and adjusted analyses, indicating those prespecified and those exploratory
Adverse events	19	All important adverse events or side effects in each intervention group
DISCUSSION		
Interpretation	20	Interpretation of the results, taking into account study hypotheses, sources of potential bias or imprecision and the dangers associated with multiplicity of analyses and outcomes
Generalizability	21	Generalizability (external validity) of the trial findings
Overall evidence	22	General interpretation of the results in the context of current evidence

Table reproduced from the CONSORT Web site 25 November 2004.

protocols but appeared in only 10% of the reports. As more journals force authors to follow the CONSORT checklist (and, better yet, provide Internet links to their protocols), this disparity should decrease.

The CONSORT group is alive and well. It periodically revises the CONSORT statement based on proposals from its members and the feedback it receives (78). For example, it has developed criteria for reporting cluster trials (79), and for reporting harm (80). In addition, a subcommittee of us is tracking down, appraising, and summarizing both individual methodological studies and systematic reviews of "Evidence Supporting CONSORT On Reporting Trials" (or ESCORT). CONSORT and ESCORT share the Web site at *http://www.consort-statement.org/*.

The 2004 Web site version of the CONSORT statement appears in Table 6–12, and its accompanying patient flow diagram is shown in Figure 6–5.

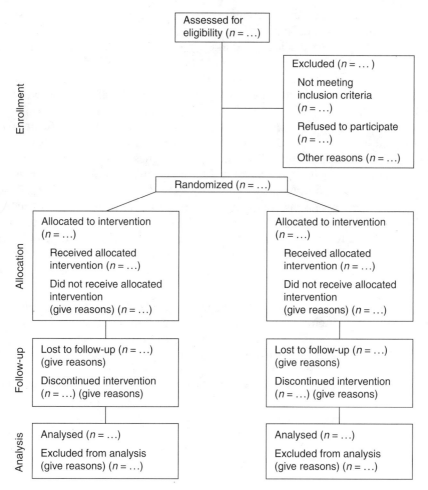

FIGURE 6–5 Revised template of the CONSORT diagram showing the flow of participants through each stage of a randomized trial.

6.11 LARGE, SIMPLE TRIALS

The first large, simple trial I know about was the 1954 trial of the Salk polio vaccine that randomized over 600,000 US school children (81). However, nearly everybody seems to have forgotten this strategy for the next 30 years. It was in 1984 that Salim Yusuf, Rory Collins, and Richard Peto described the scientific and pragmatic basis for large, simple trials (35). They presented four powerful arguments in their rationale:

1. For the major killing diseases, any treatment of overwhelming efficacy would have shown itself long ago and wouldn't need an RCT of any size to prove it. Moreover, patients with killing diseases die through a variety of mechanisms, and we shouldn't expect any single treatment to influence more than one of them. We therefore must look for only moderate but worthwhile effects of new treatments, say RRRs for death in the range of 25%. Although this might not seem an important accomplishment, if one tenth of a million women with coronary heart disease were likely to die in the next 5 years, a treatment with a RRR of 25% would save 25,000 of them.

   To confidently show (say, $P = 0.001$) this moderate but important effect, we would need to enroll about 10,000 of these women. However, we already know that the sample sizes of most RCTs are in the dozens or hundreds. These trials are far too small to be able to detect RRRs of 25% (or even 30% or 40%) when the CER is 0.10. For example, Salim Yusuf and his colleagues reported that 21 of 24 trials of long-term β blockade following myocardial infarction were too small to individually detect the 22% RRR established in a subsequent meta-analysis. Returning to our example of women with coronary heart disease, a trial of only 500 of them would be more than 90% likely to *fail* to show the efficacy of a treatment that reduced death by one-fourth. As a result, *trials of promising treatments with important but only moderate effects (on important diseases) need to be really large.*

2. For ultimately fatal diseases, preventing or delaying death provides a more convincing measure of efficacy than improving signs, symptoms, imaging, or laboratory tests. Death is simple, cheap, and unambiguous to determine. However, trials become complex and expensive when outcomes are signs (such as blood pressure in hypertension), symptoms (such as angina in coronary heart disease), diagnostic images (such as heart size in heart failure), or laboratory tests (such as tumor markers in cancer). This latter sort of trial is better suited for studying mechanisms than for determining efficacy. As a result, *trials that use death as the measure of efficacy can have very simple follow-up and adjudication procedures.*

3. For a treatment to be widely prescribed by busy clinicians to typical (i.e., not-very-compliant) patients, it has to be an easy regimen to

prescribe, to follow, and to monitor. As a result, *trials of practical treatments can have very simple interventions.*

4. We should expect to observe differences in the *degree* of responsiveness of different patient subgroups to the experimental treatment (they called this a "quantitative interaction"). However, we should not expect to observe a difference in the *direction* of responsiveness such that one subgroup would benefit from the treatment while another subgroup is totally unaffected or harmed by it (they called this a "qualitative interaction"). Moreover, if a trial is very large, even the subgroups that exhibit quantitative interactions should be equally distributed among the treatments. Two conclusions follow from this. First, really large trials needn't spend time and money on extensive baseline measurements. As a result, *really large trials can have cheap, fast, and simple procedures for enrolling patients.* Second, we are unlikely to improve the reliability of the primary analysis for efficacy by identifying and statistically adjusting for such subgroups. As a result, *really large trials can have simple analyses.*

In the 20 years since their paper, trialists around the world have successfully carried out lots of large, simple trials. I think the classic modern example is ISIS-4. In it, the investigators recruited over 58,000 patients with suspected acute myocardial infarctions in just 26 months (82).

In the eyes of most trialists and clinicians, one large, high-quality, simple trial beats any meta-analysis of several small ones of varying quality. For example, a meta-analysis of several trials on a total of about 4,000 patients concluded that magnesium administration saved lives during myocardial infarction (83). This conclusion was crushed by the just described large, simple ISIS-4 trial of 58,050 patients that revealed magnesium to be worthless in this situation.

As you'll see in the Small Trials section that follows, large, simple trials are not necessary for many chronic, nonfatal disorders in which the goals of therapy are improvements in symptoms, function, or quality of life. Moreover, some trialists (especially in the United States) argue that large, simple trials are just too simple to permit identification of mechanisms or of subgroups of patients at the extremes of risk and responsiveness.

The last two decades also have seen the laudable emergence of large, not-so-simple ("mega") trials. These trials conduct more extensive baseline studies, apply more complex treatments, use more complex designs, and monitor for nonfatal events. A recent example is the Heart Outcomes Prevention Evaluation (HOPE) factorial trial, also led by Salim Yusuf. It enrolled 9,297 patients who, for a variety of reasons, were at high risk of nonfatal and fatal cardiovascular events. Treating them with ramipril (an ACE inhibitor) produced a 22% RRR for myocardial infarction, stroke, or cardiovascular death (84). On the other hand, the point estimate of the effect of vitamin E in this trial was a 5% increase in these events, and its 95% confidence interval excluded a benefit as small as 6% (85).

6.12 SMALL TRIALS

A team of us, led by Brian Haynes, asked the question: "Among hypertensive steel workers who are neither compliant with antihypertensive drugs, nor at goal blood pressure six months after starting treatment, could a compound behavioral intervention (teaching them how to measure their own blood pressures, asking them to chart their own blood pressures and pill-taking, teaching them how to "tailor" their pill-taking to their daily habits and rituals, checking their progress every two weeks, and rewarding positive changes), provided by a high school graduate with no health professional training, compared to an 'attention placebo,' improve their compliance and blood pressure control over the next six months?" Only 38 patients entered our trial (86). We allocated them to the experimental and control groups by concealed minimization (taking into account each patients' blood pressure level, compliance, and prior exposure to instruction about their hypertension). Despite their small number (20 experimental and 18 control patients), they were enough to show, with great confidence, that the combined outcome of increased compliance and decreased diastolic blood pressure was far more likely to occur among experimental patients (70% versus 11%; $P = 0.001$).

Most of the examples in this chapter come from the large, long, complicated RCTs that occupy most of my time. This section has the purpose of showing that small RCTs are not only possible but also often sufficient to generate highly confident answers to questions about efficacy.

Small RCTs can serve three useful purposes, as summarized in Table 6–13 (87).

1. Their first purpose follows from the fact that the important number in an RCT is the number of events, not the number of patients. As a result, small trials can be large enough to provide confident, definitive answers to important questions. The record for smallness, as far as I know, is held by a crossover trial of a β blocker (pronethalol) for angina pectoris that was conducted three decades ago. As later

TABLE 6–13   **Useful Purposes Served by Small Trials**

Purpose Served	Explanation
1 Providing a definitive answer to a question about efficacy	The important number in an RCT is the number of events, not the number of patients
2 Suggesting that the "expert" emperor has no clothes	A small, indeterminate RCT can still be big enough to create uncertainty
3 Supplying randomized evidence for meta-analysis	Larger numbers generate smaller confidence intervals

RCT, randomized controlled trial.

recalled by Richard Doll (88), it required only 12 patients to generate a P value of 0.003 (89).

Those days are gone forever in angina trials because the growing array of efficacious interventions has sent CERs plummeting. For example, a recent multicenter trial of an intravenous β blocker versus "standard care," despite recruiting nine times as many patients as the pronethalol trial, failed to achieve a definitive answer (90).

There is an only semifacetious moral here for budding trialists. Pick a primitive specialty (where they've never validated any of their interventions) for your first RCT. Then, test its most promising (but unproven) intervention against a placebo for its ability to improve short-term outcomes. Specialties with a long tradition of performing RCTs are victims of their own progress. They must replace placebos with treatments they've validated in prior RCTs. This translates to decreases in CERs and ARRs. As a result, they need to perform ever larger RCTs to confidently show that this year's addition to the treatment regimen is superior to last year's, even when their RRRs are identical.

2. The second useful purpose served by small trials is to reveal that the "expert" emperor may have no clothes: that this year's experts are as full of baloney as last century's. Even small, indeterminate trials (with huge confidence intervals) can prompt us to question conventional but untested therapeutic wisdom. Consider the internal mammary artery. Surgeons now use it with considerable success as a conduit in coronary artery bypass grafting for intractable angina pectoris. Forty years ago, with that same objective in mind, they tied it off! This was because, believe it or not, they found that the simple ligation of the internal mammary artery (a very safe operation, easily performed using local anesthesia) was followed by both subjective and objective improvement of angina. Pain lessened, and electrocardiograms and treadmill tests improved in more than three fourths of the patients who underwent the procedure (91). No wonder, then, that this operation rapidly gained popularity throughout Europe and North America.

    Then R.G. Fish and his colleagues suspected that its apparent efficacy might be a "placebo effect" [if this is a new term for you, visit the section on placeboes (Section 6.8) of this chapter]. Accordingly, they told a group of preoperative patients that the procedure was experimental, had no physiological basis, and was of uncertain benefit. Only 20% (rather than the usual 75%) of their patients improved (92). Their results generated enough uncertainty in the cardiology community to conduct two simultaneous small RCTs of internal mammary artery ligation. In these trials, the operation proceeded to the point of placing a loose ligature around the isolated internal mammary artery. Then, they opened a sealed envelope that told them to tie off the arteries of a random half of patients, and to leave the other half alone. On follow-up, the sham-operated patients fared as well as those whose arteries were tied off. The "expert" emperor's nether parts were exposed to all, and the procedure was rapidly abandoned.

Although conducted to answer an important clinical question and used to justify randomized trials of coronary bypass two decades later, these two "negative" trials contained a grand sum of just 35 patients. To confidently exclude even the huge relative risk improvement of 50% in symptoms and function, however, they should have enrolled four times as many. Although they were too small to be conclusive in terms of formal statistics, these small trials changed the course of cardiac surgery. These trials not only forced the rethinking of expert opinion and the biologic rationale for the operation but also led to its abandonment.

3. Third, small trials, even when individually inconclusive, can serve as the basis for convincingly conclusive overviews and meta-analyses. For example, infusing albumin in the attempt to save the lives of critically ill burn patients was "standard" practice for decades. When three small RCTs (among 14, 79, and 70 patients, respectively) generated conflicting evidence on whether this practice actually saved or cost lives, they were combined in a meta-analysis (93). This meta-analysis generated a relative risk of dying following albumin infusion of 2.4 (95% confidence interval from 1.1 to 5.2) in burn patients. Moreover, when combined with a meta-analysis of 28 other small RCTs performed in patients with hypovolemia or hypoproteinemia, it emerged that for every 20 patients treated for one of these conditions with albumin infusions, 1 more patient would die. This startling meta-analysis of 31 trials with an average size of just 51 patients had major repercussions among clinicians (many of whom stopped using albumin in these patients) and regulators (some of whom cautioned against its further use in them). Moreover, it led to the design and initiation of a large albumin trial with a target sample size of 7,000 (over four times as many patients as all previous trials combined).

Some ethicists and trialists hold that it is inappropriate to embark on an RCT when we know that it is too small to generate a confident answer about efficacy. I disagree with this view, and discuss it, along with other special ethical issues in RCTs, in Section 5.9. However, to justify small trials on the basis of later inclusion in systematic reviews, they must be registered at their inceptions (rather than left unreported at their conclusions) so that later meta-analysts can find them.

If you have a question or comment about any of this chapter (or if you've caught us in a typo!) go to the book's website at: *http://hiru. mcmaster.ca/CLEP3*. There you also will find comments from us and other readers, chapter updates, and examples of how the authors and others use the book in teaching.

REFERENCES

1. Cox DR. Regression models and life tables. *J Roy Statist Soc B* 1972;34:187–220.
2. Silverman WA, Chalmers I. Casting and drawing lots. In: Chalmers I, Milne I, Tröhler U, eds. *The James Lind library*. [cited 2003 Sept. 25]. Available from (*http://www.jameslindlibrary.org*).

3. Black N. Why we need observational studies to evaluate the effectiveness of health care. *BMJ* 1996;312:1215–1218.

4. Writing Group for the Women's Health Initiative Investigators. Risks and benefits of estrogen plus progestin in healthy postmenopausal women; principal results from the Women's Health Initiative Randomized Controlled Trial. *JAMA* 2002;288: 321–333.

5. Heart Protection Study Collaborative Group. MRC/BHF Heart Protection Study of antioxidant vitamin supplementation in 20,536 high-risk individuals: a randomised placebo-controlled trial. *Lancet* 2002;360:23–33.

6. Kunz R, Vist G, Oxman AD. Randomisation to protect against selection bias in healthcare trials (Cochrane Review). In: *The Cochrane library*, (Issue 2): Oxford University Press, Update Software, 2003.

7. Hill AB. Suspended judgment. memories of the British streptomycin trial in tuberculosis. The first randomized clinical trial. *Control Clin Trials* 1990;11:77–79.

8. Chalmers I. Statistical theory was not the reason that randomisation was used in the British Medical Research Council's clinical trial of streptomycin for pulmonary tuberculosis. In: Weisz G, Jorland G, Opinel A, eds. *Quantification in the medical and health sciences in historical and sociological perspective*. Montreal: McGill-Queens University Press, 2005.

9. Sackett DL. The sins of expertness, and a proposal for redemption. *BMJ* 2000;320:1283.

10. van Helmont JA. *Oriatrike, or physick refined: the common errors therein refuted and the whole are reformed and rectified* [translated by J Chandler]. London: Lodowick-Loyd, 1662:526.

11. Schmidt PJ. Transfuse George Washington. *Transfusion* 2002;42:275–277.

12. Differences between the people compared. The James Lind Library (*http:// www.jameslindlibrary.org*). Accessed Wednesday 24 November 2004. © I Chalmers 2002.

13. Chalmers I, Toth B. Thomas Graham Balfour's 1854 report of a clinical trial of belladonna given to prevent scarlet fever. The James Lind Library (*http://www.jameslindlibrary.org*). Accessed Wednesday 17 November 2004. © I Chalmers 2002.

14. Kidwell CS, Liebeskind DS, Starkman S. Trends in acute ischemic stroke trials through the 20th century. *Stroke* 2001;32:1349–1359.

15. Palesch YY, Tilley BC, Sackett DL, et al. Can futile Phase III randomized trials be prevented? *Submitted* 2004 or: Tilley BC. Learning from the Past: Neuroprotective trials. Annual Meeting of the Society for Clinical Trials, Denver, Colorado, USA, 2001.

16. Sackett DL, Haynes RB, Gent M, et al. Compliance. In: Inman WHW, ed. *Monitoring for drug safety*. Lancaster: MTP Press, 1980.

17. Graham DJ, Staffa JA, Shatin D. Incidence of hospitalized rhabdomyolysis in patients treated with lipid-lowering drugs. *JAMA* 2004;292:2585–2590.

18. Schwartz D, Lellouch J. Explanatory and pragmatic attitudes in therapeutic trials. *J Chron Dis* 1967;20:637–648.

19. Sackett DL, Gent M. Controversy in counting and attributing events in clinical trials. *N Engl J Med* 1979;301:1410–1412.

20. Haynes RB, Dantes R. Patient compliance and the conduct and interpretation of therapeutic trials. *Control Clin Trials* 1987;8:12–19.

21. North American Symptomatic Carotid Endarterectomy Trial (NASCET) Collaborators. Beneficial effect of carotid endarterectomy in symptomatic patients with high-grade carotid stenosis. *N Engl J Med* 1991;325:445–453.

22. Banerjee SN, Raskob G, Hull RD, A new design to permit the simultaneous performance of explanatory and management randomized clinical trials. *Clin Res* 1984; 32:543A.

23. Sackett DL. Superiority trials, noninferiority trials, and prisoners of the 2-sided null hypothesis (Editorial). *ACP J Club* 2004;140:A-11–2.

24. Alderson P, Chalmers I. Survey of claims of no effect in abstracts of Cochrane reviews. *BMJ* 2003;326:475.

25. Dunnett CW, Gent M. An alternative to the use of two-sided tests in clinical trials. *Stat Med* 1996;15:1729-1738.

26. Ware JH, Antman EM. Equivalence trials. *N Engl J Med* 1997;337:1159-1161.

27. Sackett DL, Spitzer WO, Gent M, et al. The Burlington randomized trial of the nurse practitioner: health outcomes of patients. *Ann Intern Med* 1974;80:137-142.

28. The EC/IC Bypass Study Group. Failure of extracranial-intracranial arterial bypass to reduce the risk of ischemic stroke. Results of an International randomized trial. *N Engl J Med* 1985;313:1191-1200.

29. The EC/IC Bypass Study Group. Failure of extracranial-intracranial arterial bypass to reduce the risk of ischemic stroke. *N Engl J Med* 1985;313:1191-1200.

30. Rothman KJ, Michels KB. The continuing unethical use of placebo controls. *N Engl J Med* 1994;331:394-398.

31. Michels KB, Rothman KJ. Update on unethical use of placebos in randomised trials. *Bioethics* 2003;17:188-204.

32. Tugwell P, Pincus T, Yocum D, The Methotrexate-Cyclosporine Combination Study Group. Combination therapy with cyclosporine and methotrexate in severe rheumatoid arthritis. *N Engl J Med* 1995;333:137-141.

33. This section is condensed from a longer piece: Sackett DL. Why randomized controlled trials fail but needn't: 2. Failure to employ physiological statistics, or the only formula a clinical trialist is ever likely to need (or understand!). *CMAJ* 2001;165:1226-1237.

34. Cobb GW. Introductory textbooks: a framework for evaluation. *J Am Stat Assoc* 1987;82:321-339.

35. Yusuf S, Collins R, Peto R. Why do we need some large, simple randomized trials? *Stat Med* 1984;3:409-422.

36. Baigent C. The need for large-scale randomized evidence. *Br J Clin Pharmacol* 1997; 43:349-353.

37. Sackett DL, Straus SE, Richardson WS, et al. *Evidence-based medicine*, 2nd ed. Edinburgh: Churchill Livingstone, 2000: 111-113.

38. Antiplatelet Trialists' Collaboration. Collaborative overview of randomised trials of antiplatelet therapy—I: prevention of death, myocardial infarction, and stroke by prolonged antiplatelet therapy in various categories of patients. *BMJ* 1994;308:81-106.

39. Garg R, Yusuf S. Overview of randomized trials of ACE-inhibitors on mortality and morbidity in patients with heart failure. *JAMA* 1995;273:1450-1456.

40. Heidenreich PA, Lee TT, Massie BM. Effect of beta-blockade on mortality in patients with heart failure: a meta-analysis of RCTs. *J AM Coll Cardiol* 1997;30:27-34.

41. Schmid CH, Lau J, McIntosh MW, et al. An empirical study of the effect of the control rate as a predictor of treatment efficacy in meta-analysis of clinical trials. *Stat Med* 1998;17:1923-1942.

42. Barnett HJ, Taylor DW, Eliasziw M, et al., North American Symptomatic Carotid Endarterectomy Trial Collaborators. Benefit of carotid endarterectomy in patients with symptomatic moderate or severe stenosis. *N Engl J Med* 1998;339:1415-1425.

43. Sackett DL. Pronouncements about the need for "generalizability" of randomized control trial results are humbug. *Cont Clin Trials* 2000;21:82S).

44. McAlister FA, Straus SE, Guyatt GH, et al., Evidence-Based Medicine Working Group. Users' guides to the medical literature: XX. Integrating research evidence with the care of the individual patient. *JAMA* 2000;283:2829-2836.

45. Altman DG. *Practical statistics for medical research*. London: Chapman & Hall, 1991:443-445.

46. Detsky AS, Sackett DL. When was a "negative" clinical trial big enough? How many patients you needed depends on what you found. *Arch Intern Med* 1985;145:709-712.

47. Singer PA, Lantos JD, Whitington PF, et al. Equipoise and the ethics of segmental liver resection. *Clin Res.* 1988;36:539–545.

48. Lilford RJ, Jackson J. Equipoise and the ethics of randomisation. *J Roy Soc Med* 1995; 88:552–559.

49. Hellman S, Hellman DS. Of mice but not men–problems of the randomized trial. *N Engl J Med* 1991;324:1585–1589.

50. Freedman B. Equipoise and the ethics of clinical research. *N Engl J Med* 1987;317: 141–145.

51. Antman EM, Lau J, Kupelnick B, et al. A comparison of results of meta-analyses of randomized control trials and recommendations of clinical experts. *JAMA* 1992;268: 240–248.

52. ISIS Collaborative Group. ISIS-4. a randomised factorial trial assessing early oral captopril, oral mononitrate, and intravenous magnesium sulphate in 58,050 patients with suspected acute myocardial infarction. *Lancet* 1995;345:669–685.

53. Shapiro SH, Glass KC. Why Sackett's analysis of randomized controlled trials fails, but needn't. *CMAJ* 2000;163:834–835.

54. The US National Institutes of Health has created a useful resource for finding out more about placebo effects. It is available on the web at (*http://placebo.nih.gov/*).

55. Guess HA, Kleinman A, Kusek JA, et al., eds. *The science of the placebo.* London: BMJ Books, 2002.

56. Morton V, Torgerson DJ. Effect of regression to the mean on decision making in health care. *BMJ* 2003;326:1083–1084.

57. Walsh BT, Seidman SN, Sysko R. Placebo response in studies of major depression. Variable, substantial, and growing. *JAMA* 2002;287:1840–1847.

58. Hrobjartsson A, Gotzsche PC. Is the placebo powerless? An analysis of clinical trials comparing placebo with no treatment. *N Engl J Med* 2001;344:1594–1602.

59. Jamtvedt G, Young JM, Kristoffersen DT, et al. Audit and feedback: effects on professional practice and health care outcomes (Cochrane Review). In: *The Cochrane library,* (Issue 1). Chichester, UK: John Wiley & Sons, 2004:CD000259.

60. McCulloch P, Taylor I, Sasako M, et al. Randomised trials in surgery: problems and possible solutions. *BMJ* 2002;324:1448–1451.

61. McLeod RS. Issues in surgical randomized controlled trials. *World J Surg* 1999;23: 1210–1214.

62. Moore MJ, Bennett CL, The Southern Surgeons Club. The learning curve for laparoscopic cholecystectomy. *Am J Surg* 1995;170:55–59.

63. Devereaux PJ, Bhandari M, Clarke M, Montori VM, Cook DJ, Yusuf S, Sackett DL, Cina CS, Walter SD, Haynes B, Schunemann HJ, Norman GR, Guyatt GH. Need for expertise based randomised controlled trials. BMJ. 2005;330:88–91.

64. Kapiteijn E, Kranenbarg EK, Steup WH, et al., Dutch ColoRectal Cancer Group. Total mesorectal excision (TME) with or without preoperative radiotherapy in the treatment of primary rectal cancer. Prospective randomised trial with standard operative and histopathological techniques. *Eur J Surg* 1999;165:410–420.

65. North American Symptomatic Carotid Endarterectomy Trial (NASCET) Steering Committee. North American Symptomatic Carotid Endarterectomy Trial: methods, patient characteristics, and progress. *Stroke* 1991;22:711–720.

66. Bunker JP, Barnes BA, Mosteller F. *Costs, risks, and benefits of surgery.* New York: Oxford University Press, 1977:212–220.

67. Moseley JB, O'Malley K, Petersen NJ, et al. A controlled trial of arthroscopic surgery for osteoarthritis of the knee. *N Engl J Med* 2002;347:81–88.

68. Dimick JB, Diener-West M, Lipsett PA. Negative results of randomized clinical trials published in the surgical literature: equivalency or error? *Arch Surg* 2001;136: 796–800.

69. Urschel JD, Goldsmith CH, Tandan VR et al., Evidence-Based Surgery Working Group. Users' guide to evidence-based surgery: how to use an article evaluating surgical interventions. *Can J Surg* 2001;44:95-100.

70. Randomised trials in surgery. Letters to the Editor of the BMJ from Rajan Madhok, Helen H G Handoll, Stephen Bridgman, and Nicola Maffulli. *BMJ* 2002;325:658-659.

71. Klar N, Donner A. Current and future challenges in the design and analysis of cluster randomization trials. *Stat Med* 2001;20:3729-3740.

72. Cargill V, Cohen D, Kroenke K, et al. Ongoing patient randomization: an innovation in medical care research. *BMC Health Serv Res* 1986;21:663-678.

73. Schulz KF, Chalmers I, Hayes RJ, et al. Empirical evidence of bias: dimensions of methodological quality associated with estimates of treatment effects in controlled trials. *JAMA* 1995;273:408-412.

74. Begg CB, Cho MK, Eastwood S, et al. Improving the quality of reporting of randomized controlled trials: the CONSORT statement. *JAMA* 1996;276:637-639.

75. Moher D, Jones A, Lepage L, The CONSORT group. Use of the CONSORT statement and quality of reports of randomized trials: a comparative before-and-after evaluation. *JAMA* 2001;285:1992-1995.

76. Devereaux PJ, Manns BJ, Ghali WA, et al. The reporting of methodological factors in randomized controlled trials and the association with a journal policy to promote adherence to the Consolidated Standards of Reporting Trials (CONSORT) checklist. *Control Clin Trials* 2002;23:380-388.

77. Soares HP, Daniels S, Kumar A, et al. Bad reporting does not mean bad methods for randomised trials: observational study of randomised controlled trials performed by the Radiation Therapy Oncology Group. *BMJ* 2004;328:22-25.

78. Moher D, Schulz KF, Altman DG. The CONSORT statement: revised recommendations for improving the quality of reports of parallel group randomized trials. *JAMA* 2001;285:1987-1991.

79. Campbell MK, Elbourne DR, Altman DG, for the CONSORT Group. CONSORT statement: extension to cluster randomised trials. *BMJ* 2004;328:702-708.

80. Ioannidis JPA, Evans SJW, Gøtzsche PC, et al., for the CONSORT Group. Better reporting of harms in randomized trials: an extension of the CONSORT statement. *Ann Intern Med* 2004;141:781-788.

81. Francis T Jr, Korns R, Voight R, et al. An evaluation of the 1954 poliomyelitis vaccine trials: summary report. *Am J Public Health* 1955;45(Suppl 1.):1-50.

82. ISIS-4 (Fourth International Study of Infarct Survival) Collaborative Group. ISIS-4: A randomised factorial trial assessing early oral captopril,oral mononitrate, and intravenous magnesium sulphate in 58,050 patients with suspected acute myocardial infarction. *Lancet* 1995;345:669-685.

83. Teo KK, Yusuf S. Role of magnesium in reducing mortality in acute myocardial infarction. A review of the evidence. *Drugs* 1993;46:347-359.

84. Yusuf S, Sleight P, Pogue J et al., The Heart Outcomes Prevention Evaluation Study Investigators. Effects of an angiotensin-converting-enzyme inhibitor, ramipril, on cardiovascular events in high-risk patients. *N Engl J Med* 2000;342:145-153.

85. The Heart Outcomes Prevention Evaluation Study Investigators. Vitamin E supplementation and cardiovascular events in high-risk patients. *N Engl J Med* 2000;342:154-160.

86. Haynes RB, Sackett DL, Gibson ES, et al. Improvement of medication compliance in uncontrolled hypertension. *Lancet* 1976;1:1265-1268.

87. Sackett DL, Cook DJ. Can we learn anything from small trials? *Ann NY Acad Sci* 1993;703:25-31.

88. Doll R. Discussion. *Ann NY Acad Sci* 1993;703:31.

89. Prichard BNC, Dickinson CJ, Alleyne GAO, et al. Report of clinical trial from medical unit and MRC Statistical Unit, University College Hospital Medical School, London. *BMJ* 1963;2:1226–1227.

90. Mitchell RG, Stoddard MF, Ben-Yehuda O, et al. Esmolol in acute ischemic syndromes. *Am Heart J* 2002;144:E9.

91. Barsamian EM. The rise and fall of internal mammary ligation in the treatment of angina pectoris and the lessons learned. In: Bunker JP, Barnes BA, Mosteller F, eds. *Costs, risks and benefits of surgery*. New York: Oxford University Press, 1977:212–220.

92. Fish RG, Crymes TP, Lovell MG. Internal-mammary-artery ligation for angina pectoris. Its failure to produce relief. *N Engl J Med* 1958;259:418–420.

93. Alderson P, Bunn F, Lefebvre C, et al. The albumin reviewers. Human albumin solution for resuscitation and volume expansion in critically ill patients (Cochrane Review). In: *The Cochrane library*, (Issue 4). Chichester, UK: John Wiley & Sons, 2003.

7

TESTING QUALITY IMPROVEMENT INTERVENTIONS

Brian Haynes

Chapter Outline

7.1   Basic principles of testing health services innovations (including CDSSs) that are intended to improve patient outcomes

7.2   What you should include in protocols for health services innovations designed to improve the health of individuals

7.3   Other bits

7.4   Alternative study designs

Appendices

7.1   Diabetes Support System Trial. Patient information and consent

7.2   Types of advice to be delivered to patients and their physicians

CLINICAL RESEARCH SCENARIO

Taking care of diabetic patients has never been more rewarding—or more difficult to do well. Many efficacious treatments exist, beginning with "tight" glucose control, and continuing with prevention of cardiovascular, cerebrovascular, peripheral vascular, renal, retinal, neuropathic, skin, foot, and infectious complications. When primary care physicians become aware that their patients are having difficulties, they often refer the patients to specialty clinics for diabetes, but there's often a wait of several months for nonurgent referrals to these clinics, including the one that I work in, where a typical delay is 3 to 6 months.

It's so challenging for doctors and patients to keep track of all the recommendations, and offer them in a timely fashion to each patient, that Dereck Hunt (a student working with me at the time) and I thought a computerized clinical decision support information system might help. We built one, based on a database of studies on the diagnosis, treatment or prevention, prognosis, etiology, quality improvement, or economics of managing diabetes (1). To this, we added a "user interface" that allowed the clinician or patient to match the patient's features to the database.

The first interface required patients to use a computer and mouse to answer questions while in our clinic waiting room—not very practical for patients with low computer literacy and difficult to fit in the ebb and flow of the clinic's busy schedule. The second interface used "touch screen" software—this avoided the "mouse problem," and was acceptable to many patients, but it still clashed with the clinic schedule: even when asked to come early, patients often arrived "just-in-time" for their appointments, and doctors and nurses in the clinic didn't want to wait for patients to fill out the questionnaire, even though we were able to get it down to less than 10 minutes for most patients.

The version of the system to be tested in the protocol presented in this chapter asks patients, upon referral to our diabetes clinic, to complete a brief questionnaire (on paper, by e-mail, or at a Web site). The responses are fed into a computer program that matches the patient's responses to a database of evidence and recommendations. The computer then prepares a report for the patient and the physician with recommendations that are specific for that patient. The report has two parts, one for the patient, with lay explanations, the second for the physician, with "doctor speak" and references to the relevant evidence. The database of evidence and recommendations can also be browsed and searched on the Internet.

The objective of having patients complete the questionnaire at the time of referral is to use the several months between the date of referral and the first clinic visit to organize the documentation that is needed for an assessment, do some initial implementation, and provide the patient and doctor with some initial information about what is needed for optimal care, tailored to the individual circumstances of that patient. The hypothesis is that this will speed up the time it takes to achieve diabetes care goals and focus the diabetes clinic assessment on components of care that have not yet been fully implemented.

This computerized decision support system (CDSS) has undergone some field testing, both in a specialty clinic (2,3) and in primary care (4) but has not been assessed in a controlled trial for its effects on improving the process and outcomes of care for people with diabetes.

7.1 BASIC PRINCIPLES OF TESTING HEALTH SERVICES INNOVATIONS THAT ARE INTENDED TO IMPROVE PATIENT OUTCOMES

Innovations in the provision of health services can be developed for diverse purposes, including increasing access, effectiveness, and efficiency; reducing complexity; increasing accountability; and so on. If the purpose of the innovation is to directly improve the health outcomes of patients, that is, to increase efficacy, effectiveness, or cost-effectiveness, then the same standards should be applied as for any intervention claiming to improve health (be it a medication or procedure) that is applied directly to patients. These standards include random allocation of patients, practitioners, or practice groups to form comparable cohorts, one to receive the innovation and the other for a comparison intervention.

Logistical problems, however, can put roadblocks in meeting these standards. For example, when the intervention is a "package" of procedures, blinding of providers and patients can be difficult or impossible. The problem of "contamination" is likely to occur if patients assigned to the intervention and control groups are managed by the same providers. Indeed, some will claim that randomization is not feasible or even necessary for testing health services innovations. To these skeptics, we say: show us an intervention claim worth testing and we'll show you how to design a properly randomized trial to test it.

Staging a health services trial involves a similar range of choices as for testing any health care intervention. These choices begin with consideration of the state of evolution and testing of the intervention to date: Have the bugs been worked out? Has a pilot study been done to show that the system is reliable and acceptable to patients and clinicians and has the potential to make a beneficial difference? The choices are then filtered through the research question you have chosen. For example, are you interested at this point in:

1. whether the intervention *can* work, under relatively ideal circumstances—an efficacy or explanatory question or
2. whether it *does* work, under usual practice conditions—an effectiveness, pragmatic, or management question or
3. whether it is *worth it*—an efficiency question.

The design features follow from these choices, as shown in previous chapters, especially Chapter 5, on therapeutic trials.

7.2 WHAT YOU SHOULD INCLUDE IN PROTOCOLS FOR HEALTH SERVICES INTERVENTIONS

Your health services innovation protocol should describe at least the following features of the investigation (the order may differ depending on the circumstances, especially prior experience). Health services innovations protocols checklist:

✓ Conduct a literature review. Make it systematic, at least for the intervention.
✓ Pose the research question(s). Include the "PICOT" elements.
✓ Consider who you will want as collaborators and participants. Health care providers or their patients, or both, can be participants in health services research; we'll

call the former "collaborators" and the latter "participants" when both are involved.

✓ Employ concealed random allocation: of patients, if the provider can be blinded to the intervention; of providers, or groups of providers, if the provider can't be blinded.

✓ Recruit participants and acquire informed consent.

✓ Plan the interventions.

✓ Select measurement procedures to assess the appropriate clinical processes and events.

✓ Choose the sample size, adequate to detect clinically important differences in at least the major processes and outcomes with at least 80% power.

✓ Consider feasibility.

✓ *Conduct a literature review.*

Diabetes mellitus (DM) is a chronic disease that afflicts more than 5% of the population, with the prevalence of type 2 (DM2) being about ten times that of type 1 (DM1).

Randomized trials and systematic reviews of the trials of interventions document that the adverse consequences of diabetes can be ameliorated by the following:

- Tight glucose control for DM1 (5)
- Tight glucose control for type DM2 (6,7)
- Ramipril for patients with diabetes and one other cardiovascular risk factor (8)
- Angiotensin converting enzyme (ACE) inhibitors for patients with proteinuria (9,10)
- Tight blood pressure control (11–13)
- Tight control of dyslipidemia (14,15)
- Regular foot care (16)
- Multifactorial intervention (7)
- Influenza vaccination (17,18)

In addition to our own review, evidence concerning diabetes care has recently been exhaustively reviewed by the Canadian Diabetes Association (CDA) as the basis for their 2003 clinical practice guidelines (19).

Studies of the quality of diabetes control and ancillary care generally show less than 50% achievement of treatment goals (7,20).

A systematic review of the literature concerning CDSSs reviews reported in Chapter 2 indicates that such systems have, with considerable inconsistency, improved the quality of the processes of care in ambulatory clinical settings for chronic diseases such as HIV/AIDS, asthma, hypertension, and diabetes (21). To date, some studies have shown improvements in clinical outcomes from CDSS interventions for a variety of conditions, and two trials have done so for diabetes.

In the first diabetes trial (22), family physicians were provided with reminders for recommended care (from the American Diabetes Association guidelines) based on matching patients' characteristics in an electronic medical record. Chart audit was performed to assess the effects of the reminders on the process of care but not on patient outcomes. Median physician adherence to recommendations was 32% in the intervention group and 15% in the comparison group ($p = 0.01$). Despite the improvements seen with the CDSS, the authors were disappointed at the low rate of adherence in both groups. This study supports the notion that a CDSS can improve the process of care, albeit modestly, but does not measure effects on patient outcomes. Further, it took place in the still-rarified environment of a computerized medical record system that can support patient-specific reminders.

In the second diabetes trial (23), Norwegian general practitioner groups with computerized patient records (CPRs) were randomly allocated to have or not to have access to a CDSS to assist with the application of guideline-directed care of their patients with diabetes. Although all the participating practice groups had CPRs, the CDSS was not integrated into the CPR; rather, physicians had to initiate the CDSS computer program and compare their patient's characteristics with the guidelines. Neither the process nor the clinical outcomes of care were affected, and the CDSS was blamed for not being very "user-friendly."

Based on the CDSS systematic review, we judged that CDSSs have the potential for enhancing patient care and outcomes if they incorporate the following features: (a) timely reminders that are (b) well justified by current best evidence, (c) tailored to individual patient characteristics, (d) delivered to both patient and practitioner, and (e) followed up by a third party (e.g., a clinic nurse assigned this responsibility) for the completion of items of recommended care. A study that evaluates both the process and the clinical outcomes for CDSS for diabetes according to these features, and that has passed at least the preliminary testing for usability and acceptability in doctors' offices, appears to be justified.

The literature review in the preceding text is abbreviated from the version that would go in a research proposal, but it contains the following key elements:

- An estimate of the "burden of disease"
- An estimate of the extent to which current treatments are justified
- An estimate of the extent to which current treatments are underutilized
- An up-to-date systematic review of the relevant research concerning the intervention. In some cases it might be reasonable to focus this

review just on interventions for the condition of interest (diabetes in this case). However, sound studies of CDSSs are rare; diabetes hasn't been a common target of such studies, and one can likely learn a lot about what works and what does not from studies for other chronic disease conditions. Reviewers likely won't be impressed if you narrow the scope of the review so that there are "no prior relevant studies."
- A justification, theoretical and practical, for the features of the intervention to be tested in the proposed trial
- A self-serving statement indicating that the current proposal is just what's needed to advance the field!

✓ Pose the research question(s).

> For patients referred from primary care practices to the Diabetes Care and Research Centre (DCRC) at McMaster University, does the addition of a CDSS at the time of referral, providing evidence-based recommendations for diabetes care tailored to the circumstances of the individual patient and delivered to both the patient and referring doctor, result in increased speed and success of implementation of recommended care for diabetes, better control of diabetes and cardiovascular risk factors, increased satisfaction of patients, and increased satisfaction of referring physicians, compared with the usual referred care process?

This research question is a "mouthful," as it must be, to include the basic elements of participants, intervention, comparison group, and outcomes (PICOT). Many other questions could be asked, for example, by staging the intervention at the primary care level alone, or even in the community (a trial that we have just begun), rather than providing the service only for patients sent for referral. However, patients who are being referred are likely to have more difficulties with their diabetes than those not referred, and thus constitute a "high-risk" group with considerable room for improvement. Intervention efforts at the time of referral can thus focus on those with the most need and can potentially make it easier to detect the effects of the intervention. On the other hand, these patients may or may not constitute a "high-response" group. Indeed, they may already have received the interventions that are recommended for their care from their family physician or other specialists and may have failed to take them (for whatever reason) or failed to respond to them.

We can increase the amount of risk and increase the possibility of high response by the way we set up the eligibility criteria. Of course, we could also try to "tackle the world" in the first randomized controlled trial (RCT) of the intervention, by surveying primary care practices, or even people in communities, to find all people with diabetes, and then include all-comers in the study. Such a study would answer the different and worthy question of how useful the CDSS is "in the general population"–a management question. The choices laid out in the following text for selecting participants reflect a decision that, at this early stage of testing, it is more efficient to assess the effects of the intervention in a group that is likely to be relatively "high risk–high response." If it doesn't help in the care of such patients, it is unlikely to be useful in a setting in which a proportion of the patients need very few or none of its recommendations, or are unlikely to respond to them.

You might also want to add secondary questions to those addressed in the primary study question. These can arise from the study design (an RCT in this case) or be based on observations made among one group or the other or both. For example, an RCT-based question would be: What is the effect of the intervention on the rate of referrals? It could be that referring physicians like or dislike the computerized reminders, and this might affect their willingness to refer patents during the course of the trial. You might also ask about adverse effects: Does the intervention increase the risk for severe hypoglycemia among participants? In fact, a search for adverse effects of interventions should be included in all trials.

Descriptive secondary questions could assess such matters as the perceptions of practitioners and patients in the intervention group concerning various aspects of the intervention, to determine, for future use, what aspects they felt worked best and what suggestions they had for enhancements, especially if some aspects didn't work well.

One rule for asking secondary questions: they must not compromise answering the primary question in any substantive way, including inflating its budget to the point of nonfundability. Looking at the end of the trial for effects on referral rates would be cheap and simple, so it is easy to justify this secondary assessment. Asking doctors and patients for their perceptions and advice concerning the intervention should occur before the trial or when their participation is completed (preferably both); asking during the course of the trial could affect participation, and so would constitute "cointervention." Further, such assessments would likely be expensive, in both research staff time and paying for physician's time, thereby pushing up the trial budget and reducing its likelihood of getting funded and getting completed. If so, proceed with caution or leave this for another investigation.

✓ Consider who you will want as collaborators and participants.

Primary care doctors will be invited to collaborate in the study if they refer patients to the McMaster DCRC and if they meet the following criteria:

- The primary reason for referral is assessment and advice for DM1 or DM2.
- The patient they are referring has not been seen in the clinic for at least the previous 12 months.

Patients referred to the DCRC will be invited to participate in the study if they meet the following criteria:

- referred for assessment of DM1 or DM2
- at least one unmet recommendation for care (see the following text)
- 18 to 85 years of age and providing their own diabetes self-care
- able to speak and read English fluently (including having adequate vision to do so on their own)
- willing and able to return to the clinic for study follow-up assessments in 12 months
- willing and able to provide informed consent

Unmet recommendations for care include:

- hemoglobin A_{1c} over 7.0%
- one or more severe hypoglycemia bouts (requiring assistance from another person) in the last 6 months
- overweight and not on metformin, with no contraindication to metformin
- blood pressure of at least 140/90 mm Hg on three readings at one visit or greater than 130/85 mm Hg, averaged over at least three visits
- either low-density lipoprotein (LDL) cholesterol level greater than 4 mmol per L (155 mg/dL) or high-density lipoprotein (HDL) cholesterol level less than 1.6 mmol per L (45 mg/dL) or both
- history of coronary heart disease, stroke, peripheral vascular disease, or diabetic nephropathy, and not treated with ramipril, with no contraindication to ramipril
- diabetic retinopathy of any degree, not seen by an ophthalmologist in 12 months or more, or status of retinopathy is unknown, with no check in 24 months or more
- one or more of the following symptoms: decreased sensations in feet (on monofilament testing), absent pedal pulses, foot ulcer, or foot deformity likely to be secondary to diabetes

In health services projects of this nature, both practitioners and patients must be "onside" if the study is to proceed. If any additional work is required of the collaborating health care providers (e.g., referring physicians or their clinic staff), work will be needed "up front" *before* submitting the protocol for funding to ensure that enough physicians are willing to enter patients into the trial, not just on paper but in full knowledge of "game day" work requirements. This will generally require sounding out local practitioners and meeting directly with physicians who are potential collaborators, often best done through their leaders and networks (local academy of medicine, local primary care research groups affiliated with university departments of family medicine, and so on). The more work the physician will need to do (in finding and recruiting patients, completing forms, and following up), the more difficult the "sell" will be. The higher the recruitment and processing fees paid to physicians, the easier it will be to recruit them—but the less relevant the study will be to usual care.

The best participation by clinicians and their staff usually arises if they are:

- highly interested in the help that the project might provide for the care of their patients
- involved in the design of the procedures that will affect them
- informed about the progress of the trial on a regular basis
- expected to do procedures that are as simple and hassle free as possible and that do not disrupt their practice procedures
- fairly compensated for nontrivial time commitments

Compensation doesn't necessarily mean money—recognition of efforts and acknowledgment of good work can go a long way—but monetary compensation appropriate for time and effort spent definitely helps to encourage participation. If resources are tight, however, it is best to design procedures so that they minimize the time and burden of collaborators participating in the trial, even if this means giving up some of the objectives of the study. Even if resources are adequate, it is important to keep the demands on health professionals involved in trials low, for example, by paying for research staff to identify eligible patients, approach such patients for participation, and collect data. The reason for this is not to protect the health professionals but to guard the integrity and completeness of the data collection.

Working with the local academy of medicine and the research director for the Department of Family Medicine, we recruited more than 30 family physicians in one of the studies leading up to this investigation (3), so we now have a group of interested physicians to work with.

✓ Employ concealed random allocation.

Randomization will be according to a computer-generated randomization schedule, administered by a research assistant. The order will be concealed from patient and practitioner for the first patient referred from each practice; all subsequent patients from each practice group (including all physicians practicing at the same practice address) will be in the same study group (cluster randomization).

Allocation will be concealed by having the statistician randomly allocate participating practices, without knowledge of patient characteristics or practice names.

Randomization cannot be stratified for type 1 and type 2 diabetes because this stratification is precluded by randomizing practices rather than by patients. The analysis, however, will be stratified by these two groups.

Once assigned, randomization group cannot be blinded in this type of investigation but a number of the outcome assessments are objective, or will be assessed by staff who are kept unaware of study group allocation.

The unit of allocation for this study is a practice group because of the possibility of contamination in trials in which interventions are applied to clinicians and end points are measured for patients. For example, when individual patients are allocated to intervention and control groups within the same clinician's practice, a clinician will likely end up treating some patients with, and others without, the aid of the CDSS; knowledge gained by the clinician from the CDSS may then be applied to control patients, leading to an underestimation of the system's effect. A similar situation can occur when individual clinicians within a team or group are the units of allocation: the presence of a CDSS, or of colleagues who are using a CDSS, in the clinical setting may influence the treatment given by clinicians allocated to the comparison group. However, randomizing patients or physicians may be preferable to randomizing clinics in some situations (7), including cases where clinics differ in many respects and access to a large number of practices is limited.

It is desirable to stratify patients before randomization for variables that are likely to be related to both study outcomes and the success of intervention. In this study, including newly referred patients with type 1 and type 2 diabetes is problematic because patients with type 1 will be much younger on average than patients with type 2 and will likely differ substantially on treatments (insulin versus oral hypoglycemics) and on the numbers of ancillary recommendations. One can choose here to enroll only patients with type 1 or type 2 diabetes, or plan to include both groups, with the provision to recruit enough patients of each type to reach independent conclusions, that is, essentially run two studies at once. Fortunately, referral to our clinic has historically been about equally distributed between type 1 and 2 diabetes so that recruitment will be equally quick for the two strata.

✓ Recruit participants and acquire informed consent.

Physician Recruitment

Before the CDSS trial, physicians who refer to the DCRC clinic will be invited to join the study through face-to-face meetings with the principal investigator and by letter. They will be provided with a summary of the study protocol and be offered access to the full protocol. They will signify their intent to participate by providing a signed letter indicating that they have read and understood the study summary, that they are willing to have their patients approached by the study staff, that they are willing to receive recommendations for the care of their participating patients, and that they are willing to help their patients to follow the recommendations. These letters of agreement will be provided with the protocol when it is submitted for consideration for research funding.

Additional physicians will be recruited after the trial commences by approaching referring physicians who have not already declined to participate. Whereas it might be desirable to approach and recruit all referring physicians in advance, the clinic receives referrals from hundreds of physicians from up to 100 km away, and it is neither feasible nor necessary for this early phase investigation to recruit all physicians in advance. Nevertheless, recruiting additional physicians as the trial proceeds will enhance generalizability and increase the rate of completion of recruitment.

One could make a case for just approaching patients to participate and not asking physicians to indicate their participation in the study: the opportunity for patients to participate would then be hypothetically unfettered. However, physicians refer all patients to the clinic (i.e., no self-referral) and are instrumental to the collection of some of the baseline information about patients, as well as for implementation of some recommendations before patients are first seen at the clinic. Thus, the intervention is best viewed as a collaborative venture between referring physician, patient, and clinic.

Because the physician's personal health is not at stake, and because the physician will generally know and understand the diagnostic and treatment recommendations that will be made, there is no need for the detailed consent procedures required for patients in trials, so the procedure outlined in the preceding text is primarily aimed at ensuring that physicians are knowledgeable about the objectives and procedures of the investigation and are willing to be engaged in it. This approach is also vital to convincing funding agencies that the study is likely to be acceptable and feasible (see ✓ *Choose the sample size*, and ✓ *Consider feasibility*).

Patient Recruitment and Consent

On referral, potentially eligible patients will be given the next available appointment with the requested DCRC physician and will be immediately mailed a brochure outlining the rationale and nature of the study, accompanied by a screening questionnaire, a consent form for the study (Appendix 7.1), and a consent form to contact the patient's physician for laboratory data, if needed, along with a return mail, stamped envelope. This will be followed by a telephone call from the clinic nurse who works with the consulting physician. The nurse will review the information in the brochure, review the preliminary questions concerning eligibility (see ✓ *Consider who you will want as collaborators and participants*), and answer any questions the patient may have.

If the patient is eligible according to the eligibility questions, the nurse will invite the patient to join the study by signing the consent forms and returning them to the clinic. If necessary to establish at least one unmet recommendation for care, the nurse will contact the patient's physician's office for laboratory or blood pressure information. Complete documentation of the status of baseline variables will follow agreement of the patient to enter the study.

In health services research, unlike clinical trials, usually no "experimental" treatments or "experimental" indications for treatment are involved. Rather, patients and their primary care doctors are provided with documentation concerning current best care and support to implement it. Thus, the ethical issues mainly have to do with general aspects of participation in a research project, including disclosure of the objectives and procedures and confidentiality of information.

According to Emanuel and colleagues (24), there are seven key principles for ethical clinical research (see Table 7–1), and fulfilling these seven is necessary and sufficient for conducting clinical research.

You can judge whether we've designed the study in a way that satisfies criteria 1 to 4. We will proceed with an independent review (criterion 5) in due course, but before that we will need to develop a process for informed consent. Key principles for informed consent for clinical research in Canada appear in Table 7–2 (25).

The procedure for consent in *health services research* studies such as this one must observe the same principles, but the process is usually somewhat less demanding because no experimental treatments are involved. Rather, in our study, the objective is to improve the implementation of treatments validated in rigorous clinical trials and widely agreed by experts to represent optimal management. Ethical guidelines allow for some flexibility in the elements of consent in various circumstances, as noted in Table 7–3 (25). Some forms of health services research may not require patient consent at all, for example, clinical database research in which individual patient identifiers have been removed. Progressively more stringent privacy legislation, however, is making studies based on patient records increasingly problematic.

TABLE 7–1 Ethical Criteria for Clinical Research (24)

1. Value—Enhancements of health or knowledge must be derived from the research.

2. Scientific validity—The research must be methodologically rigorous.

3. Fair subject selection—Scientific objectives should determine communities selected as study sites and the inclusion criteria for individuals.

4. Favorable risk–benefit ratio—Risks must be minimized, potential benefits enhanced, and the potential benefits to individuals and knowledge gained for society must outweigh the risks.

5. Independent review—Unaffiliated individuals must review, approve, amend, or terminate the research.

6. Informed consent—Individuals should be informed about the research and provide their voluntary consent.

7. Respect for enrolled subjects—Subjects should have their privacy protected, the opportunity to withdraw, and their well-being monitored.

From Emanuel EJ, Wendler D, Grady C. What makes clinical research ethical? *JAMA* 2000;283:2701–2711, with permission.

TABLE 7-2   Information to Be Included in an Informed Consent (25)

1. Information that the individual is being invited to participate in a research project;
2. A comprehensible statement of the research purpose, the identity of the researcher, the expected duration and nature of participation, and a description of research procedures;
3. A comprehensible description of reasonably foreseeable harms and benefits that may arise from research participation, as well as the likely consequences of non-action, particularly in research related to treatment, or where invasive methodologies are involved, or where there is a potential for physical or psychological harm;
4. An assurance that prospective subjects are free not to participate, have the right to withdraw at any time without prejudice to preexisting entitlements, and will be given continuing and meaningful opportunities for deciding whether to continue to participate; and
5. The possibility of commercialization of research findings, and the presence of any apparent or actual or potential conflict of interest on the part of researchers, their institutions, or their sponsors.

Based on the tri-council policy statement: ethical conduct for research involving humans. Section 2. Free and informed consent [cited 2004 Sept. 23]. Available from: *http://www.ncehr-cnerh.org/english/code_2/sec02.html.*

Basic ethical principles for research are intended to be universal, but actual practices can vary considerably from country to country and within countries, according to local customs and resources, as well as evolving over time. International standards for clinical trials have been promulgated by the International Conference on Harmonization Technical Requirements

TABLE 7-3   Reason for Exceptions in Informed Consent (25)

The Research Ethics Board (REB) may approve a consent procedure that does not include, or that alters, some or all of the elements of informed consent set forth above or may waive the requirement to obtain informed consent, provided that the REB finds and documents that:

1. the research involves no more than minimal risk to the subjects;
2. the waiver or alteration is unlikely to adversely affect the rights and welfare of the subjects;
3. the research could not practicably be carried out without the waiver or alteration;
4. whenever possible and appropriate, the subjects will be provided with additional pertinent information after participation; and
5. the waivered or altered consent does not involve a therapeutic intervention.

Based on the tri-council policy statement: ethical conduct for research involving humans. Section 2. Free and informed consent [cited 2004 Sept. 23]. Available from: *http://www.ncehr-cnerh.org/english/code_2/sec02.html.*

for Registration of Pharmaceuticals for Human Use (*http://www.ich.org*), a project sponsored by the drug regulatory bodies of Europe, Japan, and the United States. The procedures for clinical trials are described under the general rubric of "Guideline for Good Clinical Practice."

Our proposal will be submitted to our local REB for assessment in preparation for its submission to a peer review funding agency. Once they have ensured that the key ethical issues are appropriately addressed, it will be sent off to the funding agency for consideration.

✓ *Plan the interventions.*

The CDSS for diabetes has been described in full elsewhere (2–4) and the database and recommendations are available in a recent book (1). The CDSS with evidence and evidence-based diabetes care recommendations has been developed as a project based on ongoing hand searching of the medical literature, with updating of the recommendations as new evidence warrants. Recommendations in the CDSS are compared with the current recommendations of the CDA (19) and only those recommendations that are supported by level 1A (systematic reviews and randomized controlled trials with adequate power) are implemented in the CDSS. New level 1A evidence not considered in the CDA recommendations will be implemented if it augments CDA recommendations.

If patients complete the paper version of the questionnaire, they will be asked to fax it to the CDSS computer, or mail it in, if need be, so that we can fax it to the computer. The computer system uses Teleform software, with optical character recognition of the patient's responses to the questionnaire.

The CDSS provides recommendations based on the information about individual patient characteristics provided in the responses to the questionnaire. For any missing or uninterpretable responses, the CDSS generates a request to be mailed to the patient, to be completed as soon as possible by faxing or mailing any additional information or by bringing it to the first referral visit. In the meantime, the CDSS generates a partial set of recommendations based on the available patient information.

A toll free "help line" will be provided for *intervention group* patients who have questions about the recommendations provided for them and about how to obtain any information they currently lack. A clinic nurse will handle the calls and provide clarification about the intent of recommendations, and their interpretation and implementation, but not additional advice.

Patients in both groups will be asked to arrive at their DCRC appointment with the recommendations they were sent, along with all of their current medications and any information that was unavailable (such as blood test results) when they first completed the questionnaire.

Once the eligibility questionnaire is complete, the nurse will work with consenting patients referred from *intervention group* practices and their family physicians to complete the baseline questionnaire. When complete, patients and their physicians will receive a set of computer-generated recommendations, tailored to the patient's own circumstances. The patient and family physician will be asked to discuss and implement as many of the recommendations as appropriate and possible before the patient's first visit to the DCRC (see examples in Appendix 7.2). Participants will be offered assistance from a DCRC clinic nurse in obtaining information to complete their questionnaires if they have any difficulty obtaining this from their physician.

Participants who are referred from *control group* practices and their physicians will receive the baseline questionnaire, which has to be completed before the first clinic visit, and a set of general recommendations for diabetes care in the form of a printed booklet including general information on diabetes and its care, specific for type 1 and type 2 diabetes, from the CDA (*http://www.diabetes.ca/Section_About/FactsIndex.asp*). The participants and the physicians will not receive any other assistance before the first clinic visit. When their baseline questionnaire is complete, specific computerized recommendations will be generated but will be concealed and stored for future reference. Thus, their care will be in the hands of the clinic nurse and physician but without the aid of the computer-generated recommendations being provided to the patient, family physician, or clinic staff.

The description above is a "bare-bones" one, backed up by appendices (two of which appear at the end of this chapter), a Web site, and references. In a research grant proposal, more detail would be provided in the text, but the basic elements are here.

Of particular importance in health services interventions, including CDSSs, is to consider whether the intervention should be "frozen" in its features for the duration of the study. Many service innovations undergo revision with time. As "moving targets," they pose challenges for testing. A common way to minimize this is to use the service in practice until it reaches a satisfactory level of maturity, having completed extensive development and field testing to "get out the bugs" before it is "ready" for an RCT.

Some methodologists hold quite another position on this matter. Tom Chalmers, for example, forcefully made the argument that "the first patient should be randomized," and all others, whenever a new procedure is introduced, until the procedure had been shown to do more good than harm. So far as we know, this dictum has never been honored, but perhaps it should be, especially for interventions that have substantial prospect for harm, such as surgical interventions, or those that are hideously expensive. As most CDSSs are neither, and if the care recommendations are based on sound research evidence of efficacy from treatments that have received regulatory approval, we'll pass on Dr. Chalmers' advice, for your consideration, "when the shoe fits," that is, when you are testing a procedure that is unproven.

The suggestion that the intervention should be mature and stable before testing in a large RCT doesn't mean that there can be no changes in the system after the study begins. For example, if new knowledge reported in the medical literature during the course of the trial rendered one or more of the recommendations in the system obsolete, then the system would need to be changed mid-stream. In this situation, the change would need to be documented, its date of implementation recorded, and any effects on the process or outcomes of care examined. An 8-year long trial of multifactorial care for patients with diabetes (7) provides an excellent example of how this can be handled: several important new studies were reported during the course of this study, showing benefits from lower goals for blood pressure, lipid level, and glucose level. The investigators incorporated these findings into the study procedures at various points during the trial, documenting the changes and timing in the final report of the study.

Abandoning trials when new evidence comes along is usually (but not always!) unnecessary and is really only a risk in trials that take a long time to complete. New evidence from other trials is seldom so definitive that it dictates a major change in practice, especially in health services research. Therefore, new evidence can often be implemented without substantively altering the question being addressed in the trial. If patients might be harmed or disadvantaged by the study intervention, compared with a new alternative, it is also possible to deal with the situation ethically by reviewing the situation with the institutional review board that approved the trial (and the trial's external monitoring board if it has one) and, with their assent, presenting the new evidence to the patients and asking for their consent to continue in the trial.

✓ *Select the measurement procedures.*

Collaborating practices will be assessed at baseline for the number of primary care physicians working together (sharing the same office area, charting facilities, and staff), size of practice, the certification level of the physicians (general practice or family medicine, in our area), time since date of latest formal postgraduate training, and number of patients referred to the DCRC during the last 2 years. The frequency of referral during the course of the trial will be monitored and any withdrawals recorded.

For patients, measurements begin with the questionnaire they were sent at the time of referral. Recommended care and status of implementation of recommendations will be determined again at the time of the first visit to the DCRC, and at the end of the follow-up period.

Other measurements for patients will be done at the first DCRC visit and include:

- date of onset of diabetes
- current diet and exercise regimen, medications, and duration
- any changes made since the time of referral

- diabetic complications [i.e., cataracts, retinopathy, neuropathy (including type), nephropathy (proteinuria and impaired creatinine clearance), coronary heart disease, cerebrovascular disease, peripheral vascular disease (claudication and amputation), and foot ulcers]
- comorbidity, including hypertension, dyslipidemia, and their treatments
- self-care, including home monitoring frequency and recording, adherence to each aspect of current prescribed regimen
- any medication allergies or intolerances
- smoking status.

Physical examination will include weight (light clothing and no shoes) and height (no shoes); blood pressure (three assessments according to Canadian Hypertension Society protocol); screening funduscopy; routine heart, lung, and abdomen examination; and skin and foot examination (including footwear, nails, ulcers, pulses, and monofilament sensation).

The main outcome assessment for the study is based on the state of implementation of recommended care for the two study groups at the first referral visit. However, it is not expected that implementation of care recommendations will be consistently complete in either group at this point. Further, the effect of recommendations that have been implemented before the referral visit is not expected to be complete. Thus, all patients will be followed for a full year from the initial date of referral, to determine the date of implementation of patient-specific recommendations for care for diabetes, control of diabetes (hemoglobin A_{1c}, frequency of hypoglycemia, or hyperglycemia requiring assistance), blood pressure, blood lipid levels, satisfaction of patients, and satisfaction of referring physicians, compared with the usual referred care process.

The details are somewhat truncated here—in a protocol for submission for research funding, a detailed description of the procedures and timing for each follow-up assessment would be needed, including measures to minimize bias. For example, measures of hemoglobin A_{1c} and blood lipid levels are done by machines and are therefore objective, not subject to the biases of investigators or patients. Measurement of blood pressure, however, is subject to bias, and should be measured by a nurse or research assistant who is not directly involved with the care of the patients and is unaware of the study group to which they have been assigned. Assessment of satisfaction of patients and their primary care providers is obviously subjective as well. Clearly, the respondents' subjective views are wanted, but their views should not be influenced or interpreted by someone who is aware of the treatment group to which they belong. A standardized, self-administered questionnaire would be appropriate in this case. If an interview is needed, the interviewer should not be aware of the group to which the patient has been assigned. The properties of all measurement instruments and procedures, objective and subjective, should be documented for reliability, validity, and responsiveness to change, preferably by citing published studies or, if necessary, by using original data you have collected.

The protocol as outlined here only calls for assessment of clinical "process" measures (implementation of care guidelines) and "intermediate" clinical care assessments (i.e., blood sugar control, blood pressure, and lipid levels). The latter can each be justified on the basis that the intensity of their control has been shown to correlate with more important clinical outcomes, such as diabetic complications and cardiovascular events (as documented in the literature review).

The results of the trial would obviously be more compelling if "major" outcome events were included, but there are two reasons why it would be inappropriate to include such events in this trial. First, the CDSS is relatively untested—in this little-tested state, it remains a "long shot" for having major effects on care outcomes, particularly considering the results of trials for other CDSSs to date. To justify the effort and expense of a major trial, one would want to have solid evidence that the CDSS is capable of changing the way care is delivered and that these changes are acceptable to patients and care providers. Second, the intervention is proposed to speed up the process of making and implementing care recommendations (using the period from time of referral to first clinic visit to identify and get started on recommendations), not to increase the number of recommendations that will eventually be made or to increase the intensity of their implementation because these are usual functions of the referral clinic and are subject to negotiation with each patient. It is conceivable that a CDSS could augment the intensity of care as well, especially if it incorporates ongoing monitoring with feedback to patients and their care providers, but these later elements are not part of the CDSS at this point. Therefore, it appears timely to conduct a relatively inexpensive and short-term "proof of concept" study at this stage of development of the CDSS.

✓ Choose the sample size.

In the CDSS trial, the primary outcome is the effect of patient-specific reminders from the CDSS on implementation of diabetes care recommendations by the time of first referral visit and by 1 year following the date of referral. In a preliminary test of the CDSS in the DCRC clinic, including mainly ongoing patients (rather than newly referred patients) (3), the number of recommendations ranged from 0 to 8, and the mean number of recommendations for implementation was 3.0 with a standard deviation of 0.3. Since then, the repertoire of the CDSS has been expanded to include up to 12 recommendations. Further, the proposed trial will include only patients newly referred. Thus, the mean number of recommendations per patient is expected to increase to 6. An "implementation score," the proportion of indicated interventions that have been completed, will be generated for each patient at the time of referral, at the first clinic visit, and at the end of 1 year of follow-up after the date of referral, and change scores will then be calculated for each of these periods for both groups.

For the first of these periods, from referral to first referral visit, it is assumed that the possible change scores (i.e., proportion of recommendations implemented) varies from -0.2 to $+0.6$ (i.e., from a reduction in proportion of recommendations met of 20% to an increase in recommendations met of 60%) and that the distribution of these change scores is uniform (a conservative assumption). From this information, the standard deviation of change scores can be calculated as follows (26): $[0.6 - (-0.2)]/($square root $12) = 0.23$. Using this estimate of the standard deviation, a two-sided α of 0.05, a β of 0.10, and assuming a minimal clinically important difference between the intervention and control group change scores of 0.2 (i.e., an absolute improvement 20% in implementation of patient-specific care recommendations), the required sample size is 30 patients per arm for each of the two strata, type 1 and type 2 patients, or 240 patients in total.

This sample size, however, must be adjusted to take into account any decrease of independence of participants within any given cluster (i.e., clinic). Cluster randomization is being used because of the possibility of contamination that would arise if physicians treated patients in both the control and intervention arms of the trial. After being reminded to perform certain diabetes-specific interventions on several occasions, physicians would likely begin to complete the same interventions for patients in the control arm of the study, thus decreasing the observed effect of the reminders.

Donner and colleagues (27–29) have demonstrated that the degree to which the sample size per arm needs to be increased can be calculated if both the cluster size and degree of within-cluster dependence, or intracluster correlation (ICC), are known. The sample size needs to be multiplied by an inflation factor (IF) to overcome this loss of independence. This factor can be calculated as IF = 1 + (cluster size − 1) × ICC. In this study, we estimate that the number of eligible patients referred from each clinic during the study period will be about seven patients with type 1 diabetes and seven with type 2. For a cluster size of seven patients per clinic per stratum, and a conservative within-cluster dependence of 0.2 (30), IF = 1 + (7 − 1) × 0.2 = 2.2. Thus, 30 × 2.2 = 66 patients are required per arm for each stratum, or about 10 clinics per arm. One additional clinic per arm will be recruited to allow for possible physician dropouts. Twenty-two clinics contributing 77 patients with type 1 diabetes and 77 patients with type 2 diabetes per group will provide adequate diversity to assess the acceptability and usefulness of the intervention in various practice settings, with adequate power to detect a moderate and clinically worthwhile effect on adherence to recommendations. As noted in the following text, 30 clinics have already indicated, in writing, an interest in participating in the study.

Some options for sample size are set out in Table 7–4. These show that the sample size chosen will be adequate even if the ICC proves to be as high as 0.3.

TABLE 7–4 Sample Size Options for a Cluster Randomized Trial with a Mean Difference between Groups of 0.2 and Standard Deviation of 0.23

Difference	Standard Deviation	Intracluster Correlation	α	Power	Patients/ cluster	Clusters/ group
0.2	0.23	0.1	0.05	0.9	7	8
0.2	0.23	0.1	0.05	0.8	7	6
0.2	0.23	0.2	0.05	0.9	7	10
0.2	0.23	0.2	0.05	0.8	7	8
0.2	0.23	0.3	0.05	0.9	7	13
0.2	0.23	0.3	0.05	0.8	7	10

You may find this description of the sample size considerations for the trial daunting, especially if you have not had any courses on statistics. "Don't try this at home" is a worthy warning in this situation, and, more importantly, a reminder that a statistician should be involved in each research project from inception. That said, the math is straightforward, especially with software packages that provide for sample size and power calculations for cluster randomized trials, such as Acluster (*http://www.update-software.com/Acluster/*) and PASS (*http://www.ncss.com/*). The more difficult bits are estimating the magnitude of the effect and, if the effect is to be measured as a continuous variable, the variance of the effect, based on the differences between the intervention and control groups. In trials, it is always these differences between the groups that are important, not the changes within the groups.

For this proposal, the key figures are the difference in the mean proportions of recommendations implemented, comparing intervention and control groups, and the variance of that difference. The figures are based on a pilot study of an earlier version of the CDSS, showing that the mean number of recommendations was three per patient. The rest is prediction and convention. If this seems like shaky ground to you, please consider that if we knew what we would find, we wouldn't need to do the trial at all!

Given that the scope of the CDSS has been expanded, it seems reasonable to expect that the number of recommendations per patient would increase. The size of the effect we will look for (set at a 20% increase in the implementation of recommendations for the intervention group compared with the control group) is based on a judgment of what's possible (given the success of CDSSs to date) and what's needed to justify the intervention, that is, a "minimally important difference."

For the variance of the differences between groups, a statistical approach to estimating variance is used, taking a "conservative" approach. The assumption is that the distribution of findings will be "uniform" with roughly equal numbers of patients with -0.2, 0, 0.1, 0.2, 0.3, 0.4, 0.5, and 0.6 as the proportion of recommendations implemented. In all likelihood, this distribution will be closer to "normal," with most people in the middle levels of 0.2 to 0.4, and with fewer people at either extreme. The normal distribution is statistically more usual, connotes less variation among the observations than for a uniform distribution, and thus makes it easier to detect differences between groups. But we've assumed a worse case in a statistical sense, a uniform distribution. This will increase the estimated sample size needed—a conservative approach so that we will recruit *at least* as many patients as needed.

We also used a conservative approach for selecting an ICC (or within-cluster dependence). Statistical tests often assume that the observations being compared are independent of one another, but this may not be the case when groups of patients are being treated by the same practitioner who is receiving recommendations for each about care to be implemented. The ICC indicates the extent to which implementation of recommendations is influenced by patients within a cluster being treated by the same practitioners. The fewer the number of clinics we recruit from (i.e., the more patients we have per cluster), the larger the ICC we can expect. Few data are available to establish exactly what ICC to use, but when studies have been done, the ICCs are generally 0.15 or less for primary care settings (29). We chose an ICC of 0.2 to be conservative.

✓ Consider feasibility.

To assess the feasibility of recruiting primary care practices to the trial, we approached the family physicians associated with the Hamilton Academy of Medicine and the Department of Family Medicine at McMaster University. Letters of support, indicating understanding and support of the study's objectives, and willingness to participate, were received from physicians from 30 practices. Based on clinic statistics for the last 3 years, these practices are expected to refer about one patient per month per practice. This will provide an adequate number of patients for the study with a recruitment period of about 6 months or less.

Patient acceptance of the questionnaires and the recommendations has been assessed in a preliminary study staged on site at the DCRC, as has the physician acceptance of the recommendations from the questionnaires (3). Acceptance was high, although patients complained that the questionnaire took too long to complete while they were waiting for their appointment. The questionnaire has subsequently been shortened. The acceptability and accuracy of the optical character recognition system has been tested, with high acceptability and an error rate of less than 3% (4).

7.3 OTHER BITS

We haven't tried to include all parts of the protocol that would need to be present for a grant application. Notably, the budget and budget justification are missing. These are too dependent on local circumstances and funding agency conditions to be of much general interest. The best way to acquire an appreciation of what is needed is to ask a colleague or mentor with similar research interests to yours, and who has had a successful grant application to an appropriate agency, for a copy of their grant application. Our local research office also provides advice on budgets and presubmission vetting of proposals. In general, we've noticed a tendency of new investigators to seriously underestimate the costs of research, so it is well worthwhile to get some advice and a helping hand.

Other missing bits include details of how the inclusion and exclusion criteria will be defined, how and when measurements will be administered, the questionnaires that will be used, and other similar details. We will certainly need to prepare and provide these before submitting an application for funding.

7.4 ALTERNATIVE STUDY DESIGNS

Campbell and colleagues (31) address the issues of testing complex packages of interventions, especially in the field of delivering health services, such as stroke units, hospital at home, implementing guidelines, and CDSSs. They suggest a four-phase framework of development and testing health services interventions, corresponding to phases of drug testing, including a preclinical or theoretical phase; Phase I, identification of the components of the intervention; Phase II, definition of the trial and intervention design; Phase III, methodological issues for the main trial; and Phase IV, promoting effective implementation of the intervention. We didn't use this framework in developing the protocol described in this chapter, although its first three elements are represented. Mark Loeb has recently described the application of this model to a cluster randomized trial of guideline-directed use of antibiotics in nursing homes (32).

REFERENCES

1. Gerstein HC, Haynes RB, eds. *Evidence-based diabetes care.* Hamilton, Ontario: B. C. Decker, 2001.
2. Hunt DL, Haynes RB, Hayward RSA, et al. Automated direct-from-patient information collection for evidence-based diabetes care. *Proc AMIA Annu Symp* 1997:101–105.
3. Hunt DL, Haynes RB, Hayward RSA, et al. Patient-specific evidence-based care recommendations for diabetes mellitus: development and initial clinic experience with a computerized decision support system. *Int J Med Inform* 1998;51:127–135.
4. Hunt DL, Haynes RB. Using old technology to implement modern computer-aided decision support for primary diabetes care. *Proc AMIA Annu Symp* 2001:274–278.
5. The Diabetes Control and Complications Trial Research Group. Lifetime benefits and costs of intensive therapy as practiced in the diabetes control and complications trial. *JAMA* 1996;276:1409–1415.

6. UK Prospective Diabetes Study Group. Intensive blood-glucose control with sulphonyl-ureas or insulin compared with conventional treatment and risk of complications in patients with type 2 diabetes (UKPDS 33). *Lancet* 1998;352:837–853.

7. Gaede P, Vedel P, Larsen N, et al. Multifactorial intervention and cardiovascular disease in patients with type 2 diabetes. *N Engl J Med* 2003;348:383–393.

8. Yusuf S, Sleight P, Pogue J et al. The Heart Outcomes Prevention Evaluation Study Investigators. Effects of an angiotensin-converting-enzyme inhibitor, ramipril, on cardiovascular events in high-risk patients. *N Engl J Med* 2000;342:145–153.

9. Viberti G, Mogensen CE, Groop LC, et al. The European Microalbuminuria Captopril Study Group. Effect of captopril on progression to clinical proteinuria in patients with insulin-dependent diabetes mellitus and microalbuminuria. *JAMA* 1994;271: 275–279.

10. Lewis EJ, Hunsicker LG, Bain RP, et al. The Collaborative Study Group. The effect of angiotensin-converting-enzyme inhibition on diabetic nephropathy. *N Engl J Med* 1993;329:1456–1462.

11. UK Prospective Diabetes Study Group. Tight blood pressure control and risk of macrovascular and microvascular complications in type 2 diabetes: UKPDS 38. *BMJ* 1998;317:703–713.

12. UK Prospective Diabetes Study Group. Cost effectiveness analysis of improved blood pressure control in hypertensive patients with type 2 diabetes: UKPDS 40. *BMJ* 1998;317:720–726.

13. Vijan S, Hayward RA. Treatment of hypertension in type 2 diabetes mellitus: blood pressure goals, choice of agents, and setting priorities in diabetes care. *Ann Intern Med* 2003;138:593–602.

14. Goldberg RB, Mellies MJ, Sacks FM, et al. The CARE Investigators. Cardiovascular events and their reduction with pravastatin in diabetic and glucose-intolerant myocardial infarction survivors with average cholesterol levels. Subgroup analyses in the cholesterol and recurrent events (CARE) trial. *Circulation* 1998;98:2513–2519.

15. Collins R, Armitage J, Parish S, et al. MRC/BHF heart protection study of cholesterol-lowering with simvastatin in 5963 people with diabetes: a randomised placebo-controlled trial. *Lancet* 2003;361:2005–2016.

16. McCabe CJ, Stevenson RC, Dolan AM. Evaluation of a diabetic foot screening and protection programme. *Diabet Med* 1998;15:80–84.

17. Govaert TM, Thijs CT, Masurel N, et al. The efficacy of influenza vaccination in elderly individuals. A randomized double-blind placebo-controlled trial. *JAMA* 1994;272: 1661–1665.

18. Nichol KL, Lind A, Margolis KL, et al. The effectiveness of vaccination against influenza in healthy, working adults. *N Engl J Med* 1995;333:889–893.

19. Canadian Diabetes Association. Clinical practice guidelines for the prevention and management of diabetes in Canada. *Can J Diabetes* 2003;27:S1–S141.

20. Harris SB, Stewart M, Brown JB, et al. Type 2 diabetes in family practice. Room for improvement. *Can Fam Physician* 2003;49:778–785.

21. Hunt DL, Haynes RB, Hanna SE, et al. Effects of computer-based clinical decision support systems on physician performance and patient outcomes: a systematic review. *JAMA* 1998;280:1339–1346.

22. Lobach DF, Hammond WE. Computerized decision support based on a clinical practice guideline improves compliance with care standards. *Am J Med* 1997;102: 89–98.

23. Hetlevik I, Holmen J, Kruger O, et al. Implementing clinical guidelines in the treatment of diabetes mellitus in general practice. Evaluation of effort, process, and patient outcome related to implementation of a computer-based decision support system. *Int J Technol Assess Health Care* 2000;16:210–227.

24. Emanuel EJ, Wendler D, Grady C. What makes clinical research ethical? *JAMA* 2000;283:2701–2711.

25. Based on the tri-council policy statement: ethical conduct for research involving humans. Section 2. Free and informed consent [cited 2004 Sept. 23]. Available from: *(http://www.ncehr-cnerh.org/english/code_2/sec02.html)*.

26. Hines WW, Montgomery DC. *Probability and statistics in engineering and management science.* New York: Ronald Press Company, 1972.

27. Donner A, Birkett N, Buck C. Randomization by cluster. Sample size requirements and analysis. *Am J Epidemiol* 1981;114:906–914.

28. Donner A. Sample size requirements for stratified cluster randomization designs. *Stat Med* 1992;11:743–750, *Stat Med* 1997;16:2927–2928.

29. Donner A, Klar N. Statistical considerations in the design and analysis of community intervention trials. *J Clin Epidemiol* 1996;49:435–439.

30. Campbell M, Grimshaw J, Steen N. Changing professional practice in europe group (EU BIOMED II concerted action). Sample size calculations for cluster randomised trials. *J Health Serv Res Policy* 2000;5:12–16.

31. Campbell M, Fitzpatrick R, Haines A, et al. Framework of design and evaluation of complex interventions to improve health. *BMJ* 2000;321:694–696.

32. Loeb MB. Application of the development stages of a cluster randomized trial to a framework for evaluating complex health interventions. *BMC Health Serv Res* 2002;2:13. *(http://www.biomedcentral.com/1472-6963/2/13)*.

APPENDIX 7.1 DIABETES SUPPORT SYSTEM TRIAL. PATIENT INFORMATION AND CONSENT

I understand that I am being asked to participate in a research study, the Diabetes Support System Trial (DSST). I have been asked because I have been referred to the Diabetes Care and Research Centre (DCRC) at Hamilton Health Sciences, McMaster University Medical Centre, for assessment of diabetes. If I choose to join the study, my participation in the study will be approximately one year.

This study has have been explained to me by [–nurse's name–], a nurse working with clinic, and with the investigator for the trial, Dr. Brian Haynes [or other DCRC doctors' names].

I understand that there is often a waiting period of several months following my referral to the clinic before I can be seen and the objective of the study is to determine whether a computerized assessment of my health information can help to put this waiting time to good use. Thus, the study is designed to speed up the rate at which my diabetes will be assessed and care recommendations will be made, encouraging me and my family doctor to work together during the time from the date of referral to the DCRC to the time when my first visit is scheduled. This assessment will:

- identify the current state of my diabetes based on the information I provide on a brief questionnaire about my medical history, diabetes-related physical examination, and laboratory tests
- compare my diabetes and its treatment with current best standards of care, according to the Canadian Diabetes Association Guidelines for 2003 (with updating as new information becomes available)
- provide recommendations for improving my diabetes, if any are needed

I understand that only approved tests and treatments will be recommended and that there are no experimental tests or treatments involved. Thus, the benefits and risks to me are those associated with current recommended diabetes care, as will be explained to me by my doctor and nurse if any recommendations for changing my care are made.

I understand that I am free to refuse to participate in the study and that doing so will not delay (or speed up) the time I must wait for my first appointment at the clinic, nor will it jeopardize the care that I will receive when I visit the clinic. I also know that if I join the study, I can withdraw at any time, also without prejudice to my care.

If I participate in the study, I understand that information about me will be kept fully confidential and that I will not be personally identified in study reports in any way. Rather, data from my care will be pooled with data from other patients so that no individual patient can be identified. Further, I will be informed of these results.

I understand that the investigation is funded by [name of funding agency], that no company that might benefit financially from the study is involved, that the investigators have no plans to commercialize the service, that the study has been reviewed by a Research Ethics Board and the funding agency for scientific merit and sound ethical practice, and that my family doctor is aware of the study and has agreed to be involved in it.

I know that I can ask questions as the trial goes along by contacting [–name of nurse– DCRC, 3V3 Clinic, McMaster University Medical Center, 1200 Main St W, Hamilton, ON L8N 3Z5 tel. 905-521-2100] or Dr. Brian Haynes, McMaster University Medical Centre, 1200 Main St W, Rm 2C10b, Hamilton, ON L8N 3Z5, tel. 905-525-9140.

I agree to participate in the Diabetes Support System Trial.

Name (*please print*): _____ Witness: _____

Signature: _____ Signature: _____

Date: _____/_____/_____ Date: _____/_____/_____

      YYYY / MM / DD   YYYY / MM / DD

APPENDIX 7.2 TYPES OF ADVICE TO BE DELIVERED TO PATIENTS AND THEIR PHYSICIANS (33)[1]

Depending on the patient's responses to the questionnaire, feedback statements based on one or more of these recommendations will be printed.

1. All patients with type 1 diabetes should be aware of the benefits and risks of intensive insulin therapy and should be offered the opportunity for intensive insulin therapy. (See details following Recommendation 17.)
2. All patients who use insulin should do regular self-monitoring of blood sugars.
3. Patients who use oral hypoglycemic agents should consider regular self-monitoring of blood sugars.
4. Patients with diabetes should have at least one ophthalmology assessment per year, including a dilated pupil examination, beginning five years after initial diagnosis of diabetes or on becoming pregnant. People with type 2 diabetes should begin checks when they are first found to have diabetes.
5. All patients with type 1 diabetes should have annual assessments to see whether there is any protein in their urine. Patients with type 1 diabetes do not need to begin having these assessments until they have had diabetes for 5 years, unless they are planning to become pregnant.
6. Patients with type 2 diabetes should have annual assessments to see whether there is any protein in their urine.
7. All patients with diabetes should do regular foot inspections.
8. All patients who have had a heart attack or a stroke or a transient ischemic attack (TIA) should take at least one aspirin every day unless there is a strong reason not to, such as allergy or other intolerance. People who have ever had angina or who have poor circulation to their legs should also consider taking daily aspirin.
9. All people who have had a heart attack should take a β blocker unless there is a strong reason not to.
10. All people with diabetes should have an annual influenza vaccination, unless there is a contraindication.
11. All people who have had a heart attack, stroke or TIA or who have angina or peripheral vascular disease should have a cholesterol assessment at least every 5 years.
12. All patients with diabetes who are between 40 and 65 years of age should have their cholesterol level checked every 5 years.
13. All patients with diabetes aged 21 years or over should have their blood pressure checked every 6 to 12 months.
14. All patients who smoke should be offered advice and help to stop smoking.

[1]Hunt DL, Haynes RB. Using old technology to implement modern computer-aided decision support for primary diabetes care. *Proc AMIA Annu Symp* 2001:274–278, with permission.

15. All people who use insulin or are on pills to control their blood sugar should have some sugar, candy, or some other source of sugar with them at all times.
16. All people with diabetes who use insulin or take pills to control their blood sugars should wear a Medic Alert or other warning bracelet or necklace, and have a card with them at all times indicating that they have diabetes and stating their medications.
17. All women with diabetes who may become pregnant should plan their pregnancy beginning well before conception.

Details for Recommendation 1

All patients with type 1 diabetes should be aware of the benefits and risks of intensive insulin therapy and should be offered the opportunity for intensive insulin therapy.

What is intensive insulin therapy?

Intensive insulin therapy is an approach to blood sugar control in which the goal is to keep blood sugars as close to normal as possible. Two methods are available:

- taking insulin three to five times a day
- using an insulin pump, a small pump that injects insulin continuously

For both approaches, it is also recommended to check one's own blood sugars three to four times per day.

Why is intensive insulin therapy recommended?

Intensive insulin therapy is recommended for patients with type 1 diabetes because it can prevent or delay some of the eye, kidney, and nerve complications associated with diabetes. The only major disadvantage is that severe low blood sugar episodes are more common. Thus, careful blood sugar monitoring is required. Intensive insulin therapy is also more demanding and expensive for the patient and the health care provider in the short term.

Is there any proof that intensive insulin therapy actually helps?

Yes! A very large, high quality study (the Diabetes Control and Complications Trial, or DCCT) found that keeping blood sugars as close to normal as possible reduces the complications of type 1 diabetes. (The UK Prospective Diabetes Study and a smaller Japanese study had similar findings for type 2 diabetes.)

How strong is this recommendation?

Very strong—the DCCT study was carried out so well that there is no doubt about the benefits of improved blood sugar control.

Recommendations from diabetes care organizations:

The Canadian Diabetes Association and the American Diabetes Association both endorse the findings of the DCCT and recommend "tight control" of blood sugars through personalized insulin therapy regimens and establishing individual blood sugar control goals for patients with type 1 diabetes.

Key References:

For patients: Intensive insulin therapy. Diabetes Evidence Module.

For health professionals: The Diabetes Control and Complications Trial Research Group. Lifetime benefits and costs of intensive therapy as practiced in the Diabetes Control and Complications Trial. *JAMA*. 1996;276: 1409–1415. (Abstracted in the Diabetes Evidence Module.)

8

EVALUATING DIAGNOSTIC TESTS

Gordon Guyatt, Dave Sackett, and Brian Haynes

Chapter Outline

8.1 Introduction

8.2 Introducing the terminology of diagnosis

8.3 Basic principles of conducting diagnostic studies

8.4 Special challenges of randomized controlled trials of diagnostic strategies

8.5 Results of randomized controlled trials of diagnostic strategies in patients with presumed operable lung cancer

CLINICAL RESEARCH SCENARIO

Some time in 1982 a Hamilton, Ontario, geriatrician named Christopher Patterson noted that he was getting confusing results when measuring serum ferritin. The lower limit of normal ferritin in the Hamilton laboratory, consistent with most labs, was 18 μg per L. Dr. Patterson was finding that when he performed bone marrow aspirations in patients with ferritin values between 19 and 50 or so, he was getting surprising results. Because these ferritin values were in the normal range, he was anticipating a relatively low probability of iron deficiency. However, he was finding iron deficiency reported from bone marrow aspirates in such patients with surprising frequency. He suspected that ferritin was behaving differently in his elderly patients than in the remainder of the population.

Dr. Patterson sought our collaboration in helping to sort out this issue. In the first discussion we had together, it became evident that while sorting out how to use serum ferritin, we could efficiently evaluate other tests advertised, and some widely used, for diagnosis of iron deficiency. These included the mean cell volume (MCV), transferrin saturation (TS), red cell protoporphyrin (RCP), and red cell distribution width (RDW).

8.1 INTRODUCTION

When making a diagnosis, clinicians seldom have immediate, easy access to the reference or "gold" standard tests—such as a biopsy or invasive imaging investigation—for the target disorders they suspect. Moreover, they often wish to avoid the risks or costs of these reference standards, especially when they are invasive, painful, or dangerous. No wonder, then, that clinical researchers examine relations between a wide range of more easily measured phenomena in the diagnostic process. In this chapter, we will refer to these phenomena as "the test or tests" of interest and distinguish them from the gold or reference standard (which one may also think of as a test).

These phenomena include elements of the patient's history, physical examination, images from all sorts of penetrating waves, and the levels of myriad constituents of body fluids and tissues. Unfortunately, even the most promising phenomena, when evaluated rigorously, almost never exhibit a one-to-one relation to their corresponding target disorders. Often, several different diagnostic tests compete for primacy in diagnosing the same target disorder.

In response to this problem, investigators have expended considerable effort at the interface between clinical medicine and scientific methods in an effort to maximize the validity and usefulness of diagnostic tests. This chapter defines and illustrates that interface. In addition, it presents some strategies and tactics for working at that interface to determine the validity, precision, and health impact of diagnostic tests.

Sensitivity Is Insensitive to Validity

Sensitivity, likelihood ratios (LRs), receiver operating characteristic (ROC) curves, and the like can (and frequently do) misrepresent a test's real value. These descriptors of diagnostic tests can (and frequently do) misrepresent a test's real value (or uselessness), just as relative and absolute risk reductions misrepresent therapeutic impact. This is because investigators often calculate these diagnostic and therapeutic descriptors for studies with design flaws that have compromised their validity.

Of what use is a study of a new cancer test that compared medical students with moribund cancer victims, gave the test results to those who were interpreting the reference standard results, subjected the medical students to the reference standard only if their diagnostic tests were positive, and never bothered to test it on a second, independent group of study participants? These four major errors would never be detected in a simple examination of sensitivity or any other test descriptor, any more than an examination of relative risk reduction would identify failure to randomize and correct for prognostic imbalance.

Throughout this chapter, we urge you to keep the following diagnostic quartet at the front of your mind (you might want to write them on your bookmark). A valid diagnostic study:

1. assembles an appropriate spectrum of patients
2. applies both the diagnostic test and reference standard to all of them
3. interprets each blind to the other
4. repeats itself in a second, independent ("test") set of patients.

The major objective of this chapter is to demonstrate how to achieve this validity. Past experience shows us this is no easy task; the methodologic quality of diagnostic test studies up to now has tended to be poor (1). Our guidelines for achieving a valid diagnostic study consider the STARD (standards for reporting of diagnostic accuracy) initiative (*http://www.consort-statement.org/stardstatement.htm*), a compilation of suggestions from an international group of methodologists concerning how authors of diagnostic test studies should report their methods and results (2).

This Chapter Is Not About How Diagnosticians Think

Clinicians seldom use just one diagnostic test to make their diagnoses. Instead, they bring together bits of their patients' histories, physical examinations, blood, and tissue samples, diagnostic images, and clinical course to arrive at their final diagnoses. Seasoned clinicians usually complete this process as a nonverbal undertaking, typically in the blink of an eye. They often have great difficulty describing to learners, how they did it and sometimes they even label it the "art of medicine."

A major focus of clinical epidemiology has been the attempt to identify and understand the "science of the art of medicine." In studying the "art of diagnosis," our focus in this chapter will be a pragmatic one. We don't know how diagnosticians "think." Instead, we will focus on what they think about, the bits of information they take from patients, and their diagnostic strategies. Then we will examine some properties of these bits of information, which, when combined in various ways, provide the best match with patients' ultimate diagnoses.

So, this chapter will employ the methods of clinical epidemiological research, not those of cognitive psychology. Our objective is to show you "external" methods for getting the diagnostic answer right, regardless of whether these methods bear any relation to any "internal" methods being applied inside a diagnostician's brain box.

Diagnostic Tests Are Not Just About Diagnosis

Before going further, we want to point out that clinicians use "diagnostic tests" for five purposes besides diagnosis.

Consider the "diagnostic test" of carotid artery ultrasound in patients with transient ischemic attacks. Certainly, you can use it to *diagnose* carotid artery stenosis. But by determining the degree of carotid stenosis, carotid ultrasound gives you three other sorts of information:

1. Carotid ultrasound can tell you the *severity* of the patient's carotid stenosis. Is it only 60% or is it almost occluded?
2. Carotid ultrasound can tell you the patient's *prognosis* for stroke and death. The greater the stenosis, the greater the risks of these awful outcomes.
3. Carotid ultrasound can predict your patient's likely *responsiveness to therapy*. Patients with low-grade stenosis are more likely to be harmed than benefited by endarterectomy, but patients with high-grade stenosis are increasingly likely to benefit from the operation.

   And consider the "TSH test" that measures the level of thyroid-stimulating hormone. Certainly, you use it in the *diagnosis* of patients with signs or symptoms suggestive of hyper- or hypothyroidism.

   Further consider another "diagnostic test" thyroid stimulating hormone (TSH), which you can use for two other purposes.
4. You could measure TSH when *screening* apparently healthy elderly individuals for subclinical hypothyroidism (although we wouldn't recommend your doing so).
5. And you must monitor TSH (and sometimes thyroid hormones themselves) in patients you're treating for hypothyroidism to *determine the proper dose and actual response to therapy* with thyroxine.

Note, however, that these uses relate to screening, determining severity, and optimally managing the patient in whom you have made a diagnosis. Some of the uses of the test relate to the patient's present state of affairs (screening, diagnosis, severity, and optimal therapy), whereas others predict her future (prognosis and likely responsiveness to subsequent therapy). Because the methods for determining the accuracy of these predictions are similar, much of what follows applies to all of these uses. These considerations raise the issue of overlap between studies of diagnosis and those of prognosis, an issue we take up in considerable detail in the introduction section of Chapter 9, on prognosis. The current chapter deals only superficially with issues of screening or of using tests to determine the severity of a patient's condition.

The issue of determining severity deserves special attention. Specialists in laboratory medicine continue to present clinicians with ranges of "normal" that are based on variability of results in normal populations. This information is of limited use in making diagnoses, and, as you shall see in the case of serum ferritin, can be very misleading. But diagnosis is not the primary way we use laboratory tests.

Rather, we often use laboratory tests to establish whether a patient has a physiologic abnormality and, if so, the magnitude of the abnormality. A patient with a low hemoglobin is anemic; a patient with an elevated aspartate aminotransferase (AST) has hepatic inflammation or necrosis; a patient with a low partial pressure of oxygen (PO_2) is hypoxemic. That the range of normal here provides considerable help in determining whether there is an underlying physiologic abnormality, and the magnitude of that abnormality, explains the continued popularity of hemoglobin, AST, and PO_2.

Anemia, hepatic inflammation, and hypoxemia are, however, abnormal physiologic states; they are not diagnoses. Having identified a physiologic abnormality, the clinician asks: "What is the explanation for this abnormality?" And for that second question, which is the topic of this chapter, the range of normal is of limited use.

There is one other aspect of diagnostic tests that this chapter does not address in detail. Recently, clinicians are increasingly using diagnostic tests as a package, as opposed to using them individually. In other words, clinicians consider a group of test results simultaneously, as opposed to sequentially. This requires knowledge of the extent of common information the tests capture. If tests capture different information, clinicians will not be misled when they assume independence. On the other hand, if test results are correlated, assuming indepence will lead to spurious under- or overestimates of the probability that the target condition is present. Estimating the extent of overlap is difficult to do intuitively, and clinical investigators have wisely chosen to use formal, statistically derived clinical prediction rules when simultaneously considering the results of a number of diagnostic tests. We consider in detail issues related to clinical prediction rules in Chapter 9, on prognosis.

Diagnosis Isn't an End in Itself

No diagnosis by itself ever made a patient better. The ultimate proof of a diagnostic test's value lies in the outcomes of the patients who submit to it. Accordingly, this chapter, in a separate concluding section with its own scenario, will discuss methods for determining whether a diagnostic test results in more good than harm. The issues here are essentially those of demonstrating the benefits and risks of a therapy, and this chapter will largely restrict itself to demonstrating how the principles of assessing therapy apply to randomized trials of diagnostic strategies (see Chapters 4, 5, and 6).

8.2 INTRODUCING THE TERMINOLOGY OF DIAGNOSIS

We debated the content and organization of this "chunk" of the chapter on the various ways of computing measures of the power of a diagnostic test. All of us were concerned that the focus on nomenclature and number-crunching might be excessive and detract from an appropriate concern with the underlying study design. In fact, ways of dealing with the numbers are less important than the issues of validity we outlined in the introduction to this chapter (we'll come back to these issues in the next section). In addition, none of us like or use "predictive values," and one of us wanted to ban them from the book. We also considered skipping all the 2-by-2 (fourfold) table stuff and going directly to multilevel LRs. Finally, we reckoned that most of you already know most of this stuff.

But the definitions and numbers remain in wide use. Therefore, while bearing all those caveats in mind, this section will identify the terms and definitions you will encounter in the literature of diagnostic tests. Those of you who are already familiar with the basics might want to jump right to the "diagnostic odds ratio." At the other extreme, if you want to consider these ideas in greater detail or at a more leisurely pace, we suggest that you go to Chapter 4 of the second edition of this book (3).

Simple Properties

Let's begin with a simple table describing the relation between a diagnostic test [say, the level of B-type natriuretic peptide (BNP) in a patient's blood serum] and a diagnosis [say, left ventricular dysfunction (LVD) on echocardiography]. An Oxfordshire (England) group of clinical investigators invited general practitioners in their area "to refer patients with suspected heart failure to our clinic." (4) Once there, these 126 patients underwent independent, blind BNP measurements and echocardiography. The first set of results from that study is shown in Table 8-1.

TABLE 8-1 Performance of B-type Natriuretic Peptide ≥18 pg/mL As a Diagnostic Test for Left Ventricular Dysfunction

		Target Disorder (LVD on Echocardiography)		Totals
		Present	Absent	
Diagnostic Test Result (Serum BNP)	Positive (BNP ≥18 pg/mL)	35 a	57 b	92 a + b
	Negative (BNP <18 pg/mL)	c 5	d 29	c + d 34
	Totals	a + c 40	b + d 86	a + b + c + d 126

From Landray MJ, Lehman R, Arnold I. Measuring brain natriuretic peptide in suspected left ventricular systolic dysfunction in general practice: cross-sectional study. *BMJ* 2000;320:985–986, with permission.

From these results, you can generate some informative measures of the accuracy of BNP in detecting LVD. Rather than trust our hand calculations, we routinely use Sharon Straus's "stats calculator" on her EBM Web site *http://www.cebm.utoronto.ca/practise/ca/statscal/*.

1. You can calculate the proportion of patients *with* LVD who also have *elevated* BNP. That calculation goes:

$$a/(a + c) = 35/40 = 0.88, \text{ or } 88\%$$

By convention, we refer to that property of "positivity in the presence of the target disorder" as *Sensitivity*.

2. You can calculate the proportion of patients who are *free of* LVD who also have *normal* BNP. That calculation goes:

$$d/(b + d) = 29/86 = 0.34, \text{ or } 34\%$$

By convention, we refer to that property of "negativity in the absence of the target disorder" as *Specificity*.

3. You can calculate the proportion of patients with *elevated* BNP who also *have* LVD. That calculation goes:

$$a/(a + b) = 35/92 = 0.38, \text{ or } 38\%$$

By convention, we refer to that property of "presence of the target disorder disease among positives" as *Positive Predictive Value* (PPV). Another term to express this value is the *Post-test Likelihood given a Positive Test Result* (PTL+).

4. You can calculate the proportion of patients with *normal* BNP who also are *free of* LVD. That calculation goes:

$$d/(c + d) = 29/34 = 0.85, \text{ or } 85\%$$

By convention, we refer to that property of "absence of the target disorder among negatives" as *Negative Predictive Value* (NPV). Clinicians more commonly think in terms of the post-test likelihood given a negative result. This likelihood is $(1 - \text{NPV})$ or $c/(c + d)$.

5. You can calculate the proportion of patients *with LVD before you even measure their BNP*. That calculation goes:

$$(a + c)/(a + b + c + d) = 40/126 = 0.32, \text{ or } 32\%$$

By convention, we refer to that "pre-test probability of the target disorder" in the total population at risk (not considering any additional diagnostic information) as *Prevalence*, because it describes the prevailing rate of the target disorder in the patients who are undergoing the diagnostic test.

6. You can calculate the odds that a patient has *LVD before you ever measure their BNP*. That calculation goes:

Pre-test Probability/(100% − Pre-test Probability) = 32%/(100% − 32%)
= 32%/68%
= 0.47

(It sometimes appears as 0.47:1 or 0.47 to 1). By convention, we refer to this as *Pre-test Odds*.

And you can convert an odds back into a probability. That calculation goes:

odds/(odds + 1) = 0.47/1.47 = 0.32, or 32%

7. You can calculate the likelihood that an elevated BNP is found in patients with, as opposed to patients without, LVD. That calculation goes:

[a/(a + c)]/[b/(b + d)] = Sensitivity/(100% − Specificity)
= 88%/(100% − 34%)
= 88%/66%
= 1.3

(it sometimes appears as 1.3:1 or 1.3 to 1). By convention, we refer to that as a *Likelihood Ratio of a positive test* (LR+) (some prefer to call it a *Positive Likelihood Ratio*, although all LRs are positive, in that they are all greater than 0).

8. You can calculate the likelihood that a normal BNP is found in patients with, as opposed to patients without, LVD. That calculation goes:

[c/(a + c)]/[d/(b + d)] = (100% − Sensitivity)/Specificity
= (100% − 88%)/34%
= 12%/34%
= 0.4.

By convention, we refer to that as a *Likelihood Ratio of a negative test* (LR−) (some prefer to call it a *Negative Likelihood Ratio*, although others point out that LRs, in that they always take values greater than 0, are never negative).

9. You can discover that if you multiply the Pre-test Odds from the population studied by the LR of a positive test result and convert the resulting Post-test Odds back to a probability, it is identical to the PPV. That calculation goes:

Pre-test odds from no. 6 above x LR+ from no. 7 above = 0.47 x 1.3
= 0.61

and

0.61/1.61 = 0.38, or 38%

(the same as you calculated in no. 3 above).

10. You can discover that if you multiply the Pre-test Odds from the population studied by the LR of a negative test result and convert the resulting Post-test Odds back to a probability, it is equal to (100% − NPV). That calculation goes:

Pre-test odds from no. 6 above x LR− from no. 8 above = 0.47 x 0.4
$$= 0.19$$

and

$$0.19/1.19 = 0.15, \text{ or } 15\%$$

and

$$100\% - 15\% = 85\%$$

(the same as you calculated in no. 4 above).

11. You can generate an overall measure of the diagnostic test's accuracy by dividing the LR+ by the LR−. As it happens, this is the same as dividing (a times d) by (b times c), which is often referred to as a "cross-products" calculation. By convention, we call the result a *diagnostic odds ratio*. From no. 7 and no. 8 above, the LR+/LR− ratio (calculated with three significant figures) is 1.32/0.371 = 3.6. And from Table 8–1 we can calculate the cross-products odds ratio of ($35 \times 29)/(5 \times 57$) = 1015/285 = 3.6.

12. You can generate 95% confidence intervals (CIs) around these accuracy measures. Once again, we rely on Sharon Straus, who has incorporated Paul Glasziou's method into her Web site: *http://www. cebm.utoronto.ca/practise/ca/statscal/.*

    The 95% CIs for the foregoing measures are shown in parentheses:

Sensitivity = 88% (74%–94%)
Specificity = 34% (25%–44%)
PPV = 38% (29%–48%)
NPV = 85% (70%–94%)
LR+ = 1.3 (1.1–1.6)
LR− = 0.4 (0.2–0.9)

You may have noticed that we haven't introduced the terms "true-positive rate" and "false-positive rate." This is because we've found inconsistencies in their construction. Sure, the obvious numerator in a "false-positive" rate is cell d of Table 8–1, but what should we use for its denominator? We've encountered three different denominators. Some folks insert ($b + d$) for its denominator, creating a number equal to (100% − specificity); others use ($a + b$), creating a number equal to (100% − PPV); and we've even encountered folks using ($a + b + c + d$) for its denominator, telling us the percentage of false-positive results in the entire study population. These are ambiguous terms and we won't use them here.

Some simple rules-of-thumb follow from these properties of diagnostic tests:

- The higher a test's sensitivity, specificity, PPV, and NPV, the more accurate that test is.
- The larger the LR of a positive test positive, the more accurate that test is.
- The farther the LR of a negative test is from 1 (the smaller it is), the more accurate that test is.
- If a test's sensitivity and the LR of a positive test are very high (say, an LR+ >20), then a negative test result pretty well rules out the target disorder. Dave Sackett's clinical clerks invented a mnemonic to remember this paradoxical property: "SnNout," which means, "When a diagnostic test has an extremely high sensitivity, a negative test result *rules out* the target disorder."
- By that same logic, if a test's specificity is very high and the LR of a negative test is very low (say, an LR− <0.05), then a positive test result pretty well rules in the target disorder. David Sackett's clinical clerks decided to call this property "SpPin," which means, "When a diagnostic test has an extremely high specificity, a positive test result rules in the target disorder."

If you apply these rules-of-thumb to BNP and LVD, you'd conclude that this diagnostic test had a good sensitivity (88%) and NPV (85%), but that its poor specificity (34%) dragged down its PPV (38%) and its LR+ (1.3), and led to an LR− (0.4) that was almost as useless as the LR+. In fact, its PPV or post-test probability (38%) was only slightly higher than its pre-test probability or prevalence (34%). And that's the way it was reported. These investigators concluded, "introducing routine measurement (of BNP) would be unlikely to improve the diagnosis of symptomatic (LVD) in the community."

However, their report also documented the effect of two other cutpoints for BNP. This led both to a counter claim on the usefulness of BNP in the subsequent letters to the editor and to an opportunity for us to describe some alternative ways of presenting information about the accuracy of a diagnostic test. When we applied a higher cut-point for a positive BNP test (≥76 rather than ≥18 in the original report) we could construct Table 8–2.

You can try your hand at calculating the various properties of the BNP at this new cut-point. Our calculations appear at the end of this section.

Multilevel Likelihood Ratios

Because the authors of the BNP study presented their results for two other cutoffs (10 pg/mL and 76 pg/mL), you can divide their test results into three groups (<10, 10–75, and >75). Although you can't any longer describe these results with binary measures like sensitivity and specificity, you can make great use of "multilevel" LRs. That is, you can describe, for any level of the test result, the likelihood that that level would be observed in a patient with, as opposed to one without, the target disorder. The calculations are as before, and the result is shown in Table 8–3.

TABLE 8-2   Performance of B-type Natriuretic Peptide ≥76 pg/mL as a Diagnostic Test for Left Ventricular Dysfunction

		Target Disorder (LVD on Echocardiography)		Totals
		Present	Absent	
Diagnostic Test Result (Serum BNP)	Positive (BNP >75 pg/mL)	26 a	11 b	37 a + b
	Negative (BNP <76 pg/mL)	c 14	d 75	c + d 89
		a + c	b + d	a + b + c + d
	Totals	40	86	126

From Landray MJ, Lehman R, Arnold I. Measuring brain natriuretic peptide in suspected left ventricular systolic dysfunction in general practice: cross-sectional study. *BMJ* 2000;320:985–986, with permission.

TABLE 8-3   Multilevel Likelihood Ratios

	Patients with LVD on Echo-Cardiography	Patients with Normal Echoes	Likelihood Ratio and 95% CI
High BNP (≥76 pg/mL)	26 (0.650)	11 (0.128)	5.1 (2.8–9.2)
Mid BNP (10–75 pg/mL)	11 (0.275)	60 (0.698)	0.4 (0.2–0.7)
Low BNP (<10 pg/mL)	3 (0.075)	15 (0.174)	0.4 (0.1–1)
Total	40 (1.000)	86 (1.000)	

From Landray MJ, Lehman R, Arnold I. Measuring brain natriuretic peptide in suspected left ventricular systolic dysfunction in general practice: cross-sectional study. *BMJ* 2000;320:985–986, with permission.

The numbers in parentheses are the proportions of patients with the various test results, calculated separately for those with and without LVD, therefore adding to 1.000 at the foot of each column. By using multilevel LRs to take advantage of the full range of BNP results, you can be slightly more optimistic about the diagnostic usefulness of higher levels. The LR for BNP results ≥76 pg per mL was 5.1. Moreover, these levels were found in 26/126 or 21% of the patients in this study, and this BNP level raised the pre-test probability of LVD in the typical patient from 32% to a post-test probability of 70%. (You can determine this from Table 8–3 for a patient with a pre-test probability of 32% and a high BNP: reading horizontally across the top row, the result is $[26/(26 + 11)] = 70\%$).

Assume that the properties of a diagnostic test are the same when applied to groups of patients with high and low prevalences of the target disorder, and you can easily apply the LR for a test result to any prevalence (pre-test odds) of the target disorder. Suppose a patient has a pre-test probability of 50% (a pre-test odds of 1:1). You don't have to reconstruct Table 8–3 for this new prevalence. You can simply multiply that patient's pre-test odds (say, 1:1) by the LR for that patient's test result (say, 80 pg/mL, with an LR of 5.1). This generates a post-test odds of 5.1, which you can convert into a post-test probability by solving $5.1/(1 + 5.1)$. This yields a post-test probability of 84%, which is much higher than you would generate with the cutoff of 10 pg per mL. For the latter case, shown in Table 8–1, you multiply 1×1.3 and get a post-test probability of LVD of only $1.3/2.3 = 0.56$ or 56%.

Likelihood Ratio Nomograms

Under this same assumption that the test properties are independent of prevalence, you can go even further and do away with calculations altogether, as shown in Figure 8–1.

Using this "likelihood ratio nomogram," you can apply any LR (the center scale) to any pre-test probability (the left-hand scale) and simply follow a straight edge over to the post-test probability (the right-hand scale). In Figure 8–1, we show this for the patient described in the previous paragraph.

Receiver Operating Characteristic Curves

If you plot the sensitivity or "hits" versus (1-specificity) or "false alarms" that result from selecting different cutoffs for the diagnostic test results, you generate a useful picture of the test's accuracy that is called an "ROC curve[1]." ROC curves nicely display the trade-offs of using one or more cutoffs for the test. We show one for our BNP in Figure 8–2.

---

[1]"Receiver" or "Response" Operating Characteristic (ROC) curves began as a helpful way of distinguishing real signals for false noises in the early days of radar.

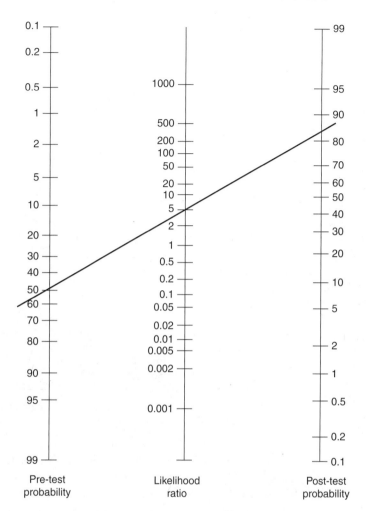

Pre-test
probability

Likelihood
ratio

Post-test
probability

FIGURE 8–1 Nomogram for converting pre-test likelihoods (*left column*) to post-test likelihoods (*right column*) by drawing a straight line from the pre-test likelihood through the likelihood ratio for the test result (5). (From Fagan TJ. Nomogram for Bayes's theorem. ***N Engl J Med*** 1975;293:257, with permission.)

An ROC curve has some useful properties:

- It illustrates the performance of a dichotomous diagnostic test when you select different cut-points to distinguish "normal" from "abnormal" results.
- It demonstrates the fact that any increase in sensitivity will be accompanied by a decrease in specificity, and vice versa.
- The closer the curve gets to the upper left corner of the display, the more the overall accuracy of the test. That is, choosing the point labelled "BNP ≥76" correctly identifies 26 affected and 75 normal patients out of the total of 126, or 80% overall accuracy (you can

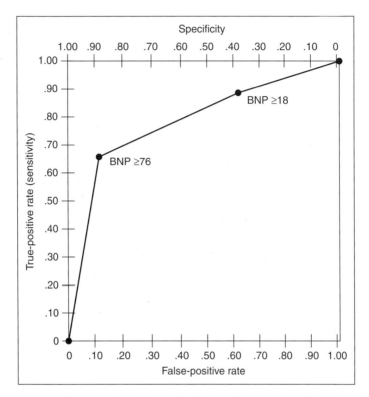

FIGURE 8–2 A receiver operating characteristic curve for B-type natriuretic peptide (BNP) as a diagnostic test for left ventricular dysfunction.

confirm this in Table 8–2.) However, choosing the point labelled "BNP ≥18" correctly identifies 35 affected but only 29 normal patients from the total of 126, which is only 51% overall accuracy (you can confirm this in Table 8–1).

- The closer the curve comes to the 45-degree diagonal of the ROC space, the less accurate the test. At 45 degrees, the test adds no diagnostic information at all.
- Getting a bit fancier, the slope of the tangent at a cut-point gives the LR for that value of the test. Notice how much steeper the tangent is for the cutoff of ≥76 than it is for the cutoff of ≥18.
- The area under the curve provides an overall measure of a test's accuracy. This property comes in handy when you are trying to decide which of two competing tests for the same target disorder is the better one. We'll come back to that when we discuss the analysis of a diagnostic test study.

Combinations of Diagnostic Tests

Clinicians almost never use single diagnostic tests in isolation. For example, Dave Sackett's team at Oxford identified 32 clinical signs for obstructive

TABLE 8-4   Likelihood Ratios for Individual Elements of the History and Physical Exam

Diagnostic Test	Likelihood Ratios for OAD for Elements Taken Individually	
	LR+	LR−
Patient said they had OAD	7.3	0.5
Patient had smoked for more than 40 yr	8.3	0.8
Patient was as old as or older than 45 yr	1.3	0.4
Maximum laryngeal height (above sternal notch) 4 cm or less	2.8	0.8

From Straus SE, McAlister FA, Sackett DL et al., CARE-COAD1 Group. The accuracy of patient history, wheezing, and laryngeal measurements in diagnosing obstructive airway disease. *JAMA* 2000;283:1853–1857, with permission.

airway disease (OAD) (6). Our physical diagnosis books recommended seeking various clusters of them, but didn't tell us how to combine their results. So, working with an international team of clinicians, we ran a Web-based study of the accuracy of a patient's history, wheezing, and laryngeal height in diagnosing OAD on simultaneous, blinded spirometry. Table 8–4 shows the LRs for individual elements of the history and physical examination.

Individually, these elements look promising, but not decisive. Might they perform better when they are combined? That depends on whether they are detecting the same (dependent or overlapping) or different (independent) aspects of these patients' conditions. When Jon Deeks did a statistical analysis that corrected for any overlap, we discovered that when all four elements were present, the LR for OAD was 220, thereby "ruling-in" the diagnosis. When none of these four elements was present, the LR was 0.13, making OAD far less likely. The area under the associated ROC curve was 0.86, which is quite good and better than the majority of diagnostic tests.

The forgoing is intended to create or refresh your memory about the basic properties of diagnostic tests, their calculation, and their conventional names. It is not intended to lull you into thinking that studies of diagnostic tests are neat, tidy, and capable of summarization in a fourfold table. The next section of this chapter addresses the process of conducting a study of a diagnostic test or tests.

Our calculations from Table 8–2 (and their 95% CIs):

Sensitivity (sens) = $a/(a + c)$ = 65% (50%–78%)
Specificity (spec) = $d/(b + d)$ = 87% (78%–93%)
Positive Predictive Value = $a/(a + b)$ = 70% (54%–82%)
Negative Predictive Value = $d/(c + d)$ = 84% (75%–90%)

Prevalence = $(a + c)/(a + b + c + d)$ = same as before, dummy!
Pre-test odds = prevalence/(1 − prevalence) = same here, too!
LR+ = sens/(1 − spec) = 5.1 (2.8–9.2)
LR− = (1 − sens)/spec = 0.4 (0.3–0.6)
Diagnostic Odds Ratio = 13

8.3 BASIC PRINCIPLES OF CONDUCTING DIAGNOSTIC STUDIES

A protocol for any study determining patients' diagnoses must attend to the following elements:

✓ Conduct your literature review.
✓ Pose your research question.
✓ Recruit your participants. Recruit a sample of patients representative of those to whom you will apply the test in clinical practice.
✓ Select your measurement procedures.
✓ Apply the gold standard. Determine whether or not the target condition is present.
✓ Select your statistical procedures. Include sample size calculation, how to represent the properties of a diagnostic test, and subgroup analysis.
✓ Measure the test's impact. Decide whether and how to measure the impact of your diagnostic test on patient outcome.

✓ Conduct your literature review

We did not, as we should have, begin our work by conducting a systematic review of studies examining the properties of tests for the diagnosis of iron deficiency. As you shall see, had we done so we might have conducted our study quite differently, or perhaps not at all. Our results, however, stimulated us to conduct the systematic review that we should have undertaken earlier in the process.

Following the primary study, the main focus of this chapter, we conducted a systematic review of studies examining the properties of diagnostic tests for iron deficiency (7). Eligible studies examined patients older than 18 years of age with low hemoglobin, explored the properties of one of the candidate tests (i.e., MCV, TS, serum ferritin, RCP, RDW, and RCP), and examined the relation between test results and findings on bone marrow aspiration.

We conducted two MEDLINE searches using methodology available in 1989 and January 1990, when we conducted the final search. The first MEDLINE search was as follows: [iron or iron (tw)] and [anemia/diagnosis or bone marrow/analysis or bone marrow/metabolism]. The second was: [iron (tw) or anemia or anemia (tw)] and [erythrocytes/analysis or erythrocytes/pathology or erythrocyte count]. In the second search, if we obtained more than 100 articles from any particular MEDLINE file, we added "diagnosis" as a subheading. We repeated these searches on all MEDLINE files between 1966 and January 1990, when we conducted the final search.

Nowadays, we would likely turn to PubMed for the MEDLINE search utilizing the sensitive filter for diagnostic tests. We would use the "related articles" feature from PubMed for any eligible studies we found, check other databases and books of recent abstracts, and contact experts in the field.

Even the limited search conducted in 1990 yielded 1,179 titles. Two team members reviewed the citations, and we retrieved any articles that either person thought might be relevant. We contacted the first author of all abstracts and requested to see a more complete report of the methods or results of each study if these were available. Two reviewers evaluated the full text of 127 potentially relevant articles and established that 55 articles were eligible.

For each relevant text, we abstracted individual patient data available in the published (or unpublished) report for two groups of patients: those who proved to be iron deficient on bone marrow aspiration and those who did not.

We present the results of this systematic review later in the chapter. First, we return to our primary study to learn its outcome and relevance to our systematic review.

✓ *Pose your research question.*

Among patients older than 65 years presenting with anemia, in whom the diagnosis is a relevant issue and in whom the underlying diagnosis remains in doubt, to what extent do values of mean red cell volume, RDW, serum iron, iron-binding capacity, serum ferritin, and RCP increase or decrease the likelihood of iron deficiency as established by a criterion or gold standard bone marrow aspiration (8)?

Conceptually, the population of interest in a study of diagnostic tests will be one in which clinicians are seriously considering the diagnosis of interest—although that diagnosis remains in doubt. We will explore the definition of the appropriate patient population at some length in the next section.

In a diagnostic test study, intervention—the second part in the triad of any research question: population, intervention or exposure, and outcome—is the test under investigation. Issues of importance in defining your intervention may include which test you are examining (e.g., the test properties of troponin I produced by different laboratories may differ) and who is interpreting the test results (e.g., test properties may appear superior when the interpreter is an expert radiologist or pathologist rather than a run-of-the-mill practitioner).

The outcome in a diagnostic test study is the reference, gold, or criterion (all synonyms) standard that definitively establishes whether a patient is target positive or target negative. Investigators face special challenges in outcome assessment when the test under investigation may actually be superior to the gold standard, when the test is sufficiently invasive that its application to all patients is ethically questionable, or when the there is no adequate gold standard to apply at or around the time of diagnostic testing. A little later in this section we explore in more detail how long-term follow-up can aid in the resolution of these challenges.

✓ *Recruit your participants. Recruit a representative sample of patients characteristic of those to whom you will want to apply the test in clinical practice.*

Our largest group consisted of consecutive patients older than 65 years presenting to Chedoke Hospital in Hamilton, Ontario, between January 1984 and March 1988 with anemia (in men, hemoglobin 12.0 g/dL or less on two consecutive occasions; in women, 11.0 g/dL or less on two consecutive occasions) who were identified through the hospital laboratory. We also included a much smaller group of patients who were admitted to St. Joseph's Hospital in Hamilton under one of the co-investigators and met study criteria. We excluded institutionalized patients, those with recent blood transfusions or documented acute blood loss, those whose participation in the study was judged unethical by their attending physician (for reasons such as impending death or severe dementia), and those we considered too ill. We didn't establish detailed criteria for definition of "too ill," "impending death," or "severe dementia." Rather, we relied on physician judgement in these areas.

How a Diagnostic Study Can Go Wrong

It seems intuitively sensible, when conducting a diagnostic test study, to scrupulously avoid misclassification of patients' true status. In other words, you will want to avoid classifying patients who are truly target negative as target positive, and vice versa. To achieve these goals, it might appear logical to recruit a target-negative population who you are certain is disease-free (such as a group of healthy young people) and a target-positive population in whom there is no doubt about their disease status (such as a group with advanced disease).

Although these choices of target-negative and target-positive populations may be appropriate while initially exploring the potential of a diagnostic test, they are almost certain to be misleading if you are trying to establish test properties for use in clinical practice. For instance, when carcinoembryonic antigen (CEA) was measured in 36 people with known advanced cancer of the colon or rectum, 35 patients (97%) showed elevated results. At the same time, much lower levels were found in people without cancer who suffered from a variety of other conditions (9). These results suggest that CEA might be useful in diagnosing colorectal cancer—or even in screening for the disease. In subsequent studies of patients with less advanced stages of colorectal cancer (and, therefore, with lower disease severity) and of patients with other cancers or other gastrointestinal disorders (and, therefore, with different but potentially confused disorders), the accuracy of CEA testing as a diagnostic tool plummeted, and clinicians abandoned CEA measurement for cancer diagnosis and screening. CEA testing has proved useful only as one element in the follow-up of patients with known colorectal cancer (10).

In an empiric study of design-related bias in studies of diagnostic tests, Lijmer and colleagues related features of the design to the power of tests, that is, their ability to distinguish between target-positive and target-negative patients (11). The systematic review of Lijmer and colleagues found that when investigators in the primary studies enrolled separate test and normal control populations, they produced misleading results. Specifically, enrolling separate test and normal populations results in a large overestimate of the power of the test to distinguish between target-positive and target-negative patients (relative diagnostic odds ratio, 3.0; 95% confidence interval [CI], 2.0–4.5).

Figures 8–3 to 8–5 illustrate what has gone wrong when investigators choose target-negative patients from groups in whom the disease is not suspected, and target-positive patients from groups in whom the diagnosis is well established. Figure 8–3 presents what is likely to happen in this situation when a test that can take a wide range of values, from the very normal to the very abnormal. Normal controls will have test results on the left end of the scale (very normal) and severely affected disease-positive

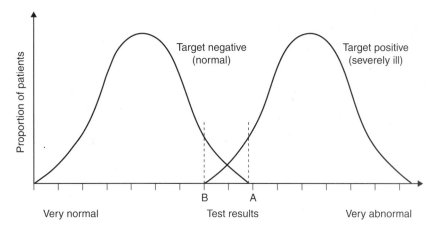

FIGURE 8–3 Minimum population overlap as a result of investigators having chosen target-negative and target-positive patients on the basis of knowing their diagnoses.

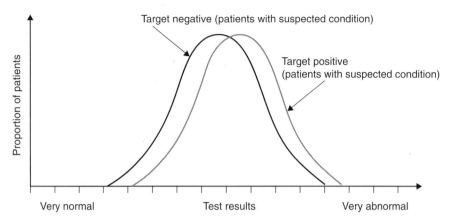

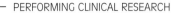

FIGURE 8–4 Target-positive patients from a population in whom diagnosis is uncertain and target-negative patients drawn from a population with competing conditions that can be confused with the target condition displaying widely overlapping results.

patients will have test results that lie on the right end (very abnormal) (Figure 8–3). The two populations will have minimal overlap and the test appears to be extremely powerful.

What will happen if, on the other hand, you choose a more appropriate population of patients for whom one is initially uncertain of the diagnoses? The target-positive patients in such a population will have less severe disease, and, thus, their results are likely to be less abnormal (Figure 8–4). The target-negative patients will be presenting with symptoms or diseases that mimic those of the target condition, and so are likely to

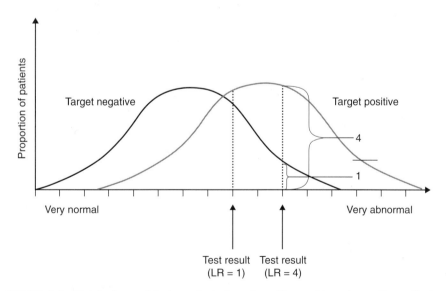

FIGURE 8–5 Distributions of test results in target-positive and target-negative patients demonstrating how likelihood ratios are the relative height of the curves at any test value.

have tests results that differ from the normal population (Figure 8-4). The consequence is far greater overlap in test results between target-positive and target-negative patients, and a test that is far less useful in distinguishing the two populations.

Bear in mind that the initial exploration of a diagnostic test may indeed enrol normal and severely diseased populations. If the results of such a study approximate those of Figure 8-3, the appropriate conclusion is not that the test is ready for clinical practice but that it shows potential. If that preliminary study shows results that approximate Figure 8-4, you needn't bother with subsequent investigations in clinically relevant populations. If a test can't differentiate the normal from the severely affected, it will surely fail to differentiate patients with mild to moderately severe disease from those with competing conditions.

What Is the Right Population?

We have established that choosing target-negative and target-positive patients from different populations is not the right way to establish the value of a test in clinical practice. There are a number of ways in which one might characterize the right population.

One way of conceptualizing the right population is that it includes a broad spectrum of the diseased, from mildly to severely (but not too severely—you'll see why in a moment) diseased, and a control population with a broad spectrum of competing conditions. An alternative approach is that you achieve the right population when you enrol the sort of patients in whom clinicians will subsequently apply the test. These will be patients who appear as if they might have the target condition, some of whom will and some of whom won't—in other words, patients who elicit diagnostic uncertainty.

How Uncertain Should You Be to Enrol a Patient?

What level of diagnostic uncertainty is appropriate? Figure 8-6 demonstrates a way of thinking about the diagnostic dilemma. The clinician estimates the probability that the target condition is present. If that probability is sufficiently low—below what we call the *test threshold*—the clinician dismisses the possibility that the target condition is the cause of the patient's presenting symptoms and moves on to other possibilities. If the probability is sufficiently high, above the *treatment threshold*, the clinician diagnoses the target condition and recommends treatment. Testing is appropriate in the intermediate range, between the test and treatment thresholds.

Using this way of thinking, studies of diagnostic tests should enrol patients for whom the probability of the target condition lies between the test and treatment thresholds. This particular conceptualization—thinking of the target population as those with a pre-test probability between test and treatment thresholds—points out the fact that thresholds may differ across groups of clinicians. For instance, we conducted a study of troponin I as a diagnostic test in the emergency department (13). We enrolled all patients

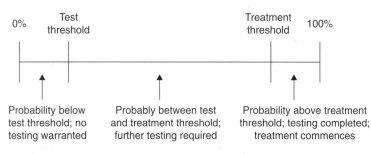

Probability of diagnosis

FIGURE 8–6   Test and treatment thresholds in the diagnostic process (12). (From Guyatt G, Rennie D. *Users' guides to the medical literature: A manual for evidence-based clinical practice*. Chicago, IL: AMA Press, 2002, with permission.)

for whom the emergency department physicians had ordered a serum troponin I because of suspected cardiac ischemia. We found that the emergency department physicians at our institution tend to have a very low threshold for ordering the troponin I test—in other words, their test threshold is probably set at a pre-test probability of less than 5%. Test properties may differ for clinician groups with a different test threshold.

Diagnostic Test Properties Can Differ by Setting

It is important to consider the setting in which to examine test properties, especially when the proposed test is an item of history or physical examination. This is because the value of the test can get "used up" as one moves from primary to secondary care settings. Take, for example, the physical signs of heat and redness in the diagnosis of deep venous thrombosis (DVT). These physical signs have shown surprisingly little utility in the diagnosis of venous thrombosis in patients referred to a thrombosis team for possible DVT (14). They may, however, have much more utility for primary care doctors or emergency department physicians in deciding which patients to consider for such a referral.

Assume—quite plausibly—that absence of heat and redness is associated with alternative diagnoses in the primary care setting and that clinicians selectively refrain from referring patients without these signs. The referred population is then enriched with patients with heat and redness. Furthermore, the patients without heat and redness who are referred are likely to have other features that make DVT more likely. The overall effect will be a loss in the diagnostic power of heat and redness in the population referred for secondary care assessment.

Changes in Prevalence Don't Change Test Properties

Changes in prevalence will not, in themselves, influence diagnostic properties. Consider Figure 8–5, which represents the distribution of test results in target-positive and target-negative populations. Figure 8–5 shows how the relative height of the distributions at any test value represents the LR at that test value. For instance, the test value at which the distributions have the same height represents a LR of 1. Figure 8–5 highlights another test result in which the height of the curve representing the distribution of results in target-positive patients is four times the height of the curve representing the distribution of results in target-negative patients. At this point, the LR of the test result is 4.

Irrespective of how many patients you sample from, the two populations (e.g., whether one draws 80% of the sample from the target positive or 80% from the target negative), the curves, and their respective heights at every point will remain unchanged. As long as this is the case, and the distribution of results in the two populations remains the same, test properties will not differ.

Changes in Spectrum Do Change Test Properties

Test characteristics will change with differences in either the distribution of disease severity in those who are target-positive, or the distribution of competing conditions in those who are target negative. With either change the shape of the curves, and thus the test properties, will differ.

Studies of exercise electrocardiography in the diagnosis of coronary artery disease provide one example of the way properties can change with different distributions of disease severity among target-positive patients. The more extensive the severity of coronary artery disease, the larger are the LRs of abnormal exercise electrocardiography for angiographic narrowing of the coronary arteries (15).

Why Is It Difficult to Keep the Distinction Between Prevalence and Spectrum Straight?

It is challenging to keep these concepts—the prevalence of the condition (the proportion of target-positive patients to the total of target-positive and target-negative patients), and the distribution of disease severity and competing conditions—clearly separated. People stumble over this distinction because changes in disease prevalence often go along with changes in disease severity.

For instance, rheumatoid arthritis seen in a family physician's office will be relatively uncommon, and most cases will be relatively mild. In contrast, rheumatoid arthritis will be common in a rheumatologist's office, and the cases will tend to be relatively severe. Tests to diagnose rheumatoid arthritis in the rheumatologist's waiting area (for instance, hand inspection for joint deformity) are likely to be very sensitive not because of the increased prevalence but because of the spectrum of disease present (i.e., degree and extent of joint deformity) in this setting.

The diagnosis of venous thromboembolism, where compression ultrasound for proximal-vein thrombosis has proved more accurate in symptomatic outpatients than in asymptomatic postoperative patients, provides another example of the association between severity and prevalence (16).

Sampling from the Right Population

Having identified a group of patients about whom physicians face genuine diagnostic uncertainty, you will next face the problem of how to sample from that group of patients. Ideally, you will include each and every eligible patient—we call this a consecutive sample of eligible patients—and you will define eligibility according to diagnostic suspicion.

If you fail to recruit a consecutive sample of patients, you risk introducing bias. If the severity of illness in truly target-positive patients differs in patients who present on weekdays versus weekends, nights, or during the holiday season, missing such patients will lead to a systematic over- or underestimate of test properties. The same is true if the spectrum of competing conditions varies across days of the week, day or night, or time of the year. Reliance on the serendipity introduced by the front-line clinicians responsible for recruiting patients may be even more dangerous. For instance, if clinicians are reluctant to expose patients to an invasive gold standard, they may exclude patients whose pre-test probability is low.

We were careful to try and enrol consecutive patients in our study of iron deficiency anemia. If, for whatever reason, enrolling consecutive patients is not possible, you should carefully describe who was more or less likely to be enrolled. You may very well wish to comment in your paper's discussion on the likelihood of bias that selective recruitment may have introduced.

Construction of Eligibility Criteria

One final note on how to construct eligibility criteria: Placing a criterion in the inclusion or exclusion criteria is sometimes arbitrary. In our iron deficiency study we could have defined more than 65 years of age as an inclusion criterion, or designated less than 65 years of age as an exclusion criterion. Similarly, we could have defined our eligible population as those residing in the community or noted residency in an institution as an exclusion criterion.

We chose to define more than 65 years of age as an inclusion criterion and residency in an institution as an exclusion criterion. Why? Because we were uninterested in identifying all patients younger than 65 years and then ultimately listing them as excluded patients. On the other hand, we were ready to document all anemic patients older than 65 years of age and then note the institutionalized patients as excluded.

So, we suggest you make the decision about what to place in inclusion criteria and what to place in exclusion criteria on the basis of what you are ultimately intending to document and report.

Summary of Patient Selection Issues

Table 8–5 summarizes a number of messages for the investigator that follows from this reasoning. We have already emphasized the importance of careful consideration of the population from which you will draw

TABLE 8-5 Implications of the Vulnerability of Test Properties to Differences in the Distribution of Disease Severity in Target-positive Patients and Differences in the Distribution of Competing Conditions in Target-negative Patients

- Carefully consider the population from which you draw your patients.
- Consider the filter through which your patients have passed before becoming eligible for your study.
- Beware that test properties may differ in subpopulations within your sample, and so consider subgroup analyses.
- If possible, recruit a consecutive sample of patients presenting with the diagnostic dilemma.
- Be cautious in interpretation of your results, particularly with regard to the populations to which your results are generalizable.

your patients. If the tests under study are items of history and physical examination, the filter through which patients have passed becomes particularly important. As we have pointed out, diagnostically powerful items of patient history and physical examination can get "used up" as patients move from primary to secondary and tertiary care settings. We will deal with subgroup analysis in the statistical analysis section of this chapter.

Finally, we urge caution in addressing the generalizability of your test results. Studies of diagnostic tests are logistically challenging, and obtaining funding is less easy than for therapeutic studies. As a result, investigators seldom conduct large studies of diagnostic tests. You and your colleagues are unlikely to meet the ideal in which you enrol a number of centers and conduct your study across a variety of settings, ultimately testing the reproducibility of your findings across centers and settings. What you can do, however, is acknowledge the limitations of your study and remind readers that confidence in your results must await replication in apparently similar settings (to say nothing of testing in apparently different settings).

✓ Select your measurement procedures.

All patients had the following laboratory tests: hemoglobin, MCV, RDW, serum iron, iron-binding capacity, serum ferritin, and RCP. The complete blood count was carried out using a Coulter S + IV. Serum iron and iron-binding capacity were measured according to the methods of the International Committee for Standardization in Hematology (17). Serum ferritin was measured using a radioimmunoassay described in detail previously (18). RCP was measured using a previously described micro method (19).

What Test to Test?

In considering a diagnostic test study, you may face some relatively mundane considerations of test choice. Recently, for instance, we had to decide on which manufacturers' version of troponin we would test in patients presenting with symptoms of possible cardiac ischemia (11).

Other choices are more challenging and more interesting. We may think of tests as the machines that process laboratory specimens, or produce images by use of x-rays or ultrasound. The laboratory machine will not, however, produce anything of use without a technician to run the specimen through, and the x-ray or ultrasound images are useless without a clinician or radiologist to interpret them. Particularly in the latter situation—the clinician or radiologist interpreting an image—the test properties are likely to be dependent on the skill of the interpreter. Thus, in a sense, if you choose to examine test properties in radiographs that were interpreted by a group of radiology residents, you are evaluating a different test than if you choose radiologists with extensive specialized training and long experience with that particular diagnostic test (20).

Consider, for instance, a study that looked at the diagnostic properties of helical computerized tomography (CT) scan for acute appendicitis (18). The investigators reported that "the scans were interpreted immediately by residents or staff members of our Emergency Radiology Division." When the residents had read the initial scan, an attending radiologist subsequently checked the accuracy (and agreed in all but 1 of 100 patients enrolled).

The investigators do not tell us how often it was the staff or the residents interpreting the scans, nor do they indicate the experience of the interpreters. Might results have differed had the radiologists made all the initial interpretations? What about the radiologists' experience with the test?

Helical CT scan to diagnose appendicitis is a relatively straightforward test that does not require special skill, and the answer here may be that we needn't be particularly skeptical about the residents' interpretation or wonder about superior test properties that highly skilled interpretation might provide. The more sophisticated the test, and the more the conduct and interpretation is likely to differ with the clinicians involved, the more important is the choice of interpreter.

Who to Choose As the Test Interpreter?

Assume you are in a situation in which whether a resident on-call, a run-of-the-mill staff physician, or a highly skilled individual interprets a test will influence its properties. Whom should you choose for your study? Whomever you choose, should you require a minimal amount of experience with the test before allowing a clinician to participate? Depending on your choice, you will be asking a different study question. "What are the test properties of ultrasound when interpreted by ...."—and fill in the rest with resident, run-of-the-mill staff, or super expert.

One could make an argument for any of the three. Many would contend that the inexperienced resident will not provide a fair evaluation of the test. On the other hand, if the target audience for your study are clinicians who will often be ordering the test in off-hours and relying on residents' interpretation, the accuracy of interpretation under these circumstances may be exactly what they want to know.

This formulation highlights the choice between asking an explanatory question (in this case, how does the test perform under optimal conditions when interpreted by exceptionally skilled individuals?) and a management or pragmatic question (how does the test perform when interpreted by ordinary clinicians in day-to-day practice?). The choice between explanatory and management is not a yes or no because there is a continuum between explanatory and management studies. For instance, insisting that a staff radiologist interpret the test will be intermediate in the explanatory-management spectrum between the expert and whoever happens to be around, such as an on-call resident. In the study of helical CT scan for diagnosis of appendicitis, surgeons likely had to act on the basis of the initial interpretation rather than on the interpretation of a more senior individual checking the result hours later. Thus, had the investigators wanted to take an extreme management approach they would not have bothered having the residents' readings checked by staff (or at least would have reported the results using the residents' readings as well as those of the staff).

What Should the Test Interpreters Know?

A second choice involves the information you wish to make available to the individual interpreting the test. Intuitively, and as usually practiced, investigators wish to know the independent contribution made by a test to the diagnostic process. Thus, investigators generally ensure that the individual interpreting the test does so without any other information about the patient (except perhaps the basic reason why the test has been ordered).

That is not, of course, what actually happens in clinical practice. Radiologists seek as much clinical information as possible. At minimum, they require a requisition that provides basic clinical details. Often, when the clinical situation is complex, clinicians recognize they can get the most informative interpretation by visiting the radiologist before or at the time she or he looks at the image and providing a detailed account of the clinical context.

Thus, in the extreme of a management diagnostic study, one would allow the test interpreter to have the same sort of information about the patient they would ordinarily have available in day-to-day clinical practice. Even if you choose to allow availability of clinical information, you have to decide between standardized details or whatever the clinician feels is appropriate in the clinical context. The former choice allows the reader to know exactly what is provided, but moves the question away from the extreme management design. The latter provides the answer to a management question but raises potential applicability issues. "Were the radiologists provided with the same detail of information," a clinician reading your report might ask, "as occurs in my clinical setting?"

What Test to Test: Resolution

There is no right answer about which test to test. The choice depends on what you think will be most useful to the clinical community and your own curiosity and interests. What is important is to realize the range of choices regarding who interprets the test and what information is provided to the interpreter, and to make the choice consciously and carefully. In the helical CT scan study, the investigators apparently did not realize the importance of the issue because they do not tell us what information was available to the radiologists when they interpreted the test results. They do tell us, however, that the test results formed the basis of clinical management. This suggests that the interpreters were given the clinical information that referring clinicians generally convey in routine practice.

Specifying Test Technique

You should take care to conduct your test according to accepted standards as defined by experts in the field. When the time comes to report your results, you should specify how you conducted the test in sufficient detail to ensure that others will be able to reproduce your results. In our study of iron deficiency diagnosis, for example, we stated the laboratory methods used for each test and cited the relevant publication.

Reproducibility

You can make a case for demonstrating the reproducibility of your test. Doing so will ultimately help the clinician reader of your report to be confident that you conducted your test according to accepted standards and achieved the anticipated performance. If your reproducibility proves superior to what one would ordinarily expect in clinical practice (due to special training and calibration of the participating radiologists, for instance) the readers of your paper may legitimately question whether the test will perform as well in their setting as it has in yours.

If you do measure reproducibility, you should quantitate chance-corrected, or chance-independent agreement using statistics such as kappa (21,22), phi (23,24), or an intra-class correlation coefficient that compares variance between patients to the total variance, including both between- and within-patient variance [for a clinician-friendly explanation of these concepts, see (25)].

Blinding

Generally, blinding of the individual conducting or interpreting the test to the gold standard is critical for the validity of a study of diagnostic tests. We need only think of our own experience in hearing previously inaudible murmurs after receiving the results of the echocardiogram, or noting previously invisible nodules on the chest radiograph after receiving results of the CT scan of the chest, to realize the importance of blinding. In the iron deficiency study, blinding of those conducting the test presented no difficulties because the test was completed before the results of the gold standard became available.

✓ *Apply the gold standard. Determine whether or not the target condition is present.*

A bone marrow aspiration was undertaken and interpreted by a hematologist (MA) blind to the results of the laboratory tests. The bone marrow slides were air-dried, fixed with methanol, and Prussian blue staining was applied (26). The first 65 marrow aspirations were also interpreted by a second hematologist (also blind), and discrepancies resolved by consensus. The results of the aspiration were classified as iron absent, reduced, present, or increased. Chance-corrected agreement between the two hematologists reading the marrows was calculated using a weighted kappa, with quadratic weights. The weighted kappa statistic quantifying chance-corrected agreement for the 65 marrows that were interpreted by two hematologists was 0.84.

To determine the properties of a diagnostic test requires comparison with a gold, reference, or criterion standard accepted as the definitive determination of whether patients are target positive or negative. Typically, another test that is more time consuming, expensive, difficult, or invasive than the test under consideration will provide this standard. In this section, we will deal with a number of design features crucial for valid diagnostic studies, as well as some challenging situations you may confront in dealing with limitations of your gold standard.

How Should You *Not* Construct Your Gold Standard?

On occasion, there is no single test that will constitute the gold standard for a target condition. When this is the case, investigators typically construct a composite measure that, for them, represents the gold standard. For instance, one study evaluated the utility of tests for diagnosing pancreatitis (27). There is no single clinical or pathological measure that defines pancreatitis, and so investigators constructed a gold standard that relied on a number of tests, including tests for serum and urinary amylase. This is quite reasonable, except for the fact that serum and urinary amylase were two of the tests the investigators were evaluating. This "incorporation bias" will inevitably create a spuriously sanguine assessment of test properties, and is something you should scrupulously avoid.

To Whom Should the Gold Standard Be Applied?

The short answer is, "to everyone." In some instances, administrative or logistical errors may prevent performance of the gold standard in all patients. For instance, in our study of iron deficiency anemia, out of 259 bone marrow aspirations, 24 proved uninterpretable, leaving 235 (91%) available for comparison with test results.

If (as is likely in this instance) unavailability of the gold standard is a random event unrelated to test results, loss of patients for comparison with the test will increase random error and thus reduce the power of your study but will not cause problems with bias. Serious trouble can arise, however, when test results bear on who gets the gold standard.

Verification Bias

The most common situation when clinicians will behave differently according to test results—performing the gold standard on patients whose test results increase the probability of disease and refraining from performing the gold standard in those whose test results decrease the probability of disease—will be when the gold standard is invasive. Clinicians may be hesitant to perform an invasive procedure in patients whom they perceive to have a low probability of the target condition. This situation, sometimes called "verification bias" (28,29) or "workup bias" (30,31), threatened the validity of the prospective investigation of pulmonary embolism diagnosis (PIOPED) study that examined the usefulness of ventilation–perfusion (V/Q) scanning in the diagnosis of pulmonary embolism (PE) (32). Patients with V/Q scans interpreted as "normal/near normal" and "low probability" were less likely to undergo pulmonary angiography (69%) than those with more positive V/Q scans (92%). This is not surprising because clinicians might be reluctant to subject patients with a low probability of PE to the risks of angiography.

Fortunately, long-term follow-up provides a potential solution to this problem, particularly when you are most concerned about the pragmatic consequences of making a particular diagnosis. For instance, the PIOPED investigators applied a second reference standard to the 150 patients with low probability or normal/near normal scans who failed to undergo angiography (136 patients) or in whom angiogram interpretation was uncertain (14 patients); they would be judged to be free of PE if they did well without treatment. Accordingly, they followed every one of these patients for 1 year without treating them with anticoagulants. Not one of these patients developed clinically evident PE during this time, from which we can conclude that clinically important PE (if we define clinically important PE as requiring anticoagulation to prevent subsequent adverse events) was not present at the time they underwent V/Q scanning.

Estimating What Might Have Happened

Statistical techniques are available to estimate what the results might have been, had gold standard assessments been available for such patients. For instance, Punglia and colleagues studied 6,691 men who underwent prostate-specific antigen-based screening for prostate cancer. Of these men, 705 (11%) subsequently underwent biopsy of the prostate. Unfortunately, the likelihood of having the biopsy depended on the test result (33). Under the assumption that the chance of undergoing a biopsy depends only on the prostate specific antigen (PSA) test result and other observed clinical variables, the authors used a mathematical model to estimate adjusted ROC curves (28). Adjusting for verification bias significantly increased the area under the ROC curve (i.e., the overall diagnostic performance) of the PSA test, as compared with an unadjusted analysis (0.86 versus 0.69, $P < 0.001$, for men younger than 60 years of age; 0.72 versus 0.62, $P = 0.008$, for men as old as 60 years or older) and suggested a different optimal cut-point.

The key assumption of this method is that the chance that a man will undergo prostate biopsy depends only on observed variables (e.g., the age, the PSA level, or the results of digital rectal examination; the variables the authors had at their disposal) and not on the presence or absence of cancer, which cannot be directly observed. This assumption can be easily questioned, particularly when the investigators have not measured the full range of possible predictor variables. Because these techniques require having potentially unavailable information at ones' disposal, and involve regression modeling, they are fraught with uncertainty. Far superior to these approaches is ensuring that all patients, irrespective of their test results, receive the gold standard assessment (either the definitive test or long-term follow-up).

Ensuring Your Standard Is As Gold As Possible

As we noted, when you consider the test under investigation you can make arguments for measuring or not measuring reliability and for using run-of-the-mill or expert test interpretation. This is not the case for the gold standard. Here, you will want to be as definitive as possible. That means getting the most expert interpretation you possibly can. Ideally, it also means showing that your experts are really as good as they claim, or as you hope.

In our study of iron deficiency anemia, a senior hematologist interpreted all the bone marrow results. Not content to simply trust this individual's accuracy, we asked another hematologist to interpret a subset of the bone marrow aspirates. In the 65 specimens read by both hematologists, we were able to document chance-corrected agreement (kappa statistic) of 0.84. This near-perfect agreement reassured us of the caliber of our gold standard.

What If Your Test Is More Gold Than the Standard?

You may be facing the intriguing situation in which you suspect your test is actually superior to the gold standard. If you are right, any comparison with a standard that is more brass than gold will lead to an underestimate of the diagnostic power of the test you are evaluating. What are you to do?

One strategy for dealing with this problem is to use long-term follow-up as a gold standard. Ultimately, most conditions declare themselves unequivocally. If they do not, it almost certainly wasn't worth diagnosing them in the first place.

For instance, while the PIOPED investigators accepted angiography as their gold standard, they didn't have the results of the test in some patients. Their solution to the problem was, in these patients, to rely on long-term follow-up as the ultimate gold standard. In untreated patients, the investigators presumed that those with no clinical events on long-term follow-up didn't have pulmonary emboli in the first place. This assumption might have been incorrect, but even if it was, those patients with pulmonary emboli destined to not recur would be better off undiagnosed (and thus not exposed to the bleeding risk of long-term warfarin therapy).

While relying on long-term follow-up as a gold standard will, in most instances, help you deal with the problem, the suspicion that your test is superior to the gold standard may test your ingenuity. For instance, investigators examining CT virtual colonoscopy as a test for screening patients for colon cancer suspected the new test might be superior to conventional colonoscopy. Long-term follow-up for occurrence of colon cancer would have been fraught with problems, including logistic issues. Instead, the investigators performed the index test, virtual colonoscopy, on all eligible patients. Patients then underwent standard invasive colonoscopy. After the colonoscopist completed the evaluation of a given segment of the colon, a study coordinator revealed the results of the virtual colonoscopy for the previously examined segment. If a polyp measuring 5 mm or more in diameter was seen on virtual colonoscopy but not on the initial optical colonoscopy, the colonoscopist closely reexamined that segment and was allowed to review the images obtained on virtual colonoscopy for guidance. This "segmental unblinding" resulted in the creation of an enhanced reference standard and allowed for the assessment of false negative results on optical colonoscopy that would otherwise have been recorded as false-positive results on virtual colonoscopy.

✓ *Select your statistical procedures. Include sample size calculation, how to represent the properties of a diagnostic test, and subgroup analysis.*

The following is from the paper we published describing the results of our iron deficiency anemia study:

> "Receiver operating characteristic (ROC) curves for each test were generated. The area under the curves were compared using the method of Hanley and McNeil (34). Since the ROC curves in this study were all generated from the same cohort of patients, we used the correction factor which reflects the correlation between the tests (35). Using the same cut-points, likelihood ratios for each category were calculated."
>
> "To determine the independent contribution of each test to the diagnosis, and whether a combination of tests could improve diagnostic accuracy, stepwise logistic regression procedures were used. The status of iron stores (present or absent) was used as the dependent variable, and the values of the diagnostic tests (dichotomized using the cut-point which maximized accuracy) as the independent variables."

The following is from a follow-up grant we submitted to obtain funds to complete the study and the analysis:

"The area under each ROC curve will be calculated, and the areas compared. ROC curves will be constructed for clinically sensible subgroups, and the areas under the curves obtained (we recognize that the sample size may severely limit the power of such subgroup analysis, but the analysis may nevertheless be enlightening)."

More from the results of the published paper:

"Thirty-six percent of our patients had no demonstrable marrow iron and were classified as being iron deficient. The serum ferritin was the best test for distinguishing those with iron deficiency from those who were not iron deficient. No other test added clinically important information. The likelihood ratios associated with the serum ferritin were as follows: >100 μg per L, 0.13; >45≤100, 0.46; >18≤45, 3.12; and ≤18, 41.47. These results indicate that values up to 45 increase the likelihood of iron deficiency, whereas values greater than 45 decrease the likelihood of iron deficiency. Seventy-two percent of those who were not iron deficient had serum ferritin values greater than 100, and in populations with a prevalence of iron deficiency of less than 40%, values of greater than 100 reduce the probability of iron deficiency to less than 10%. Fifty-five percent of those who were iron deficient had serum ferritin values of less than 18, and in populations with a prevalence of iron deficiency of greater than 20%, values of less than 18 increased the probability of iron deficiency to greater than 95%."

Ideally, you will plan to collect your data in one group of patients, establish the test properties in that population, and confirm the results in a second population. If you do adhere to this ideal plan, it raises complex issues of sample size calculation and analysis, which we deal with in our chapter on prediction and clinical decision rules (Chapter 9). Indeed, if you take this route, you will simultaneously have to hold in your mind the issues of this chapter as well as the issues related to clinical decision rules.

As it turns out, conducting a high-quality diagnostic test study is very challenging at every step of the way, from formulating the proposal, through obtaining funding, to carrying out the proposal. You can gain an idea of the challenges involved in considering that in 2003 ACP Journal Club published reports of 86 randomized trials, but only seven diagnostic test studies. Remember too, to gain entrance to the lofty ranks of ACP Journal Club, a diagnostic test study needn't address the issue of internal replication.

Because the challenges of conducting diagnostic test studies are so formidable, and to avoid redundancy with the prognosis chapter, we will assume that you are going to accept the limitation that your study is not going to involve internal replication, and you will leave it for someone else to replicate your findings. This means that ultimately you will include a paragraph in the "limitations" section of your discussion stating why you elected not·to do an internal replication of any sort, and acknowledging that (unless your study is itself a replication of your own prior work, or someone else's) clinicians should be cautious about the use of your findings in clinical practice until someone has produced similar results in another setting.

Sample Size Calculation

We would have happily reported here exactly how we did our sample size calculation in the iron deficiency study. The grant, however, was funded in 1984, probably submitted the year before, and the details are not recoverable. We do, however, remember the essential approach we took, and would still recommend the same simple approach for choosing sample sizes for diagnostic test studies.

Our strategy relies on deciding on the CIs around the sensitivity and the specificity one wishes to achieve. Let us say, for instance, that you would like to ensure that the 95% CIs are no wider than ±10%. You then decide whether target-positive or target-negative patients will be less frequent, and focus on that group.

In our diagnostic test study we were aware that a minority of our patients would be iron deficient. We therefore focused our sample size calculation on these patients.

Wishing to be conservative, we assumed a sensitivity of 50%—the reason being that this will yield the widest CI (for a given sample size, as values of sensitivity or specificity, or any proportion, diverge from 50%, the CIs narrow). Using the following formula, we then ascertained the sample size needed to produce a 95% CI of ±10%:

$$95\% \text{ CI} = \pm 1.96 \times \sqrt{pq/n}$$

where p is the proportion of target-positive patients with a positive test result (in this case 0.5) and q is $(1 - p)$ (the proportion of target-positive patients with a negative test result, in this case also 0.5). So, having specified that $pq = 0.25$ (0.5×0.5) one can determine the value of n such that $1.96 \times \sqrt{pq/n} = 10\%$ (the 95% CI that one hopes to achieve).

The value of n, then, is the number of target-positive patients one needs to recruit. As it turns out, to achieve a CI of 10% with a 50% sensitivity we needed to enrol approximately 100 target-positive patients. We started to recruit, planning to stop when we reached this specified number. In any study that takes this approach, the total sample size will depend on the ratio of target-positive to target-negative patients in one's population. For instance, if we were right in our estimate that one third of those enrolled would be target-positive, we would end up with 100 target-positive and 200 target-negative patients, a total sample size of 300. As it turns out, we ran out of money, and stopped recruitment somewhat shy of our goal of 100 iron-deficient patients.

One could criticize this approach in that if one is going to eventually calculate LRs one should estimate sample size on the basis of that analysis. Technically, that is correct. We would argue, however, that there is an inevitable arbitrariness in sample size estimation that increases the merit of keeping things simple. We continue to recommend the approach to choosing a sample size for a diagnostic test study that we described above.

Describing What Happened

The STARD group has recommended that diagnostic test studies include a flow diagram summarizing the study design and results (see Figure 8–7). The suggested diagram, while attractive, is fully appropriate only in situations when the test result can assume only two values, traditionally designated as positive and negative. In the introductory section of this chapter we reviewed the various ways of presenting diagnostic test results. You will recall that whenever possible, using as many cut-points as possible will maximize the power of your test, and its usefulness to the clinician. Thus, if your test permits more than one cut-point, you will not be using sensitivity and specificity, and the STARD diagram of Figure 8–7 will be of limited use to you.

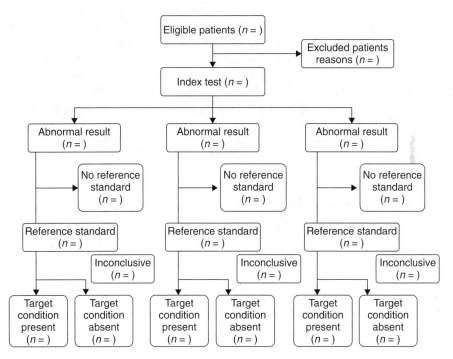

FIGURE 8–7 Prototype of a flow diagram for a study on diagnostic accuracy. (From Bossuyt PM, Reitsma JB, Bruns DE et al., STARD steering group. Towards complete and accurate reporting of studies of diagnostic accuracy: the STARD initiative. *BMJ* 2003;326:41–44, with permission.)

TABLE 8-6   **Reasons for Exclusion of Patients Found to be Anemic on At Least One Hemoglobin Determination**

Reason for Exclusion	Number of Patients Excluded
Patient judged too ill, demented, or terminal	212
Patient or family refused consent for bone marrow aspiration	200
Not anemic on second haemoglobin determination	200
Recent transfusion	152
Previous bone marrow aspiration had revealed diagnosis	108
Institutionalized	95
Miscellaneous	108
Total	1,075

From Guyatt GH, Oxman A, Ali M, et al. Laboratory diagnosis of iron deficiency anemia: an overview. *J Gen Intern Med* 1992;7:145-153, with permission.

The STARD diagram does, however, raise several important issues that you should not ignore, however many cut-points you use. First, when you conduct your study, you need to keep track of patients who met your inclusion criterion, but whom you rejected because they also met an exclusion criterion. Consider Table 8-6, which comes from the report of our study of iron deficiency anemia. As it turns out, we excluded 1,075 patients who met our inclusion criteria. This may appear a little depressing, given that only 235 patients (19%) ultimately contributed to the main results. Documenting all of these ultimately ineligible patients also involved appreciable resources. We could have saved ourselves some of the work and produced a table that raised fewer questions about the generalizability of our study by defining some of the exclusion criteria as inclusion criteria. For instance, we could have eliminated 108 patients by defining our eligible group as those without prior bone marrow aspiration and another 95 by specifying residency in the community as an eligibility criterion. On the other hand, we would argue that Table 8-6 gives clinicians a vivid sense of the process of our study and a useful feel about the nature of the patients whom community laboratory results suggest, on at least one occasion, are anemic.

A second issue raised by Figure 8-7 is that there may be instances in which you obtain a test result, but fail to obtain a gold standard. For instance, in our study of iron deficiency anemia we documented 259 conducted bone marrow aspirations, but 24 of these were too poor to be interpretable. The STARD investigators suggest that authors report the results in these patients. Although we did not include the results of laboratory measures possibly indicative of iron deficiency in those for whom bone marrow results were not available in our paper, we agree with the STARD investigators that it is a good idea and would do so were we writing our research report today.

Your test may, on occasion, yield indeterminate, uninterpretable, or inconclusive results. If it does, as the STARD diagram indicates, you should report the gold standard findings in such patients. Such patients may have common characteristics. For instance, patients with chronic obstructive pulmonary disease or pneumonia are more likely to have uninterpretable or indeterminate V/Q scans. If this is so, such patients may be more or less likely to be suffering from the target condition. If that is the case, the indeterminate result actually provides diagnostic information. This argues strongly for including "test results indeterminate, uninterpretable, or inconclusive" as a diagnostic category and for reporting the LR associated with this "test result."

Choosing Cut-points

Ideally, you would have as many cut-points as possible (in fact, one would have a LR associated with each unique test result–a point to which we will return). This is because the true underlying LR will be different with each value of the test result. If you were to group all patients with serum ferritin values of 18 to 45 in a single category, as we did, you would assume that a value of 19 carries the same importance in terms of increasing the likelihood of iron deficiency as a value of 44. This is, of course, not so.

Table 8–7 presents the serum ferritin results of our study of iron deficiency anemia. Applying the results, one would infer that a result of 19 had a LR of 3.12 and a result of 17 had an LR of 41.47. Similarly, one would infer that a value of 44 had an LR of 3.12 and a value of 46 an LR of 0.46. This is, of course, not so. The true underlying LRs would increase smoothly as serum ferritin dropped from 44 to 19 and values at either extreme of this range would approximate values at the lower and upper part (respectively) of the adjacent intervals.

So why didn't we use additional cuts? Unfortunately, as you use progressively smaller ranges here, the number of observations will decrease, and the estimates of LRs will become unstable and therefore untrustworthy. So, the investigator faces competing objectives: the smaller the range,

TABLE 8–7   Likelihood Ratios for Serum Ferritin

Interval	Number Iron Deficient	Number Not Iron Deficient	Likelihood Ratio
Ferritin			
≤18	47	2	41.47
>18≤45	23	13	3.12
>45≤100	7	27	0.46
>100	8	108	0.13
Total	85	150	

From Guyatt GH, Oxman A, Ali M, et al. Laboratory diagnosis of iron deficiency anemia: an overview. *J Gen Intern Med* 1992;7:145–153, with permission.

the more specific the LR becomes for values in that interval; but the larger the range, the more stable and trustworthy becomes the LR representing the average LR for all values in that interval.

How should you balance these competing objectives? In general, we have kept narrowing the intervals until we have started to see counter-intuitive patterns of LRs that lose the smooth gradient of increasing or de-creasing values. For instance, had we cut at 18, 30, and 45 we may have seen results such as those depicted in the hypothetical Table 8–8.

It is biologically implausible in the extreme that the LRs would behave in this way—decreasing, then increasing, then decreasing again as serum ferritin increased. But if you have few enough observations, chance will start to produce results such as these. The rule then: keep decreasing the range of LRs until one sees counter-intuitive results (i.e., one loses the smooth gradient of increasing LRs as test results increase or decrease). Choose the number of cuts that maximizes the number of intervals without losing that smooth gradient.

Having established that principle, what cut-points should one choose? The decision is somewhat arbitrary. To make it less so, we suggest three rules. First, if there are existing standard or traditional cut-points, choose these. In our laboratory, and in many others, the cut-point of 18 was used to distinguish "normal" from "abnormal." Second, choose a cut that approximates the value at which the LR changes from less than 1.0 to greater than 1.0. In our ferritin data, as far as we could tell, a value of 45 approximated that threshold. Third, choose numbers that represent intu-itive boundaries for people (numbers such as 10, 25, 50, and 100). That rule provided the basis of our choice to use a cut-point of 100.

The problem with the extent to which cut-points are arbitrary is that it makes it almost certain that you will capitalize on the play of chance. The only way of avoiding doing so is to decide on your thresholds before your data are available. You should indeed strive to meet this goal—the

TABLE 8–8 Hypothetical Likelihood Ratios for Serum Ferritin

Interval	Number Iron Deficient	Number Not Iron Deficient	Likelihood Ratio
Ferritin			
≤18	47	2	41.47
>18≤30	12	8	2.65
>30≤45	11	5	3.89
>45≤100	7	27	0.46
>100	8	108	0.13
Total	85	150	

From Guyatt GH, Oxman A, Ali M, et al. Laboratory diagnosis of iron deficiency anemia: an overview. *J Gen Intern Med* 1992;7:145–153, with permission.

problem, although, is that your *a priori* choices may not work very well with your data. To the extent that your choice of cut-points is data driven, the necessity of replication becomes more compelling. This is one of the issues that you should deal with in the discussion section of the report of your study.

The Likelihood Ratio Line

If you have sufficient observations, you can go beyond the multiple cut approach and construct an LR line that describes the relation between the test result and the LR across the entire range of test values. Following our iron deficiency observational study, we conducted a systematic review of all such studies (7). We identified 55 eligible studies that examined the relation between results of tests for iron deficiency and the presence or absence of iron in the bone marrow aspiration. These 55 studies included results for serum ferritin in 2,579 patients. Largely from figures in the studies, we estimated results of serum ferritin and recorded whether iron deficiency was present, for all the 2,579 individuals. Figure 8–8 depicts the LR line that we generated from these data. As you can see, this line has a completely smooth curve representing the relation between ferritin result and the LR, thus eliminating the problem of biologically implausible increases or decreases in LRs between categories.

Generating such an LR requires statistical modeling, and you will need the help of a statistician for this exercise. A description of alternative approaches to this modeling is beyond the scope of this text. We used one strategy based on generating a best-fit model (36) to generate the

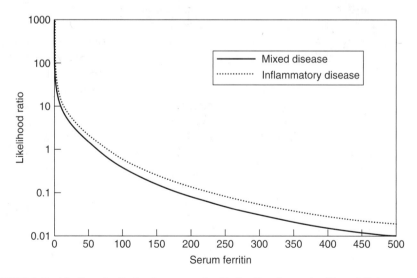

FIGURE 8–8 Likelihood ratio line for serum ferritin for the diagnosis of iron deficiency anemia. (From Guyatt GH, Oxman A, Ali M, et al. Laboratory diagnosis of iron deficiency anemia: an overview. *J Gen Intern Med* 1992;7:145–153, with permission.)

serum ferritin LR line. This approach led to the following equation for estimating the LR at any given level of serum ferritin:

$$L = e^{(6.5429 - 1.6985 \times \ln(x))},$$

where L is the likelihood ratio, and x is the serum ferritin value.

If you happen to have sufficient data, we would encourage you to get the help required to generate an LR line. What constitutes a sufficient amount of data will depend on the exact nature of what you have available, but if you have more than 100 target-positive and 100 target-negative patients, you may discuss the possibility with your statistician colleagues.

Receiver Operating Characteristic Curves

Clinicians need LRs to make optimal use of diagnostic tests. ROC curves represent a complementary approach that plots the relation between sensitivity and (1–specificity) at different threshold values. We described some of the properties of ROC curves in the introductory section of this chapter. Historically, one reason for using ROC curves was to help choose the optimal cut-point. However, we know that multiple cut-points and LRs provide much more complete and useful information about test properties, so this particular purpose has become irrelevant.

ROC curves continue to provide a useful visual representation of the power of the test. In addition, the area under the curve provides a single number that captures the power of the test. Finally, if you are interested in comparing the relative performance of more than one test directed at the same diagnostic problem, ROC curves provide one very helpful way of addressing the issue of whether apparent differences in the power of two or more tests are likely to be due to chance (34).

In our study, for instance, comparison of ROC curves demonstrated that ferritin was far more powerful than other tests. Areas under the ROC curve were 0.91, 0.79, 0.78, and 0.72 for seurm ferritin, transferrin saturation, MCV, and RCP, respectively. Whereas the difference between the serum ferritin and the other three tests proved statistically significant ($P \leq 0.001$ in each case), any differences seen in the other four curves were explained by chance ($P \geq 0.1$). We also used this approach to address the power of the test in relevant subgroups (e.g., those with a hemoglobin of fewer than 10.0 versus greater than 10.0) and found no differences in the area under the curve for these subgroups.

Although we don't consider the presentation of ROC curves as mandatory, we suggest, because of all the valuable information they can generate, you consider including them in the article in which you present your data.

Does a Test Independently Contribute to Diagnostic Power?

In our anemia study we evaluated multiple tests, including serum ferritin, transferrin saturation, and MCV. You may also be interested in whether, given initial diagnostic information (which will typically include history, physical examination, and perhaps also prior laboratory or imaging investigations), a particular test provides additional information. For instance, we established that ferritin was the most powerful test. It nevertheless remained important to determine whether, given the availability of ferritin results, MCV or transferrin saturation results could more precisely define the probability that iron deficiency explained the patient's anemia.

Logistic regression methods are well suited for addressing this sort of question. The dependent variable in such a regression will be the patients' status on the gold standard, target condition present or absent. As we describe in the chapter on analyzing data (Chapter 15), rather than using a stepwise approach in which you leave it to the computer to decide on the order of the variables and the order in which they enter the model, you will want to specify the order. If you have information from history and physical examination, you will likely want to specify that this information enters the model first. The reason is that it is inexpensive to collect, and indeed mandatory. Thus, the appropriate goal for an investigator regarding a laboratory or imaging investigation is to establish the extent to which it adds information above and beyond history and physical examination. Using a similar logic, if you have tests that are inexpensive and noninvasive, they should enter the model before more expensive and invasive tests.

In the models we generated, serum ferritin provided important information beyond clinicians' estimates of pre-test likelihood (37), and no other test provided additional information above and beyond serum ferritin (7). Thus, on the wards and in out-patient clinics, we now discourage simultaneous ordering of serum ferritin and iron and iron-binding capacity. The result of the latter test not only adds no new information but may in fact be misleading if it leads to "double-counting" of the results. This double-counting is always a risk when clinicians examine the results of more than one test when results are not independent.

✓ *Measure the test's impact. Decide whether and how to measure the impact of your diagnostic test on patient outcome.*

In 1986 a group of thoracic surgeons, radiologists, and clinical epidemiologists became interested in the optimal approach to the diagnosis of metastatic disease in patients with apparently operable lung cancer. In patients with mediastinal disease (diagnosed by mediastinoscopy) the recurrence rates after resection are very poor, suggesting that patients with a positive mediastinoscopy are not well served by thoractomy with resectional surgery. Mediastinoscopy is, however, an invasive procedure that can be associated with complications. The advent of CT scan made surgeons wonder whether the imaging procedure could obviate the need for mediastinoscopy in some patients. As an alternative to mediastinoscopy, some authorities began to suggest undertaking a CT scan and, only if nodes were enlarged, to perform the mediastinoscopy. If nodes were not enlarged, the suggestion was to go straight to thoractomy.

A systematic review summarized more than 40 studies that had addressed the sensitivity and specificity of CT scanning in this context (38), but the impact of the alternative management strategies (mediastinoscopy on all versus selected mediastinoscopy) on patient-important outcomes remained uncertain. We argued that the only way of sorting this out was to conduct a trial in which investigators would randomize patients to the alternative diagnostic strategies and measure the frequency with which thoracotomy without cure (the adverse outcome that medistinoscopy was intended to prevent) occurred. We persuaded a peer-reviewed granting agency that we were right and launched the randomized trial.

Following the completion of this first trial, we used exactly the same logic to argue for a randomized trial in which patients without demonstrable mediastinal disease and no apparent distant metastases were randomized to go straight to surgery or have imaging evaluation for bone metastases (bone scanning) or abdominal and brain metastases (CT scan). Again, a peer-reviewed agency judged the proposal meritorious, and we conducted the trial.

Why Is Accuracy Not Enough?

One can conceptualize a hierarchy in the assessment of diagnostic technologies from, at the outset, a demonstration of technical capability to, at the summit of the hierarchy, a demonstration that application of the technology improves patient-important outcomes and is cost effective (39). Demonstrating diagnostic accuracy is an intermediate stage in this hierarchy.

There are a number of reasons that a test may be accurate and still not provide an important addition to clinical practice. First, the test may not change clinicians' estimate of the probability of the presence of the target condition enough for them to alter management. For instance, before we conducted our study, some thoracic surgeons felt that even after a "negative" CT scan, the probability of mediastinal metastases was still too high to forego mediastinoscopy. For these clinicians, the results of CT scanning didn't matter—whether positive or negative, the next step was still a mediastinoscopy.

Second, there may be no effective therapy available, or the therapy that one would generally apply might be of uncertain benefit. The administration of clofibrate following the diagnosis of hypercholesterolemia probably cost some patients their lives (40); the administration of the antiarrythmic agents encainide and flecainide following demonstration that the drugs could virtually obliterate aysmptomatic ventricular arrhythmias almost certainly did so (41). In both cases, patients would have been better off without the diagnostic tests that led to application of a harmful therapy. Nonstress testing that monitors fetal heart rates clearly adds diagnostic information and eases the anxiety of the attending obstetricians, but it does not change perinatal morbidity or mortality (42,43).

These examples make it evident that the ultimate standard of the usefulness of a diagnostic test is not its accuracy but rather whether it improves patient-important outcomes. The only definitive way of establishing impact on outcomes is to conduct a controlled trial in which patients are randomized to alternative diagnostic strategies.

When Should You (Not) Consider a Randomized Controlled Trial of a Diagnostic Technology?

Adequately powered, methodologically rigorous randomized trials are generally challenging to mount and expensive to implement. Research resources are limited. These considerations suggest that we should exercise care in choosing which diagnostic tests to subject to the ultimate standard of usefulness.

In most instances, randomized trials of diagnostic tests are either not appropriate or a poor use of research dollars. First, if the test improves the diagnosis of a condition with a clearly beneficial therapy, there is no question about its usefulness. Chest radiographs clearly aid in the diagnosis of pneumonia, and patients with bacterial pneumonia do better with antibiotic treatment. No ethics committee would permit a randomized trial of chest radiographs in patients with suspected pneumonia and (in contrast to many of the decisions of such committees) they would be right. The usefulness of a test is even more evident when therapy is not only effective but also has substantial down sides. While patients with pulmonary embolus benefit from warfarin therapy, those without clinically important clot suffer substantial risk from unnecessary warfarin administration. Thus, tests such as V/Q scanning that accurately distinguish patients with and without embolus needn't be evaluated through randomized trials. Funding of our randomized controlled trials (RCTs) of alternative diagnostic strategies in patients with presumed operable lung cancer required a convincing case that the link between test result and improved patient outcome was uncertain.

The case for RCT evaluation becomes compelling as tests become more expensive and invasive. It might be interesting to address whether patients are any better off with testing in a whole host of situations in which clinicians regularly order laboratory investigations such as hemoglobin, electrolytes, or renal function tests. The relatively benign nature of the tests and their relatively low resource consumption argue against investing research dollars in a trial addressing the impact of this testing on patient outcomes. Granting agencies looked with favor on our proposals for evaluating diagnostic strategies for apparently operable lung cancer because of the relatively large expense of tests such as mediastinoscopy and CT scanning, the relative invasiveness of some of the tests themselves (mediastinoscopy) or follow-up investigations that might follow a positive test (adrenal biopsy), and the invasiveness of the procedure that testing was designed to avoid (thoracotomy).

A final situation in which randomized trials of diagnostic tests are imperative is when the test is used for screening. The inevitable harms of screening (i.e., raising anxiety, unnecessary investigation as a result of false positives, and cost) and the risk of misleading conclusions as a result of length and lead time bias strongly suggest that we should be extremely reluctant to undertake widespread dissemination of screening tests without randomized trials that demonstrate improvement in patient-important outcomes.

8.4 SPECIAL CHALLENGES OF RANDOMIZED CONTROLLED TRIALS OF DIAGNOSTIC STRATEGIES

All the issues that Dave Sackett discusses in this book's comprehensive chapters on conduct of RCTs (Chapters 4, 5, and 6) apply to RCTs of diagnostic tests. There are a number of issues particularly relevant to trials of diagnostic strategies that we will review briefly here.

Conceptualization of the Intervention

No test, by itself, will ever benefit a patient. For patients to be better off, subsequent treatment has to differ depending on the test result. In our RCT of mediastinoscopy versus CT scan–directed management, patients with a positive CT scan went on to mediastinoscopy and those with a negative CT scan went straight to thoracotomy. In the second trial, those in the imaging arm went to thoracotomy only if the battery of investigations were negative. Positive results led to futher testing or outright cancellation of surgery.

This is the reason that we generally talk about RCTs of diagnostic strategies, rather than diagnostic tests. The point also highlights that your protocol should be very specific about how clinicians will respond to test results. Tests will only be beneficial if clinicians understand the importance of results and act accordingly. So, for instance, our imaging studies offered detailed guidance for clinicians faced with positive test results. For instance, what follows is our specification for how clinicians were to handle a positive CT of the liver:

> Only lesions that are both multiple and characteristic will not require histologic confirmation. If histologic confirmation is required, because, for example, the liver is the only suspected site of metastases, then material must be obtained by aspiration techniques with either CT or ultrasonographic guidance. For patients in whom the diagnosis of metastatic disease is made on the basis of characteristic liver CT scan, a repeat scan will be conducted in 3 months time to confirm the diagnosis. In addition, patients will be followed to determine if their clinical course is consistent with metastatic disease to the liver, and, when they die, autopsy will, if possible, be obtained.

Concealment of Randomization

Concealment of randomization is relatively straightforward in a blinded drug study. When, as in RCTs of diagnostic strategies, blinding is not possible, how to conceal randomization becomes a crucial issue. We believe that the only acceptable strategy is central randomization. Alternatives such as opaque, sealed envelopes are not immune to tampering. Central randomization, typically by telephone, involves confirming eligibility criteria, obtaining unique patient identifying information, and then providing the caller with the patient's allocation to experimental or control condition. Computerized telephone randomization is available. Internet randomization is a feasible alternative.

Screening Studies

One way to consider screening is as a subcategory of diagnosis. Because screening-eligible patients often do not present seeking care, because screening programs subject large numbers of people to the deleterious consequences of screening so that a small number may achieve putative benefits, and because the links between screening and benefit are invariably tenuous, the confidence that screening benefits outweigh risks almost invariably requires an RCT.

There are two fundamental designs of screening studies (see Figure 8–9) (44). In one design, patients are randomized to receive the screening test or to not receive the screening test. This is the design that, for instance, randomized trials in breast cancer prevention have typically used. The advantages of this design include the fact that it definitively tells you what occurred in all screened patients and that it potentially allows assessments of

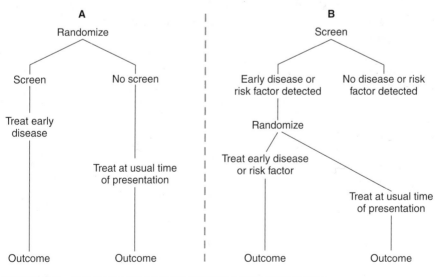

FIGURE 8–9   Designs for randomized controlled trials of screening.

benefits and downsides (false reassurance, for instance) in those who screen negative.

In the second design the screening process occurs before randomization. Patients who screen negative are not followed. Those who screen positive are randomized to receive or not receive an intervention. The major advantage of this design is its efficiency. One needn't follow the majority of those screened—those who screen negative on the test. This design is only feasible when the net benefit of treating target-positive patients remains uncertain. You could not, for instance, screen for breast cancer and randomize women with a positive mammogram to a full diagnostic workup versus watchful waiting.

Choosing Measures of Outcome

The usual counsel to measure and report all patient-important outcomes that the alternative management approaches may influence applies to randomized trials of diagnostic technologies. The choice of outcomes may require particularly careful thought in studies of diagnostic strategies, depending on what exactly the test is designed to achieve.

For instance, most cancer trials measure, as their primary outcomes, total mortality and disease-free survival. When we did our trials of diagnostic strategies for presumed operable lung cancer we did not anticipate the more aggressive strategies would impact these outcomes—or if they did, they would do so in such a small proportion of patients that sample sizes required to detect these effects would be well outside of the bounds of feasibility. The radiological investigation in the study of possible mediastinal tumor spread was designed to avoid mediastinoscopy—an invasive procedure—with the possible adverse consequence of increasing the number of patients destined to recur who underwent thoracotomy. In other words, a patient whose mediastinoscopy would have been positive (had it been done) but who had a negative CT scan and went straight to thoractomy could be considered to have had "unnecessary" surgery. The study surgeons preferred the term "thoracotomy without cure" to "unnecessary thoracotomy." When, however, we also considered patients with what proved to be benign disease who underwent thoracotomy, it proved difficult to argue that the thoracotomies were other than unnecessary.

In the second study, the additional investigations were designed to avoid thoracotomies without cure. Patients with spread of their disease to bone, brain, liver, or adrenal would not benefit from a thoracotomy. The primary outcome of both studies, unnecessary thoracotomy or thoracotomy without cure, was unconventional, and followed directly from consideration of exactly what the testing strategy was designed to achieve.

Studies of diagnostic strategies must also attend to complications associated with invasive tests. Undergoing an invasive test can itself be considered an adverse outcome because of the inevitable associated anxiety, pain, and discomfort. Thus, in the second study, we recorded and highlighted the additional invasive tests in the full investigation arm of the RCT.

Another outcome specific to randomized trials of diagnostic technology is the reassurance that negative test results may provide. For example, Sox and associates found that patients with noncardiac chest pain experienced less short-term disability when randomized to receive, versus not receive, testing with creatine phosphokinase and electrocardiogram (45). One can by no means rely on such reassurance. McDonald and colleagues found that 21 of 39 patients (54%) referred for echocardiogram with possible cardiac symptoms or a murmur continued to experience anxiety about their heart despite normal findings on the test (46). The flip side of this reassurance is the anxiety generated by labelling a person who receives a positive result of a screening test as having a potentially important health problem.

8.5 RESULTS OF RANDOMIZED TRIALS OF DIAGNOSTIC STRATEGIES IN PATIENTS WITH PRESUMED OPERABLE LUNG CANCER

Readers may be curious about the results of the studies used as examples in this section. In the first study of 342 patients randomized to mediastinoscopy, 315 (92%) actually underwent the procedure, in comparison to 153 of 343 (45%) in the CT scan group. The relative risk for thoracotomy without cure in those with underlying cancer associated with being in the CT group was 0.95 ($P = 0.34$, 95% CI 0.75–1.19). The relative risk of having a thoracotomy among patients who ultimately proved to have benign disease was 0.42 ($P = 0.05$, 95% CI 0.12–1.13). The relative risk of "unnecessary" thoracotomies (thoracotomies without cure and thoracotomies in those who proved to have benign disease) was 0.88 ($P = 0.15$, 95% CI 0.71–1.1). The mediastinoscopy strategy cost $708 more per patient (95% CI $723–$2,140). While the wide CIs preclude a definitive recommendation from this study, we concluded that the CT strategy is likely to produce the same number of, or fewer, unnecessary thoracotomies in comparison to doing mediastinoscopy on all patients, and is also likely to be as expensive, or less so.

In the second study, the relative risk of thoracotomy without cure (the combination of open and close thoracotomy without resection, incomplete resection, and thoracotomy with subsequent recurrence) in the full versus the limited investigation group was 0.80 (95% CI 0.56–1.13, $P = 0.20$). Forty three of 318 patients (14%) in the full investigation group and 61 of 316 patients (19%) in the limited investigation group underwent an apparently complete resection at thoracotomy but the malignancy subsequently recurred (relative risk 0.70, 95% CI 0.47–1.03, $P = 0.07$). Patients in the full investigation group were more likely to have avoided thoracotomy because of extrathoracic metastatic disease discovered before surgery than those in the limited investigation group (22 versus 10 patients, relative risk 2.19, $P = 0.04$, 95% CI 1.04–4.59). The total number of negative invasive tests was 6 in the full investigation group and 1 in the limited investigation group (relative risk 6.1, $P = 0.10$, 95% CI, 0.72–51.0) and the total number of invasive tests 11 versus 6 (relative risk 1.84, $P = 0.23$, 95% CI, 0.68–4.98).

The full investigation strategy cost $823 less per patient (95% CI $2,482–$725). Again, the wide CIs preclude definitive recommendations. We nevertheless concluded that full investigation for metastatic disease in non-small cell lung cancer patients without symptoms or signs of metastatic disease may reduce the number of thoracotomies without cure.

REFERENCES

1. Reid MC, Lachs MS, Feinstein AR. Use of methodological standards in diagnostic test research. Getting better but still not good. *JAMA* 1995;274:645–651.

2. Bossuyt PM, Reitsma JB, Bruns DE, et al, STARD steering group. Towards complete and accurate reporting of studies of diagnostic accuracy: the STARD initiative. *BMJ* 2003;326:41–44.

3. Sackett DL, Haynes RB, Guyatt GH, et al. *Clinical epidemiology: a basic science for clinical medicine*, 2nd ed. Boston, MA: Little, Brown and Company, 1991:69–152.

4. Landray MJ, Lehman R, Arnold I. Measuring brain natriuretic peptide in suspected left ventricular systolic dysfunction in general practice: cross-sectional study. *BMJ* 2000,320:985–986.

5. Fagan TJ. Nomogram for Bayes's theorem. *N Engl J Med* 1975;293:257.

6. Straus SE, McAlister FA, Sackett DL, et al., CARE-COAD1 Group. The accuracy of patient history, wheezing, and laryngeal measurements in diagnosing obstructive airway disease. *JAMA* 2000;283:1853–1857.

7. Guyatt GH, Oxman A, Ali M, et al. Laboratory diagnosis of iron deficiency anemia: an overview. *J Gen Intern Med* 1992;7:145–153.

8. Guyatt GH, Patterson C, Ali M, et al. Diagnosis of iron deficiency anemia in the elderly. *Am J Med* 1990;88:205–209.

9. Thomson DM, Krupey J, Freedman SO, et al. The radioimmunoassay of circulating carcinoembryonic antigen of the human digestive system. *Proc Natl Acad Sci USA* 1969; 64:161–167.

10. Bates SE. Clinical applications of serum tumor markers. *Ann Intern Med* 1991;115: 623–638.

11. Lijmer JG, Mol BW, Heisterkamp S, et al. Empirical evidence of design-related bias in studies of diagnostic tests. *JAMA* 1999;282:1061–1066.

12. Guyatt G, Rennie D. *Users' guides to the medical literature: A manual for evidence-based clinical practice*. Chicago, IL: AMA Press, 2002.

13. Hill SA, Devereaux PJ, Griffith L, et al. Can troponin I measurement predict short term serious cardiac outcomes in patients presenting to the emergency department with potential cardiac symptoms? *Can J Emerg Med* 2004;6:22–30.

14. Anderson DR, Wells PS, Stiell I, et al. Thrombosis in the emergency department: use of a clinical diagnosis model to safely avoid the need for urgent radiological investigation. *Arch Intern Med* 1999;159:477–482.

15. Hlatky MA, Pryor DB, Harrell FE Jr, et al. Factors affecting sensitivity and specificity of exercise electrocardiography. Multivariable analysis. *Am J Med* 1984;77:64–71.

16. Ginsberg JS, Caco CC, Brill-Edwards PA, et al. Venous thrombosis in patients who have undergone major hip or knee surgery: detection with compression US and impedance plethysmography. *Radiology* 1991;181:651–654.

17. International Committee for Standardization in Haematology. The measurement of total iron and unsaturated iron binding capacity in serum. *Br J Haematol* 1978;38:281–287.

18. Luxton AW, Walker WHC, Goldie J, et al. A radioimmunosassay for serum ferritin. *Clin Chem* 1977;23:683–689.

19. Piomelli S, Young P, Gay G. A micro method for free erythrocyte protoporphyrin: the FEP test. *J Lab Clin Med* 1973;81:932–940.

20. Rao PM, Feltmate CM, Rhea JT, et al. Helical computed tomography in differentiating appendicitis and acute gynecologic conditions. *Obstet Gynecol* 1999;93:417–421.

21. Fleiss JL. Measuring agreement between two judges on the presence or absence of a trait. *Biometrics* 1975;31:651–659.

22. Donner A, Klar N. The statistical analysis of kappa statistics in multiple samples. *J Clin Epidemiol* 1996;9:1053–1058.

23. Cook RJ, Farewell VT. Conditional inference for subject-specific and marginal agreement: two families of agreement measures. *Can J Stat* 1995;23:333–344.

24. Meade MO, Cook RJ, Guyatt GH, et al. Interobserver variation in interpreting chest radiographs for the diagnosis of acute respiratory distress syndrome. *Am J Respir Crit Care Med* 2000;161:85–90.

25. McGinn T, Guyatt G, Cook R. Measuring agreement beyond chance. In: Guyatt G, Rennie D, eds. *Users' guides to the medical literature: A manual for evidence-based clinical practice.* Chicago, IL: AMA Press, 2002.

26. Dacie SV, Lewis SM. *Practical haematology*, 4th ed. London: Churchill Livingstone, 1984:107–109.

27. Kemppainen EA, Hedstrom JI, Puolakkainen PA, et al. Rapid measurement of urinary trypsinogen-2 as a screening test for acute pancreatitis. *N Engl J Med* 1997;336:1788–1793.

28. Begg CB, Greenes RA. Assessment of diagnostic tests when disease verification is subject to selection bias. *Biometrics* 1983;39:207–215.

29. Gray R, Begg CB, Greenes RA. Construction of receiver operating characteristic curves when disease verification is subject to selection bias. *Med Decis Making* 1984;4:151–164.

30. Ransohoff DF, Feinstein AR. Problems of spectrum and bias in evaluating the efficacy of diagnostic tests. *N Engl J Med* 1978;299:926–930.

31. Choi BCK. Sensitivity and specificity of a single diagnostic test in the presence of work-up bias. *J Clin Epidemiol* 1992;45:581–586.

32. The PIOPED Investigators. Value of ventilation/perfusion scan in acute pulmonary embolism. Results of the prospective investigation of pulmonary embolism diagnosis (PIOPED). *JAMA* 1990;263:2753–2759.

33. Punglia RS, D'Amico AV, Catalona WJ, et al. Effect of verification bias on screening for prostate cancer by measurement of prostate-specific antigen. *N Engl J Med* 2003;349: 335–342.

34. Hanley JA, McNeil BJ. The meaning and use of the area under a receiver operating characteristic (ROC) curve. *Radiology* 1982;143:29–36.

35. Hanley JA, McNeil BJ. A method of comparing the areas under receiver operating characteristic curves derived from the same cases. *Radiology* 1983;148:839–843.

36. Albert A. On the use and computation of likelihood ratios in clinical chemistry. *Clin Chem* 1982;28:1113–1119.

37. Patterson C, Guyatt GH, Singer J, et al. Iron deficiency anemia in the elderly: the diagnostic process. *Can Med Assoc J* 1991;144:435–440.

38. Dales RE, Stark RM, Sankaranarayanan R. Computed tomography to stage lung cancer. *Am Rev Respir Dis* 1990;141:1096–1101.

39. Guyatt GH, Tugwell P, Feeny DH, et al. A framework for clinical evaluation of diagnostic technologies. *Can Med Assoc J* 1986;134:587–594.

40. Committee of Principal Investigators. WHO cooperative trial on primary prevention of ischemic heart disease using clofibrate to lower serum cholesterol: mortality follow-up. *Lancet* 1980;2:370–385.

41. Echt DS, Liebson PR, Mitchell LB, et al. Mortality and morbidity in patients receiving encainide, flecainide, or placebo. The cardiac arrhythmia suppression trial. *N Engl J Med* 1991;324:781–788.

42. Brown VA, Sawers RS, Parsons RJ, et al. The value of antenatal cardiotocography in the management of high-risk pregnancy: a randomized controlled trial. *Br J Obstet Gynaecol* 1982;89:716–722.

43. Flynn AM, Kelly J, Mansfield H, et al. A randomized controlled trial of non-stress antepartum cardiotocography. *Br J Obstet Gynaecol* 1982;89:427–433.

44. Barratt A, Irwig L, Glasziou P, et al. Recommendations about screening. In: Guyatt G, Rennie D, eds. *Users' guides to the medical literature: A manual for evidence-based clinical practice.* Chicago, IL: AMA Press, 2002.

45. Sox HC Jr, Margulies I, Sox CH. Psychologically mediated effects of diagnostic tests. *Ann Intern Med* 1981;95:680–685.

46. McDonald IG, Daly J, Jelinek VM, et al. Opening pandora's box: the unpredictability of reassurance by a normal test result. *BMJ* 1996;313:329–332.

9

DETERMINING PROGNOSIS AND CREATING CLINICAL DECISION RULES

Gordon Guyatt

Chapter Outline

9.1   Why study prognosis?
9.2   Prognosis versus diagnosis
9.3   Clinical prediction rules
9.4   Basic principles of conducting prognostic studies

CLINICAL RESEARCH SCENARIO

Critically ill patients managed in intensive care units (ICUs) are at increased risk of gastrointestinal (GI) bleeding. This is true even for patients without previous problems with gastric or duodenal ulcers, or with other GI pathology. In the late 1980s, stress ulcer prophylaxis with histamine H_2-receptor antagonists (drugs that reduce acid secretion in the stomach) was widely used in ICUs to prevent GI bleeding in critically ill patients. Clinicians were increasingly aware that the incidence of serious bleeding had apparently decreased markedly and suspected that it might be low enough that prophylaxis was no longer warranted for all patients. As a result, they raised questions about the advisability of stress ulcer prophylaxis. Specifically, clinicians questioned what subgroups of critically ill patients (if any) still had a risk of bleeding that was sufficiently great that they should receive stress ulcer prophylaxis. We set out to address this issue.

9.1 WHY STUDY PROGNOSIS?

There are two fundamental reasons why clinicians need to know a patient's prognosis. One is that, irrespective of management decisions, patients often are interested in knowing how well, or badly, they are likely to fare. Certain diagnoses, such as a diagnosis of cancer, carry with them almost inevitable questions about how long a patient is going to live. Clinicians must be prepared to address patients' questions about their fates, or prognosis.

The second fundamental reason why clinicians need to know a patients' prognosis is that it may alter their recommended management plan. If a patient's risk of the adverse outcome that the treatment is designed to prevent is sufficiently low, a therapeutic intervention may not be warranted. The reason is that all interventions carry with them a burden of cost, inconvenience, and adverse effects. Furthermore, the opportunity for benefits varies from patient to patient, depending on their prognosis. The research scenario that introduced this chapter provides an example: In the late 1980s, clinicians began to suspect that the incidence of stress ulceration in patients with GI bleeding was sufficiently low that, at least in some critically ill patients, the cost, inconvenience, and side effects of stress ulcer prophylaxis were too great to warrant prophylaxis.

As the risk of the adverse outcomes that treatment is designed to prevent decreases, and the risk of treatment-induced adverse outcomes increases (I'll call such events "treatment toxicity"), patients become progressively less enthusiastic about a potential therapeutic intervention. When the probability of adverse outcomes becomes sufficiently low, or when the treatment toxicity becomes sufficiently great, patients begin to cross a threshold beyond which they would decline even effective therapy. Thresholds differ in individuals, but as the incidence of adverse events in untreated patients decreases further, or as toxicity rises further, more and more patients would decline therapy designed to lower their risk. Eventually, even those who value the benefits highly and are less concerned about adverse effects no longer find the benefits worth the risks.

9.2 PROGNOSIS VERSUS DIAGNOSIS

In what ways are studies of prognosis and diagnosis similar? Both types of studies often have the same purpose: to identify patients who have a higher or lower probability of a particular condition (diagnosis), outcome (prognosis), or responsiveness to therapy. For instance, in patients with carotid stenosis who benefit from carotid endarterectomy, as the number of cardiovascular risk factors [age more than 70 years; systolic blood pressure greater than 160 or diastolic less than 90; stroke or transient ischemic attacks (TIAs) in the last 30 days; stroke rather than TIA; carotid stenosis more than 80%; ulceration on angiography; history of hypertension, heart failure, myocardial infarction (MI), dyslipidemia, claudication, or smoking] increases, the risk of a subsequent stroke increases. As the risk of stroke increases, the potential benefits of endarterectomy increase. Table 9–1 presents data from a randomized trial of carotid endarterectomy about the relation between the number of risk factors, the magnitude of benefit in terms of the absolute risk reduction that patients can expect from endarterectomy, and the number of patients one needs to treat with endarterectomy to prevent a stroke (1).

TABLE 9-1 Relation between Risk Factors and Risk Difference with Carotid Endarterectomy in Patients with Cerebrovascular Disease (1)

Number of Risk Factors	Number of Patients in Trial	Risk Difference (%)	Number Needed to Treat
0–5	305	3.8	27
6	153	9.8	10
7 or more	201	19.4	5

From North American Symptomatic Carotid Endarterectomy Trial Collaborators. Beneficial effect of carotid endarterectomy in symptomatic patients with high-grade carotid stenosis. *N Engl J Med* 1991;325:445–453, with permission.

In certain clinical situations, the distinction between prognosis and diagnosis blurs completely. For instance, when a clinician asks "does this patient with chest pain in the emergency room have a myocardial infarction," the real, underlying question of interest may be "does this patient have a risk of adverse events sufficiently great that the patient requires admission to the hospital."

It isn't difficult to think of other instances in which distinctions between prognosis and diagnosis blur. For instance, although most clinicians think of troponin I as useful in the diagnosis of acute MI, it may also provide information about the long-term prognosis of patients presenting with acute coronary syndrome (2). Consider the prognostic value of preoperative characteristics in estimating the likelihood of cardiac events after noncardiac surgery. Clinicians only need to follow patients for a few days to determine whether they have attained the outcome of interest. Moreover, long-term follow-up is often a component of the reference standard in many diagnostic test studies. For instance, investigators have used long-term follow-up to establish a diagnosis of "no pulmonary embolus" in patients who did not undergo a pulmonary angiogram at the time of presentation with possible pulmonary embolus (3).

Another similarity lies in the nature of the relation between the predictor variable (the diagnostic test or the prognostic factor) and the outcome (disease present or absent, or outcome present or absent). The association between the diagnostic test and the disease is seldom, if ever, causal. That is, the high troponin, or low serum ferritin is a consequence of the pathological processes of MI and iron deficiency, and not the cause. The same is true when troponin is used to predict outcome, or for other common prognostic variables such as lung or cardiac function, or functional capacity. Prognostic variables such as smoking, high blood pressure, or high serum lipids may, on the other hand, have an etiologic link to the outcomes with which they are associated.

In what ways do prognostic and diagnostic studies differ? Diagnostic studies geared to establish test properties for clinical practice should restrict themselves to populations with an intermediate probability that the target condition is present. If the probability is too low—below a "test threshold"—it may not be worth ordering the test, particularly if it is expensive or invasive. If the probability is too high—above the "treatment threshold,"—the clinician should not bother with further testing but rather go ahead and treat. Thus, there is little point in enrolling patients at very high or very low risk in studies of diagnostic tests unless, of course, one cannot identify characteristics that distinguish between high- and low-risk patients. Prognostic studies, however, may enrol a wider spectrum of patients, including those with very low and very high probabilities of the outcome of interest.

Diagnostic test studies typically focus on an individual laboratory or radiological test, or a small number of tests. Prognostic studies typically address a number of prognostic factors, often starting with demographic variables (such as age and sex) and including markers of disease severity (such as physical examination findings and disease staging). However, investigators may focus on the prognostic usefulness of tests ordinarily considered as bearing primarily on diagnosis. Classical diagnostic test studies do not usually address the independent contribution of the diagnostic test to the diagnostic process, whereas prognostic studies often use techniques such as multivariable regression to cast light on the independent contribution of each prognostic factor.

Diagnostic test studies usually compare the test results to a "gold," reference, or criterion standard ascertained at the same time as, or shortly after, testing. Prognostic studies, by their nature, involve following patients over time to determine whether the outcome of interest occurs. Diagnostic test studies report results in terms of likelihood ratios (LRs) or (less usefully) sensitivity and specificity. Prognostic studies typically report relative risks, odds ratios, or survival curves and their associated hazard ratios.

Thus, despite many similarities in basic study design, the issues in prognostic and diagnostic test studies are often different enough that we considered it worth having separate chapters addressing these issues.

9.3 CLINICAL PREDICTION RULES

Clinical prediction rules, when properly developed, may take studies of prognosis to a higher level. Clinical prediction rules include simultaneous consideration of several factors in predicting the prognosis of individual patients. They may also be developed for use with patients for whom clinicians have not yet established a firm diagnosis. In the latter case, they may predict the result of either an intermediate test, such as plain x-ray, or a more definitive test or diagnostic pathway.

To illustrate this, consider patients presenting to an emergency department with chest pain suggestive of an acute coronary syndrome. In such patients with acute coronary syndrome, the nature of the patients' pain, the electrocardiogram, and cardiac enzymes all play a major role in deciding on the likelihood of acute MI. Once the clinician has established that a particular patient does indeed have an MI, she must simultaneously consider age, degree of cardiac dysfunction, and presence of arrhythmias in deciding on how likely the patient is to be alive a year from presentation. Thus, a clinical prediction rule can help make a diagnosis or can assist in the management of the patient once the diagnosis is made.

The task of simultaneously considering a number of variables in deciding on the probability of a diagnosis, or the likelihood of a subsequent adverse event, represents a considerable cognitive challenge. In particular, clinicians are at risk of double-counting. That is, they may fail to fully take into account that, to the extent that one variable is correlated with another, a patient's status on the second variable will add relatively little diagnostic or prognostic information. For instance, when considering whether patients who are anemic are iron deficient, it might be tempting to think that a low mean cell volume suggests iron deficiency and that a low serum ferritin strengthens the case. As it turns out, however, the information is redundant, and mean cell volume adds nothing once you've considered the serum ferritin. If clinicians treat the tests as if they are independent, they risk over- or underestimating the likelihood of iron deficiency.

Considering the magnitude of the cognitive challenge, the possibility naturally arises that mathematical models that simultaneously consider all relevant variables will do a better job than the clinicians' intuition. When we say "simultaneously consider," we mean that they avoid the problem of "double-counting" the results of tests that are correlated with one another. All such models provide an estimate of the likelihood of a diagnosis (such as myocardial infarction or ankle fracture) or of future adverse events (such as a poor outcome in patients presenting with syncope, or the need for reoperation in patients with tibial fracture). Thus, such models have received appellations that include "clinical prediction rules" or "clinical prediction guides." The term "guides" may be more appropriate for models that simply generate estimates without dictating a course of action. On the other hand, some argue that "rules" is a good term because it emphasizes the necessity for rigorous and replicable application of each component of the diagnostic or prognostic strategy.

Some models go one step further than models (by any name) that simply generate estimates: They prescribe a particular course of action. For instance, the Ottawa Ankle Rule tells clinicians that, in patients presenting with ankle injuries, if they find no tenderness in specific areas and if the patients can bear their own weight, the likelihood of an underlying fracture is very low. The rule does not, however, stop there. It also tells clinicians that, in such low-risk patients, they needn't order radiographs. One term for such prescriptive models is "clinical decision rules."

9.4 BASIC PRINCIPLES OF CONDUCTING PROGNOSTIC STUDIES

A protocol for any study determining patients' prognosis must attend to the elements outlined in the following checklist:

✓ Conduct your literature review.

✓ Pose your research question.

✓ Recruit your participants. Recruit a representative sample of patients who do not have the outcome of interest at the time of initial observation and who are, preferably, at an identifiable, common, and early point in their disorder or exposure.

✓ Choose what you will measure. Record all patient characteristics that might show substantial associations with the outcome of interest.

✓ Use measurement strategies. Use accurate and unbiased measurement of the outcome of interest.

✓ Select your statistical procedures. Include sample size and analysis.

✓ Select your presentation and interpretation methods.

Note that this checklist is almost identical to that for diagnostic test studies, reflecting the very close relation between the goals and methods of these two types of studies.

Planning for the study that will provide the focus for this discussion began 15 years ago. My colleague, Dr. Deborah Cook, led all aspects of the work, from inception to completion. Our team submitted the grant in 1988, the granting agency funded the study in 1989, and the journal article reporting the results appeared in 1994 (4). We have learned a lot since then, and the narrative of the study will often focus on what we would have done differently if we were conducting the study today.

✓ *Conduct your literature review.*

In 1987, when we began planning our study, intensivists regularly administered stress ulcer prophylaxis with H_2-receptor antagonists to critically ill patients. The results of a number of randomized trials supported this practice, and, in 1991, our group published a systematic review and meta-analysis that we had conducted while our prognostic study was getting underway. The review demonstrated a 50% reduction in patient-important bleeding with prophylaxis (5).

Despite this strong evidence in support of prophylaxis, in the late 1980s, clinicians began to question its routine use because of the increasing evidence that the incidence of serious bleeding from stress ulceration was decreasing. Our review (which was fully systematic or comprehensive for the randomized trials, but not for the observational studies) found an incidence of serious bleeding of 2.6% in 27 randomized trials. We identified only three studies in adults, published between 1984 and 1987, that had prospectively evaluated the independent contribution of a variety of patient characteristics to risks of bleeding.

Whereas our search for observational studies was not comprehensive or systematic, we have repeated the search using the sensitive "Clinical Queries" for prognosis in PubMed (*http://www.ncbi.nlm.nih.gov/entrez/ query/static/clinical.html*), which utilizes the following search string: "incidence" [Medical Subject Headings (MeSH)] OR "mortality" (MeSH) OR "follow-up studies" (MeSH) OR 'mortality" (SH) OR prognos* (WORD) OR predict* (WORD) OR course (WORD). This search failed to reveal additional relevant articles. If your goal is to be comprehensive, you can pursue other useful strategies once an initial search has identified most of the relevant articles. For each of these articles, you can use Science Citation Index (particularly useful for older articles), to find newer studies and reviews that cite the older studies, or use the "Related Articles" feature of PubMed.

✓ *Pose your research question.*

In the report of the study, we described our project this way:

"We undertook this prospective study to determine the incidence of clinically important GI bleeding in a heterogeneous group of critically ill patients and to identify patients at sufficiently low risk of bleeding to obviate the need for prophylaxis."

In this book, we are proposing that you make explicit what we felt was implicit in this statement. The statement we made in the published paper (in the shaded box at the beginning of this section) places the question squarely in the "clinical decision rule" category. That is, if we succeeded in answering the question, we would be providing clinicians with management advice: "In this particular subgroup of patients, you should withhold prophylaxis." As we proceed with this discussion we will review the particular challenges implicit in this framing (issues that we were not fully aware of at the time and that resulted in limitations in our study design, and the analysis and interpretation of the data).

Consideration of clinical decision rules highlights the need for investigators to be vividly clear on the question they are addressing and the alternative designs that flow from that question. Clinicians might ask, "Should clinicians prescribe H_2-receptor antagonists in particular subgroups of critically ill patients, in relation to their risk of GI bleeding?" This question, however, is too vague. There are two ways one can shed light on the optimal management of critically ill patients who may be at risk of GI bleeding. One way would be to conceptualize the issue as a question of prognosis; the other would be to conceptualize the question as one of therapy. In the prognostic conceptualization, one attempts to identify a subgroup at sufficiently low risk that prophylaxis is not warranted and another group at higher risk in whom prophylaxis is appropriate. This formulation suggests an observational prognostic study as the appropriate design.

Within the prognostic conceptualization, there are at least three ways of structuring the question. Table 9–2 presents the range of possibilities.

The formulation in the second column of Table 9–2 uses an implicit approach to the issue of exploration of possible subgroups with different prognoses—that is, the possibility that there are important predictors of outcome.

One can make the exploration of prognostic factors explicit in one of two ways. The third column of Table 9–2 builds the issue into the description of the patients. Alternatively, as in the fourth column of Table 9–2, one can frame the exposure not as time but as the prognostic factors. The final column suggests an alternative strategy for addressing the management problem: a randomized clinical trial in which investigators would randomize patients to receive H_2-receptor antagonists or placebo.

Any time an investigator hopes to end up with a clinical decision rule prescribing a particular management strategy (as opposed to a clinical prediction guide or a rule that simply generates a probability of a diagnosis or a subsequent adverse outcome) the question of whether to do an observational study or a randomized trial should arise. When the comparable effect of the intervention in terms of relative risk reduction across a range of differing pretest probabilities is reasonably secure, the prognostic study should suffice. If this is not the case, one should seriously consider the clinical trial. Indeed, at the time we designed the study we debated whether we should conduct a randomized trial. Our complete uncertainty about the event rates we might expect (and the possibility that they might be low enough to make the study completely unfeasible) decided the issue.

What Treatment Should Patients Receive in a Prognostic Study?

A final issue that confronted us was in the definition of the population. Note that, in the preceding text, we specified that patients were not receiving stress ulcer prophylaxis. That makes sense in terms of finding a group with a risk low enough to withhold prophylaxis. After all, if one identified a very low-risk group in whom clinicians had administered prophylaxis, the natural objection would be, "Sure, the risk is low, but that may be because of the H_2-receptor antagonists the patient received. If they hadn't received prophylaxis, their bleeding risk may have been much higher."

Specifying that a patient not receive prophylaxis becomes problematic, however, as soon as one considers the clinician who believes that her patient needs to have the bleeding risk reduced. After all, we knew at the time we started the study that H_2-receptor antagonists were effective in reducing bleeding. Under such circumstances, is it ethical to withhold prophylaxis?

TABLE 9–2 Framing Questions Addressing the Issue of Who Should Receive Stress Ulcer Prophylaxis

	Simple prognosis	Prognostic factors in population specification	Prognostic factors as exposure	Randomized trial
Patient	Critically ill adults not receiving stress ulcer prophylaxis	Critically ill adults not receiving stress ulcer prophylaxis varying in a number of characteristics (ventilated or not, coagulopathy or not, renal failure or not, and so on)	Critically ill adults not receiving stress ulcer prophylaxis	Critically ill adults not receiving stress ulcer prophylaxis
Exposure or Intervention	Time	Time	Mechanical ventilation, coagulopathy, renal failure, and so on	H_2-receptor antagonists versus no prophylaxis or placebo
Outcome	Patient-important bleeding from stress ulceration	Patient-important bleeding from stress ulceration	Patient-important bleeding from stress ulceration	Patient-important bleeding from stress ulceration

We could have dealt with this problem in two ways. First, we could have asked clinicians to assume that all their patients were at a sufficiently low risk that prophylaxis would not be warranted. In keeping with that assumption, clinicians would then withhold prophylaxis in all their patients. Alternatively, we could have restricted our sample to patients in whom clinicians were comfortable withholding prophylaxis. We will return to this choice in the next section in which we describe the selection of participants for a prognostic study.

✓ *Recruit your participants.*

Recruit a representative sample of patients who do not have the outcome of interest at the time of initial observation, preferably at an identifiable, common, and early point in their disorder or exposure.

> We considered consecutive patients older than 16 years of age admitted between June 1990 and July 1991 to four university-affiliated medical–surgical ICUs for enrollment. Patients were ineligible if they had upper GI bleeding (i.e., hematemesis, a nasogastric aspirate containing gross blood or coffee ground material, hematochezia, or melena) within 48 hours before or 24 hours after admission, prior total gastrectomy, facial trauma or epistaxis, brain death, a hopeless prognosis, or had been discharged within 24 hours. Limited resources at three centers forced us to enrol random subsets of eligible patients and close entry at weekends during part of the study period.
>
> We encouraged attending physicians to withhold stress ulcer prophylaxis in all patients except those with head injury, greater than 30% body surface burns, organ transplants, endoscopic or radiographic peptic ulcer or gastritis in the prior 6 weeks, or upper GI bleeding 3 days to 6 weeks before admission.

Articles in the published literature often report ranges of observed frequency of adverse outcomes so wide that they provide the clinician with no useful information. For instance, reported recurrence rates after passing a first urinary stone range from 20% (6) to 100% (7). The reported risk of recurrence after a febrile seizure ranges from 1.5% to 76.9% (8). Differences in sample selection go a long way in explaining such discrepancies, and they have led to oft-cited criteria suggesting that investigators should enrol patients at an early and uniform time in the course in their illness (9). In our study, we selected patients at the common point of admission to the ICU and excluded those who were bleeding at the time of their admission.

Critics have also made much of distortions created when investigators conduct studies of patients presenting to tertiary care centers. Typically, such patients fare badly in comparison to patients presenting to primary-care and secondary care institutions whom the clinicians decide not to refer. Clearly, primary care clinicians using data from studies in tertiary care centers will be giving their patients an excessively gloomy outlook.

Not only will patients in tertiary centers have a poorer prognosis but also the prognostic factors that were powerful in a primary or secondary care population may lose their prognostic power in the tertiary population if that factor is associated with the likelihood of referral. For instance, age may be powerfully associated with adverse outcomes. If primary care physicians selectively fail to refer either the youngest or oldest patients, the age distribution of patients in the referral center will be narrower. Age will therefore lose some of its predictive power.

What then if you are a clinician working in a tertiary care center? If you use data from an entire cohort of patients identified in primary care at the onset of a condition, you may be paying attention to prognostic factors that do not discriminate, within your setting, between patients destined to have good and poor outcomes. Should you not then use prognostic information from studies of patients presenting to centers similar to your own?

Different Practice Settings: the Solution

The solution to the problem of different practice settings lies in ensuring that the population enrolled is representative of the underlying population to whom you would like to apply the results. If you would like to apply results to patients affected severely enough to warrant specialist consultation, then enrolling patients presenting to such a setting would be appropriate.

The solution is not, however, without problems. Most referral centers provide primary care for the local communities they serve. Accordingly, the patients they follow, if considered together, have mixed prognoses. The solution to this situation is obvious: For questions of prognosis at the primary-care level, restrict the study population to patients from the local catchment area. For questions of prognosis of referred patients, only those patients referred from outside the catchment area would be considered.

Whereas this problem is at least theoretically solvable, other sticking points remain. Criteria for referral onward may differ depending on locality. Typically, if the threshold for referral is low, patients who are less sick with a better prognosis will appear in the secondary care or tertiary care population. A higher threshold for referral will produce a population with a gloomier outlook.

This problem is not restricted to secondary care contexts. Different patient populations may exhibit different thresholds for consulting their primary care provider. A parent may react to a febrile seizure that is a few seconds long with neglect. The parents' financial status and the cost of a visit to a clinician, or the distance required to travel or competing demands on time and energy may profoundly influence the decision whether to seek professional help. These factors may vary systematically across populations, leading to substantial variations in thresholds across those populations.

Could the solution be to conduct population-based studies in which investigators endeavor to identify all incident cases and follow them forward? Such studies may or may not face enormous logistical difficulties. Planners of health services are likely to find them useful. Clinicians, however, will find them less helpful. For instance, knowing that as many as

50% of patients who die from an MI do so before arrival at the hospital will not help the clinician to provide prognostic information to patients who do make it as far as the hospital.

The Inevitable Filter, and What Investigators Can Do About It

These reflections make it evident that patients enrolled in virtually all prognostic studies have passed through some sort of filter. Thus, the best that investigators can do is to characterize that filter as explicitly as possible and describe the characteristics of the patients enrolled in the prognostic study as comprehensively and precisely as possible. The inevitability of this filter explains, to a considerable extent, the difficulties in generating robust clinical prediction models generalizable across settings, a point to which we shall return.

In addition to characterizing their inevitable filter, and their patients, investigators can also avoid obvious filters that would bias their patient samples to the point where they are applicable to virtually no other settings. One obvious mistake is to try and work backwards. For instance, several studies of the risk of renal stone recurrence focus on currently symptomatic patients and ask them if they have had stones previously. In such studies, those with multiple recurrences have far higher likelihood of being included than those with only a single episode, biasing estimates of recurrence rates upwards. Similarly, in a study of the risk of bowel cancer in patients with ulcerative colitis, some patients were included in the cohort because they had developed cancer, inevitably creating an overestimate of recurrence rates (10,11). The underlying principle dictates that investigators ensure that patients who do and who do not develop outcomes have an equal chance of inclusion in the ultimate study cohort.

Another way to violate this principle is to enrol patients on the basis of their returning to a clinical setting for follow-up. Such an approach may bias results in either direction. If the sickest patients (particularly those who die) can't make it to clinic, the study will yield a rosy estimate of prognosis. If those who are doing well don't bother to show up, the estimate will be pessimistic.

An increasingly popular and attractive strategy for enrolling cohorts and examining prognosis is to use a large administrative database. Such databases will, in general, minimize problems with filters that distort the nature of the population. Their problems, in regard to estimating prognosis, lie in limited, incomplete information and in inaccuracies. Although inaccuracies may include problems in initial classification of patients, the classification of comorbidity is likely to be more problematic, and we will return to this issue in the next section.

Prognosis and Treatment: the Unnatural History

People once referred to studies of prognosis as "natural history" studies. Implied in the "natural" was an absence of treatment, or at least minimal interventions. Medical science has advanced to the point where there are few conditions for which we can offer patients no treatment of benefit (or failing that, one that ultimately proves harmful!).

As a result, for most studies of prognosis, many patients are receiving effective treatment. Moreover, whether patients are taking effective treatment becomes a prognostic factor. This is not necessarily problematic, as long as you remember not to interpret the magnitude of the association between treatment and outcomes in an observational study as the magnitude of the treatment effect.

For instance, one observational study of prognosis after MI found that thrombolytic therapy was associated with reduction in the relative risk of death by more than 50% (12). Randomized trials tell us that the actual relative risk reduction with thrombolysis is approximately 25% and that risk reduction is more or less constant across patients with different levels of baseline risk. The reason for the apparently larger treatment effect in the observational study was that patients given thrombolysis were less sick to start with—that is, they had a better underlying prognosis. Such findings serve as a poignant reminder of the gap between documenting association and establishing causation.

In the ICU bleeding risk study, treated patients presented another difficulty. Our goal was to define a group at sufficiently low risk that prophylaxis was not necessary. However, if patients were already receiving prophylaxis, their underlying risk without prophylaxis would be higher than that which we observed in our study.

Could we have solved this problem by restricting our enrollment to patients in whom clinicians did not administer prophylaxis? We could not have done so because use of that filter would likely have biased our results. Presumably, clinicians administered prophylaxis to those at higher risk. Estimates generated from the prophylaxis-free patients would thus be biased downwards. When clinicians applied such estimates to the entire population, they would be underestimating risk.

We dealt with this conundrum by enrolling all patients, but encouraging clinicians to withhold prophylaxis. Then, when we had the results, we used the results and other data to estimate what might have happened if no patient received prophylaxis. Our major finding was that in unventilated patients without coagulopathy, bleeding risk was very low—0.1%.

✓ *Choose what you will measure.*

Record all patient characteristics that might show substantial associations with the outcome of interest.

We recorded the age, sex, admitting diagnosis, and Acute Physiology and Chronic Health Evaluation (APACHE II) score in all eligible patients within 24 hours of admission (13). Daily evaluations included assessment for sepsis [all three of: core temperature >98.6°F (>38.5°C) or <89.6°F (<35.0°C), white blood cell count >15,000 per mm^3 (>15.0 × 10^9/L) or <3,000 per mm^3 (<3.0 × 10^9/L), and positive blood culture]; hypotension (either systolic blood pressure <80 mm Hg for 2 hours or more, or a decrease in systolic blood pressure of ≥30 mm Hg); renal failure [creatinine clearance <40 mL per min, oliguria (<500 mL urine per day), or serum creatinine >2.8 mg per dL (>250 μmol/L)]; coagulopathy [any one of: platelet count <50,000 per μL (<50 × 10^9/L), an International Normalized Ratio of greater than 1.5 (prothrombin time >1.5 times control), or partial thromboplastin time >2.0 times control]; hepatic failure [any two of: serum bilirubin >8.8 mg per dL (>150 μmol/L), serum aspartate aminotransferase >500 IU per L, serum albumin <41 g per L (<25 μmol/L), or clinical signs and symptoms of hepatic coma]; Glasgow Coma Scale (GCS) less than 5; administration of heparin or coumadin; glucocorticoids (>200 mg hydrocortisone or equivalent per day); aspirin or nonsteroidal antiinflammatory drug; respiratory failure (need for mechanical ventilation for at least 48 hours); active enteral feeding; and prophylaxis for stress ulceration (two or more doses).

To the extent that patients in two or more subgroups have a different prognosis, they are ill served when clinicians provide them with the same information about their ultimate fate. For instance, patients younger than 60 years have, on average, half the risk of dying after MI than those older than 60 years. Any useful study of prognosis after MI must, therefore, provide information specific to patients who differ by age.

The tasks for the investigator include identifying all potential risk factors, deciding how they will be measured, and deciding how to deal with them in the analysis. A thorough review of the relevant literature will elucidate the risk factors that previous investigators have found associated with the outcome of interest. Conversations with clinicians who deal frequently with the patients of interest may suggest additional prognostic factors. At times, investigators have used formal expert panels to identify the most plausible predictors. For example, investigators used the expert panel approach to derive the initial 34 physiologic variables included in the APACHE mortality prediction model.

This process highlights one of the limitations of using a large administrative database to generate a predictive model: You are limited to the variables in the database. If a key predictive variable is missing, your model will be less powerful than it would have been had you been able to measure all potential prognostic factors.

✓ *Use measurement strategies. Use accurate and unbiased measurement of the outcome of interest.*

Potentially, research personnel can interview patients, if they are in a state to be interviewed, and make direct measurements of risk factors of interest. For most prognostic studies, this approach will be prohibitively expensive. The next best alternative is to abstract information from patients' charts. Here, the investigator can specify rules to deal with ambiguous situations (if there is more than one value on a chart, for instance, which do you use?), and train research personnel in data abstraction. Investigators should measure the reliability of data abstraction. Ideally, you will measure interrater reliability (i.e., chance-corrected or chance-independent agreement) using statistics such as kappa (14,15), psi (16,17), or an intraclass correlation coefficient that compares variance between patients to the total variance, including both between- and within-patient variance [a chapter in the Users' Guide text provides a clinician-friendly explanation of these concepts (18)]. Confidence intervals (CIs) tell readers about the precision of the estimates of agreement. For instance, in a recent study of predictors of reoperation after tibial fracture, we documented substantial agreement between two observers in the assessment of the radiographic cortical continuity and fracture type (kappa = 0.75, 95% CI 0.68–0.83 and kappa = 0.78, 95% CI 0.62–0.90, indicating agreement of 75% and 78% beyond that expected by chance, respectively) (19). If the interrater reliability is high, one can be confident that the intrarater reliability is at least as high, and is usually higher.

Use of an administrative database is still less expensive and has the additional major advantage of allowing access to very large numbers of patients (see Table 9–3). One disadvantage that we have already noted is that the database may not record all the important prognostic factors. A second disadvantage is the potential inaccuracy of the data.

Unfortunately, some databases yield suboptimal quality data. Comparisons of prospective recording of data (20), as well as independent chart audit (21), have sometimes demonstrated substantial inaccuracies in administrative databases. Databases are particularly vulnerable to inaccuracies in recording information about prognostic variables such as the presence of hypertension, diabetes, or a smoking history. If you intend to use administrative databases, you would be wise to check the quality control procedures, and the evidence of accuracy, of the databases. At the same time, the three major advantages of administrative databases noted in Table 9–3 may, for some investigations, outweigh the more numerous downsides.

TABLE 9–3 Using Administrative Databases for Prognostic Studies

Advantages	Disadvantages
Inexpensive	May not have measured important prognostic factor
Large numbers of patients	Accuracy of data may be limited
Blinding to outcome of those documenting predictors ensured	Model may work well but fail in clinical practice because of errors by doctors using prognostic model
Those recording outcomes unaware of the study hypothesis	Those recording outcome never blinded to prognostic factors
	No informed consent for your study
	Lack of flexibility; data is given, can't tailor to study

If your intent is to develop a prediction rule for clinicians to use in day-to-day practice, you face an additional set of measurement challenges. Will clinicians record information accurately? If the rule requires them to add up "points" associated with the presence or absence of prognostic factors, will they do so accurately? Even if they meet these criteria, does the prediction rule add anything to clinician's intuitive judgment of the probability of outcome events? Another type of study would be needed to determine this.

These considerations suggest that, ideally, you will not accept that demonstration of the accuracy of a prediction rule warrants recommending it for the clinical arena. Rather, you must demonstrate that the rule leads to superior prediction. You can do so observationally by recording clinicians' intuitive estimates of the probability of outcome and by comparing these predictions to those of the rule. But, if you wish to demonstrate that application of the rule improves outcomes, you must move from an observational study design to a randomized trial, and address the issues we outline in the therapy chapters of this book (Chapters 4–6) or in the quality improvement chapter (Chapter 7).

In our study of bleeding risk in the ICU we hired research personnel to abstract data. We failed, however, to document the reproducibility of their data collection. Despite the fact that we ultimately suggested a decision rule, we made no attempt to collect the clinicians' intuitive estimates of bleeding risk and thus to document that our rule did a better job. We are far from alone in these omissions, but do not condone their occurrence, and will do better if we tread this path again; the standards for doing this type of research continue to improve.

Blinding

Blinding is an issue whenever the data are subject to interpretation. This is not usually the case with machine-measured laboratory data (such as serum creatinine) and with physical states (such as alive or dead). With other data, blinding observers of outcome to predictor variables is important, and blinding those who measure potential predictors to outcomes is also important.

Ideally, when results are subject to interpretation, those establishing the patients' status regarding prognostic factors should be unaware of whether patients suffered the outcome of interest (and vice versa—those recording the occurrence of outcomes should be unaware of prognostic features). Ensuring that this criterion is met may, however, prove logistically challenging and involve commitment of substantial resources. Is blinding, in this context, worth the effort and cost?

Although the issue of blinding has been examined for randomized trials, we know of no empirical data addressing this question for prognostic studies. When data are collected prospectively, blinding of those who record potential baseline predictors to outcome is ensured. Similarly, if ascertainment of outcome is not subject to interpretation, blinding of the outcome assessor is not necessary. My intuitive impression is that—even when these guarantees are not in place—unblinded recording of prognostic variables will usually not introduce substantial bias. One relatively easy safeguard that you can use is to leave data collection personnel unaware of study hypotheses. In administrative databases, those who record outcome data will always be unblinded (and those who record predictor data, always blinded), but will be unaware of the hypotheses of future investigators making use of the database.

One instance in which the issue is more important is in testing clinicians' use of prediction rules. Here, you must ensure that the information you obtain is the clinicians' bottom-line estimate using the rule prior to their determining the presence or absence of the target condition, or the occurrence of the target event.

In our study of bleeding risk in critically ill patients, we made no attempt to have separate data collectors, blind to other information, or collect prognostic and outcome data. With little increase in resources, we could have made efforts to ensure that data collectors were unaware of the specific study goals.

Categorization of Prognostic Factors

For some potential prognostic factors, there is only one way to deal with the data. Factors such as age and sex leave little latitude and thus present no special challenges.

For many other prognostic factors, however, the situation is not so simple. Consider, for instance, measuring the prognostic factors of renal failure (measured by serum creatinine) or mental status (measured by GCS). These variables have sufficient categories that one can consider them as continuous variables. Alternatively, you could choose a number of cuts (GCS 1 to 5, 6 to 10, etc.). Finally, you could dichotomize the variable (GCS <5 versus ≥ 5).

Furthermore, variables such as creatinine and GCS change over time. How can you deal with this issue? Three basic approaches are to choose a single point in time (such as admission to the ICU), dichotomize the variable, and treat it in a ever–never fashion (the patients are classified as "coma positive" if they had a GCS score of <5 any time during their stay in the ICU), or use a sophisticated analysis in which time of occurrence of coma is considered (treating the variable as a time-dependent covariate).

What are the relative merits of these choices? Treating the variable as a continuous time-dependent variable maximizes use of the available data, likely leads to the most powerful statistical model, and sometimes yields important insights. We will come back to this issue when we examine options for statistical analysis. For now, we will note that in our study of prognostic factors for bleeding in the ICU we took one of the simplest approaches, classifying continuous variables that change over time as "ever–never."

Measuring Risk Factors for a Clinical Decision Rule

To determine how well a clinical decision rule functions in real-world practice, you will need the clinicians who will be applying the rule to evaluate each patient's status on the predictor variables. All of us recognize that clinicians are liable to make errors or oversights or do not apply the measurement rules properly. This is exactly the point. In deciding whether to disseminate a clinical prediction rule, we should be aware of how it actually functions in day-to-day practice. Errors and oversights will compromise rule accuracy, but if that is what actually happens in clinical practice, we should certainly know about it.

Individual clinicians may think that they will do better than their colleagues and can apply the rule's performance when prognostic factors are measured and recorded by investigators rather than clinicians. However, just as everyone thinks they are above-average drivers, our judgements that we are above-average clinicians are suspect. In any event, as educators and teachers, we should be using the performance of decision rules in clinical practice in our decisions about instruction and dissemination.

Strategies for Accurate and Unbiased Measurement of the Outcome of Interest

Outcome criteria, developed prior to the study, consisted of overt bleeding (defined as hematemesis, gross blood or coffee grounds in the nasogastric aspirate, hematochezia, or melena) and clinically important bleeding [defined as overt bleeding plus one of the following within 24 hours of onset of the bleed, in the absence of other causes: spontaneous decrease in systolic blood pressure of >20 mm Hg, increase in heart rate of >20 beats per minute and a decrease in systolic blood pressure of >10 mm Hg on orthostatic change, or decrease in hemoglobin level of >2 g/dL (>20 g/L) and subsequent transfusion, after which time the hemoglobin level does not increase (the number of units transfused −2 g/dL)]. The foregoing criteria were applied by three adjudicators not involved in the patients' care, with a fourth adjudicator and repeated reviews for disagreements.

Agreement among adjudicators on the presence of overt versus clinically important bleeding was 81% after the first review (kappa = 0.71) and 100% after the second reading. Agreement was 100% on the source(s) of bleeding.

Issues in the accurate and unbiased measurement of outcomes are similar to the issues in accurate and unbiased measurement of prognostic factors. However, investigators legitimately devote more attention to minimizing both bias and random error in outcome measurement.

One strategy to ensure accuracy of outcome measurement is to choose a "hard" outcome. The hardest possible outcome—and the only one that is likely to be free of measurement error—is all-cause mortality. Assessors will seldom err in the decision about whether someone is alive, and if you are successful in following up all patients, you should be confident that this aspect of your study is sound.

Other outcomes are almost as free from measurement error. Assuming that the data is abstracted from medical records (and does not rely on patients' memory), ascertaining whether a patient has been hospitalized or discharged from hospital, begun dialysis, or has had a reoperation following initial nailing of a tibial fracture may be subject to oversight or coding errors but should not be fraught with errors of judgement. For all-cause mortality and these other hard outcomes, administrative databases with a high degree of quality control should provide accurate information. If you are abstracting from charts, all you have to worry about is oversight and coding errors.

Many other outcomes involve judgement, and the possibility of biased assessment enters. Just as those who assess the presence or absence of predictors should ideally be unaware of whether the outcome is present or absent, those making decisions about outcomes should be unaware of predictor status. Once again, however, investigators have not addressed the impact of blinding in prognostic studies.

Reducing random error in ascertainment of outcome is important. Although random error should be equally likely to increase or decrease the strength of association for continuous outcomes, this is not true for binary data. For yes–no outcomes, random misclassification will systematically reduce the strength of association. Table 9–4A presents a data set demonstrating a relative risk of 2.0 for an adverse outcome when a risk factor is present. What will the data look like if outcome assessments are subject to a 20% random misclassification rate (in other words, 20% of those with an adverse outcome are classified as having no adverse outcome, and 20% of those without an adverse outcome are misclassified as having the adverse outcome)? Table 9–4B provides the answer. The apparent relative

TABLE 9–4   Random Misclassification Rate

A: No Random Misclassification

	Adverse outcome present (%)	Adverse outcome absent (%)
Risk factor present	40	60
Risk factor absent	20	80

Relative risk: $40/100 \div 20/100 = 2$

B: 20% of Observations in 2A Subject to Random Misclassification

	Adverse outcome present (%)	Adverse outcome absent (%)
Risk factor present	44	56
Risk factor absent	32	68

Relative risk: $44/100 \div 32/100 = 1.375$

risk decreases from 2.0 to 1.375. In general, then, random misclassification reduces the strength of association between a prognostic factor and the outcome of interest.

In using an administrative database, it is important to ascertain that quality control mechanisms are in place. Ideally, you will be able to find out the reliability and accuracy of the outcome data in which you are interested. If you are abstracting your own data, formal adjudication becomes desirable.

We have dealt with the issue of adjudication in some detail in the therapy chapters (4 and 5) and will not repeat that discussion here. In brief, basic strategies include detailed rules for deciding whether the outcome is present or absent, training of adjudicators, documentation of adjudicator reliability, and establishing a mechanism for resolving disagreements. Our study of GI bleeding provides a good example of an outcome that is subject to disagreement, and for which detailed criteria and documentation or reliable measurement were important.

Strategies for Ensuring Completeness of Follow-up

Ensuring complete follow-up is a challenge in well-resourced randomized trials. Seldom do investigators conducting prognostic studies have funding to conduct the detective-style hunt that is often necessary to optimize follow-up. Fortunately, the degree of loss to follow-up that could destroy a randomized trial is much less likely to impact significantly on a prognostic study.

Consider, for instance, the recently completed Women's Health Initiative randomized trial in which women were randomized to receive an estrogen–progesterone combination or matched placebo. Of 16,683 women who enrolled, 583 (3.5%) were lost to follow-up. That looks very good, until you consider that one of the crucial outcomes, major cardiovascular events, occurred in only 288 patients—about half the number of those lost to follow-up. The absolute difference in number of events between treatment and control was only 44. Much was made of the "significant" difference in cardiovascular events between the two groups—it reached the usual threshold P value of 0.05—but a difference of only a few events among patients in the two groups who were lost to follow-up would render differences between treatments nonsignificant. Considering all this, the 3.5% loss to follow-up appreciably weakens inferences about cardiovascular events.

In prognostic studies, event rates are typically much greater than in randomized trials. Because it is the ratio of event rates to loss to follow-up that determines the significance of the number lost to follow-up, higher event rates mean a greater tolerance for loss to follow-up. If event rates are even of the order of 20%, a loss to follow-up of 3.5% is unlikely to seriously threaten inferences based on study results. The more crucial numbers in prognostic studies (as in randomized trials) are the number of events, not the number of patients.

This is not to say that investigators in prognostic studies can be cavalier about loss to follow-up. You should check to see what documentation your candidate administrative database can provide about their success in follow-up. If you are conducting your own prospective or retrospective cohort study, you should marshal whatever resources you have available to implement the strategies described in detail in the therapy section to ensure optimal follow-up.

✓ *Select your statistical procedures. Include sample size and analysis.*

We conducted a forward stepwise logistic regression analysis on the 12 potential risk factors evaluated daily plus the following: age; APACHE II score; head injury; multiple trauma; transplant recipient; status 1 week or less after cardiovascular, thoracic, abdominal, pelvic, orthopedic, neurosurgical or peripheral vascular procedure; surface burn; peptic ulcer, or gastritis within 6 weeks of ICU admission; and upper GI bleeding 3 days to 6 weeks prior to admission. Variables significantly ($P < 0.05$) associated with clinically important bleeding in a simple regression analysis were entered into a multiple logistic regression analysis and tested for interaction. The analysis was repeated for the subset of patients who did not receive prophylaxis. All statistical tests were two-tailed.

The key initial decision in the analysis of a prognostic study is how one treats the dependent variable (in the case of the example, whether the patient had a GI bleed). The options are to treat the outcome as a yes–no event or to consider the time to occurrence in a life table or survival analysis. We will begin by assuming that you will decide (as we did in our study of GI bleeding) to take the simpler approach in which all you consider is whether the outcome occurred, or did not.

Analysis with Outcome as Yes/No Event, Univariable Analysis

Although investigators have suggested intriguing alternatives [such as discriminant function analysis (22), recursive partitioning (23), and neural networks (24)], regression analysis has stood the test of time as the standard approach to the problem of establishing independent predictors of an outcome of interest. In the case of a binary outcome, the technique is referred to as "logistic regression" (*logistic* because the technique relies on logarithms). Logistic regression explores the relation between an independent or predictor variable (which can be binary, categorical—i.e., three or more discrete categories in which an observation may be classified—or continuous) and a dependent or outcome variable that is yes–no.

In univariable (sometimes called "univariate"[1] or "simple") logistic regression, you consider only a single independent variable and examine the magnitude of the relation with the dependent variable, and whether the

---

[1]If one is being technically precise, "univariate" refers to one outcome or dependent variable, and "multivariate" refers to an analysis using more than one outcome or dependent variable. However, the proper technical usage is the exception rather than what one usually finds reported

apparent relation might be explained by chance. The major limitation of the approach is that independent variables in a series of univariable regressions may be correlated with one another (sometimes referred to as "covariation").

If clinicians were considering two or more such correlated variables and were treating them as if they were independent, a misleading impression of the likelihood of the outcome event would result. For an obvious example, if you considered both that a patient was 80 years old (increasing the likelihood of the outcome) and that the patient was born in 1924 (which contains the same information), you would overestimate the probability of the outcome of interest.

In our study of ICU patients, we found ten univariable predictors of important GI bleeding (see Table 9–5). As described in subsequent text, and as Table 9–5 (25) shows, not all turned out to be independent predictors.

Analysis with Outcome as Yes–No Event, Multivariable Analysis

You can deal with the problem of covariation among the independent variables by conducting multivariable (or "multiple" or "multivariate") analysis in which we construct a model that simultaneously considers all the independent variables.

There are a variety of ways of constructing such models. One fundamental strategy is to avoid any restrictions or constraints on the model. The term used for this approach is a "stepwise" regression.

You can conduct a "forward" stepwise analysis or a "backward" stepwise analysis. In the forward procedure, the most powerful predictor of outcome enters first. The independent variable that explains the greatest

TABLE 9–5   Risk Factors for Clinically Important Bleeding among 2,252 Patients Admitted to an Intensive Care Unit (25)

Risk Factor	Simple Regression		Multiple Regression	
	Odds Ratio	P Value	Odds Ratio	P Value
Respiratory failure	25.5	<0.001	15.6	<0.001
Coagulopathy	9.5	<0.001	4.3	<0.001
Hypotension	5.0	0.03	3.7	0.08
Sepsis	7.3	<0.001	2.0	0.17
Hepatic failure	6.5	<0.001	1.6	0.27
Renal failure	4.6	<0.001	1.6	0.26
Enteral feeding	3.8	<0.001	1.0	0.99
Steroid administration	3.7	<0.001	1.5	0.26
Organ transplant	3.6	0.006	1.5	0.42
Anticoagulant therapy	3.3	0.004	1.1	0.88

From Guyatt GH, Rennie D, eds. *Users' guides to the medical literature: A manual for evidence-based clinical practice.* Chicago, IL: AMA Press, 2002:527, with permission.

proportion of the residual variance (the variance of variability unexplained after entering the first variable) enters next, and so on, until all variables are entered.

Alternatively, you can do a backward procedure in which all variables initially enter the model. You then test the models with all variables but one, testing how the model behaves with each variable omitted in turn. You then drop the variable explaining the least variance (assuming that it does not cross whatever threshold we have chosen for explaining a statistically significant proportion of the variance) from the model. You repeat the procedure with the remaining variables, omitting each one in sequence. The procedure is complete when a statistically significant decrease in the proportion of variance explained occurs when you omit the last remaining variable.

Limitations of Stepwise Approaches, and a Solution

When two or more independent variables are highly correlated ("multicollinearity"), stepwise approaches may give misleading results (26). For instance, assume that variable A is truly related to the outcome of interest, but is highly correlated with variable B. For instance, low glomerular filtration rate, reflected in serum creatinine level, is associated with drug accumulation and adverse reactions. Blood urea nitrogen (BUN) is highly correlated with creatinine. In a particular instance, chance may lead to variable B being more strongly associated with the dependent variable than variable A. In such a situation, the final model will retain B but not A. To use the example, although BUN is not truly the determinant of the adverse reaction, in a particular data set, chance may lead to a stronger association of BUN than creatinine with adverse reactions. BUN may therefore remain in the final model generated by stepwise approaches, and creatinine disappears.

Putting constraints on the regression may deal effectively with this problem. Ideally, investigators will use their understanding of the underlying biology to create a hierarchy among the independent variables. As the model is being constructed, those variables postulated to be, on biological grounds, more plausibly causally linked to the dependent variable, are forced into the model first. In the example in the preceding text, A is forced into the model before B—creatinine before BUN. This is likely to result in a final model that includes A but not B—creatinine but not BUN.

In general, we recommend that you avoid conducting stepwise analyses without restraints. Rather, you should always generate a priori hierarchies of association and conduct analyses that reflect these hierarchies. The reason is that, whether you are interested in prediction alone or in making causal inferences, the effect of random error in stepwise regression without restraints is liable to generate a misleading model.

Analyses that Consider Time to Event

Adverse outcomes, the typical dependent variables in prognostic models, do not all happen at the same time. In general, predicting time to event is more informative than simply predicting whether an event occurs or does not occur. When the adverse outcome is death, time to event is conceptually the only issue of interest. After all, we do not need predictive variables to tell us if we are going to die (the sad story is that the ultimate death rate is always 100%) but when the unfortunate event is likely to occur.

Statisticians have developed regression models based on survival analysis (most notably, the Cox model) that allow investigators to determine the extent to which independent variables predict not only whether an event will occur but also how soon it will occur. In general, such models are preferable to simpler models relying only on whether an event does or does not occur.

One major advantage of survival models is that they allow consideration of the timing of occurrence of independent variables. For instance, patients may not be ventilated, or may show evidence of coagulopathy, at the beginning of their stay in the ICU. Ventilation may become necessary, or coagulopathy may develop, during their stay. The most powerful of models would include the timing of the occurrence of potential predictors—so-called time-dependent covariates.

Use of time-dependent covariates can uncover fascinating and important relations. For instance, in another study in which Deborah Cook led our group, we examined the predictors of ventilator-associated pneumonia in the ICU (27). Independent predictors of ventilator-associated pneumonia in multivariable analysis included a primary admitting diagnosis of burns [risk ratio, 5.09 (95% CI, 1.52–17.03)], witnessed aspiration [risk ratio, 3.25 (95% CI, 1.62–6.50)], and paralytic agents [risk ratio, 1.57 (95% CI, 1.03–2.39)]. Using time-dependent covariates we found that mechanical ventilation in the previous 24 hours [risk ratio, 2.28 (95% CI, 1.11–4.68)], rather than more distant exposure to mechanical ventilation, was associated with to increased risk. Perhaps most interesting, exposure to antibiotics early in the patient's ICU stay conferred protection [risk ratio, 0.37 (95% CI, 0.27–0.51)], but later exposure did not.

The downside of using time-to-event analysis is the complexity of the underlying model. In making predictions in clinical practice, it is unrealistic to think that clinicians will go beyond an ever–never framework in attempting to estimate the likelihood of an adverse event occurring within a particular period of time.

Limitations of Regression Modeling—Sample Size and Number of Events

Unless you have a large data set in which many patients suffered the outcome of interest, you often have a problem as you contemplate how to approach the multivariable logistic regression. Models require an adequate number of outcome events for each predictor—a rule of thumb dictates ten outcome events for each independent variable. Therefore, if you are interested in testing 25 potential predictors, your data set would need to include at least 250 outcome events.

If you violate this assumption, you are likely to produce an unstable model. By unstable model, we mean one in which, given differences in just a few observations, the model generated would be quite different. Too few events in relation to the number of independent variables can also lead to biased estimates. Furthermore, if the independent variables are highly correlated ("multicollinearity" is the technical term), the requirements in terms of multiple events per independent variable may be even greater. Finally, the guideline of ten events per independent variable is just that—a guide. Some authorities have suggested even more stringent criteria, up to 25 events per independent variable.

Usually, investigators will measure more predictor variables than the number of outcome events can accommodate. Investigators generally address the problem by conducting initial univariable regressions with each independent variable. Only variables that demonstrate significant associations with the dependent variable pass the threshold that permits their inclusion in the subsequent multivariable analysis. Arguments can be made for different threshold P values between 0.05 and 0.20.

In our prognostic study of bleeding in the ICU, we conducted univariable analyses on each of 20 independent variables. Of these, ten proved significant at a 0.05 threshold (i.e, respiratory failure, coagulopathy, hypotension, sepsis, hepatic failure, renal failure, enteral feeding, steroid administration, organ transplant, and anticoagulant therapy). We entered these ten variables in a multiple regression analysis. In this analysis, only two (i.e., respiratory failure with an odds ratio of 15.6 and coagulopathy with an odds ratio of 4.3) remained significantly associated with bleeding. This implies that the ten variables predictive in the univariable analysis had substantial correlations with one another.

Note that we did not construct *a priori* hypotheses about the hierarchy of predictors or conduct a regression in which we entered variables in order according to that hierarchy. If we were to conduct the analysis again, we would generate *a priori* hypotheses about which predictors are most important and would enter these variables first in our regression.

That is not the only limitation of our analysis. We had only 33 events (major GI bleeds). Theoretically, to conduct a multiple regression analysis with ten independent variables, we should have had 100 events. What might we have done to deal with this situation (and what, in general, might you do)?

First, we could have raised the threshold of variables in the univariable analysis to enter the multiple regression. However, we already chose a relatively strict criterion of 0.05, and a stricter criterion could have led to the omission of potentially powerful predictors.

Alternatively, we could have grouped variables into categories according to an intuitive notion of their relation with one another. This would have been tricky because the variables don't fit well into categories. But, by stretching, we might have created the following categories: respiratory failure, hepatic failure, and renal failure; coagulopathy, anticoagulant therapy, sepsis, and hypotension; and enteral feeding, steroid administration, and organ transplantation. We could have then constructed three models, one for each category of variables. Had we got lucky (and our questionable regression in which we included all ten variables suggests we would have), each of the three regressions would yield only one significant predictor. The three predictors could then enter a final model.

Our study had another problem. We would like to have recorded outcome rates when no patients received prophylaxis, but this may have been unethical, and was certainly impractical. In this respect, we remain happy with how we dealt with the problem. The following text from the paper describes our approach to dealing with patients who received prophylaxis for prevention of stress ulceration.

> Patients not ventilated for more than 48 hours and without coagulopathy, who comprised 62% of the study group, were at an extremely low risk of clinically important bleeding (0.1%, or at worst, 0.5% when the upper limit of the confidence interval is considered). Of the 1,405 patients in this group, 283 (20.0%) received prophylaxis. A conservative estimate, based on synthesis of the available data, is that if no patient had received prophylaxis, twice the number of patients (or at worst, 1%) might have bled. If prophylaxis reduces this risk by 50%, one would need to administer prophylaxis to more than 900 low-risk patients to prevent one episode of bleeding. These results support the view that the risk of bleeding in patients without these two risk factors is low enough that prophylaxis can be safely withheld.

Further Limitations of Regression Approaches—Replicability

Prediction models are notorious for not performing well when applied to a new setting. There are three reasons why even rigorously derived clinical prediction rules may perform substantially less well in a new setting. First, the prediction rules derived from one set of patients may reflect associations between given predictors and outcomes that occur primarily because of the play of chance. Authors sometimes refer to this phenomenon as overfitting. Indeed, one would predict some degree of overfitting in virtually every model, leaving us reconciled with losing at least some of the model's predictive power in a new sample of patients. That is, even if, in a new study, the sample is drawn from the same population, the same clinicians are making the measurements, and the study design is otherwise identical, the model generated by the first sample is unlikely to work as well when applied to the second.

Second, predictors may be idiosyncratic to the population, to the setting, to the clinicians using the rule, or to other aspects of the design of an initial study. If that is so, the rule may fail in a new setting.

Finally, because of problems in the feasibility of rule application in the clinical setting, clinicians may fail to implement a rule comprehensively or accurately. The result would be that a rule succeeds in theory but fails in practice.

Statistical methods can deal with the first of these problems. For instance, you can split the population into two groups, using one to develop the rule and the other to test it. The first half is often called the training set or derivation set and the latter half, the test set or validation set. Typically, 60% or two thirds of the data are used for training and 40% or one third for testing. An obvious requirement of this approach, however, is that both the derivation and validation sets have the appropriate balance of predictors and outcome events–1 to 10 or more.

Alternatively, you can use more sophisticated statistical methods built on the same logic. Conceptually, these approaches involve removing one patient from the sample, generating the rule using the remainder of the patients, and testing it on the patient who was removed from the sample. You repeat this procedure, sometimes referred to as a "bootstrap technique," in sequence for every patient under study (28). Note that these procedures help only with the "play of chance" problem; if you have studied an idiosyncratic population, for instance, no amount of statistical confirmation will make a model more applicable to a new setting.

Although statistical validations within the same setting or group of patients reduce the chance that the rule reflects the play of chance rather than true associations, they fail to address the other two threats to validity–idiosyncratic populations and clinicians' failure to implement the rule effectively. The only way you can be confident of the persistent prognostic power of a prediction guide is finding that it works in a number of new populations, applied in each case by a new set of clinicians.

In our study of GI bleeding, we didn't try even the split-half or bootstrap methods to test our model. A critical reader of our work would have been skeptical about the likelihood of the findings holding up in a new population, and our publication did not meet the criteria for clinical prediction rules of ACP Journal Club (*http://www.acpjc.org/shared/purpose_and_procedure.htm*). Indeed, in a subsequent study on a new population of critically ill patients, all of whom were ventilated, Dr. Cook and her colleagues found that a multiple regression model suggested elevated serum creatinine clearance and lack of enteral nutrition, rather than coagulopathy, elevated the risk of serious GI bleeding (29).

You should attend to the limited inferences from any individual prognostic study. We will address this issue explicitly in the next section.

Sample Size Calculation

As with any other study, if you are considering prognostic studies you will often have access to a limited population–or at least, the prospect of limited resources to access the large potential population. If you have access to a large administrative database, the population that is accessible may be very large, but it may stretch your resources to analyze all of it. Calculation of sample size involves exploring the consequences of the population you have available, however small or large, for answering the question(s) you've posed.

A simple and transparent way of specifying sample size is to use the rule of needing ten outcomes for each independent variable. If this leads to an unfeasible sample size, you can hypothesize that only a prortion of the variables you test will prove significantly related to the outcome of interest. For instance, if you anticipate recruiting 1,000 patients of whom 10% will have events, and you wish to test 20 independent variables, your sample size will be insufficient by half. However, if you plan to enter into your multiple regression only variables significant in the univariable regression, and if you anticipate that only half your variables will prove significant in the univariable regression, then your sample size is adequate. If your database includes 100,000 patients with 1,000 events, you could theoretically manage 100 variables, or, say, plan for a ratio of one independent variable for 25 outcome events. More likely, however, you will be able to find the resources for analyzing only a fraction of the data, so you will want to adopt a random sampling strategy that suits your study questions, and here is where you will definitely want to get sound statistical advice.

When the Dependent Variable is Categorical or Continuous

This discussion has dealt in detail with the common situation in which the dependent variable in a prognostic study is dichotomous (i.e., dead or alive, stroke or no stroke, and return to work or not return to work). We have outlined an extension of this, in which clinicians consider the time to occurrence of this event. Occasionally, however, the outcome may be categorical, and if so, either ordered or not ordered.

For instance, in another study of ICU patients led by Deborah Cook, we were interested in variables associated with one of three possible decisions: no resuscitation order (assumed resuscitate), explicit order to resuscitate, and explicit order not to resuscitate (30). When the outcome is a nonordered categorical one such as this, polytomous (alternatively termed polychotomous) regression methods are extremely useful (31). You can set one level of outcome as a reference point and then calculate odds ratios associated for each independent variable associated with the relative likelihood of the other levels.

For instance, here we calculated one set of odds ratios for patients with an explicit directive to resuscitate with reference to patients with no explicit directive. The second set of odds ratios was calculated for patients with an explicit directive of do-not-resuscitate with reference to patients with no explicit directive. To provide an example: Being older than 75 years did not increase the odds of having an explicit resuscitation directive relative to no directive, but it had a large effect on the likelihood of having a do-not-resuscitate directive relative to no directive (odds ratio 8.8, 95% CI 4.4–17.8).

Dependent variables may also be continuous, such as if one is predicting exercise capacity or quality of life. Under these circumstances, linear regression (so termed because it assumes a linear relation between independent and dependent variables) is the analytic tool of choice.

✓ *Select your presentation and interpretation methods.*

There are many options for the presentation of the results of a prognostic study. You should consider the needs of your target audience in deciding how to present your results.

When the dependent variable in a regression equation is a continuous variable such as exercise capacity or quality of life, one reasonable way of capturing the power of the prediction model is to calculate the proportion of variance explained. If we were able to explain 100% of the variance with a set of predictors, knowledge of a patient's status on those predictors would allow you to specify that patient's score on the outcome measure with complete accuracy. The proportion of variance explained tells us how close we are to this ideal (and unattainable) situation.

A second useful approach is to present the magnitude of change in the dependent variable one can expect with a particular change in the independent variable. For instance: "for every increase in the forced, expired volume of 1 L in 1 second, you can anticipate an increase in the 6 minute walk test distance of 108 m" (32).

The proportion of variance explained is not very useful when the dependent variable is dichotomous or categorical. Odds ratios and relative risks effectively capture the power of the individual predictors. For instance, in predicting risk factors for important bleeding in the ICU, we found that the odds ratio associated with mechanical ventilation in the multivariable model was 15.6. Ideally, you will present not only the odds ratio or relative risk but also the confidence interval around the point estimate (which we did not do in our bleeding risk paper). For instance, in our study of predictors of a no resuscitation order, we found that patients with an APACHE score of more than 30 had odds of 9.9, with a 95% confidence interval from 4.5 to 21.7, for a no resuscitation order, relative to those with an APACHE score of less than ten.

The fact that human beings typically think in terms of risks and not in terms of odds can make presentation of results as odds ratios very misleading when event rates are high. For instance, consider a risk factor that increases the event rate from 98 in 100 to 99 in 100. The relative risk of 1.01 comes much closer to capturing our intuitive notion of what has happened than does the odds ratio associated with these data, 2.02.

Capturing the magnitude of predictive power of the entire model when the dependent variable is dichotomous is more challenging. One possibility is to create a receiver operating characteristic (ROC) curve, which plots sensitivity against 1—specificity for different cut-points. The area under the curve reflects the power of the model (33). One way of understanding the ROC curve in this context is that if you randomly select one person with the outcome of interest and one without, the area under the ROC curve presents the probability that the model will predict a higher likelihood of the outcome for the individual who actually suffered the event of interest (34). This depiction makes it evident that an area under the ROC curve of 0.5 represents a useless model because in such a model the probability of predicting a higher likelihood for the person who had the event is equal to the probability of predicting a lower likelihood for the person who had the event (both are 50:50). An area of 0.8 represents a reasonably powerful model.

Calibration is another indicator used to describe the performance of a prediction model that generates a continuum of risk. Calibration is the trustworthiness of the probabilities generated by the model. For instance, in a model that predicts the likelihood of dying, if out of 2,000 patients the mortality prediction model assigns 100 patients an 80% risk of mortality, then 80 out of 100 of those patients should die. You should be able to translate the probabilities generated by the model into the actual frequencies of events. One way to test calibration is to organize patients according to risk level. For example, when estimating mortality you can construct ten strata or deciles according to the predicted risk level (10% ... 20% ... and so on). You can then compare the observed with the expected numbers of deaths in each stratum of patients (35). If the model predicts the numbers of observed and expected events equally well across strata, we say it is well calibrated. It is possible that a rule will predict well for those with 90% probability of mortality but is not accurate for those with a predicted 20% mortality risk, in which case we would say it is not well calibrated. A formal goodness-of-fit statistical test is used to evaluate the calibration of the model across each decile of risk.

The Application of Clinical Prediction Guides

The most important finding of our study was that a simple decision rule predicts bleeding risk and allows more selective use of stress ulcer prophylaxis, avoiding unnecessary exposure to potential adverse effects. As noted earlier, patients not ventilated for more than 48 hours and without coagulopathy, who comprised 62% of the study group, were at an extremely low risk of clinically important bleeding. These results supported the view that the risk of bleeding in patients without these two risk factors is low enough that prophylaxis can be safely withheld, substantially reducing the use of prophylactic agents in the critically ill.

On the other hand, this study supported the use of prophylaxis in the subset of ICU patients who have a coagulopathy or are ventilated for more than 48 hours. The risk of bleeding among these patients was 3.7% despite the fact that more than half of the patients received prophylactic therapy of some type.

Perhaps the best we can hope for in terms of impact on the clinician from the presentations discussed so far are impressions such as the following.

- "We know a lot about how to predict bleeding."
- "We don't know very much about how to predict bleeding."
- "For ventilated patients, I'd better watch out for bleeding."

In the last decade or so, investigators have tried to offer clinicians much more than these general impressions. Clinicians function in the enormously complex world of clinical decision making using heuristics, or rules of thumb, that offer simplified rules of practice (36). Clinical prediction guides (or decision rules) attempt to add to clinicians' store and use of these heuristics.

In doing so, these guides must present clinicians with something other than regression coefficients. Simplicity is the key. In our paper on predicting GI bleeding, we went beyond presenting the results of the regression (and in so doing, moved the target journal from an intensive care specialty journal to a high-profile general medical journal). Having discovered from the regression analysis that mechanical ventilation and coagulopathy were the two key, powerful, independent predictors of bleeding, we calculated bleeding rates in patients free of these risk factors and in those with at least one of these risk factors present. In patients who remained free of mechanical ventilation or coagulopathy throughout their ICU stay, the risk of bleeding was 1 in 1,000. For those with at least one risk factor, the risk was 37 in 1,000. The rule that follows is to intervene in those who are mechanically ventilated or who suffer from a coagulopathy and withhold prophylaxis in other patients. Simple, and memorable.

Yes, simple and memorable, but possibly wrong. As already mentioned, we didn't conduct any internal validation of the rule (such as split-half replication or bootstrapping), nor did we specify that our rule should be tested in a new population before clinicians apply it in their practices. We did not note that clinicians may err in deciding who meets the criteria for a coagulopathy. We also did not point out that the ultimate test of the rule would be a trial in which ICUs were randomized to an arm in which clinicians made decisions to intervene on the basis of whatever guides their usual practice, and an arm in which a variety of strategies encouraged clinicians to prescribe prophylaxis for patients with either mechanical ventilation or a coagulopathy, and no others.

Despite these limitations, our prediction guide has merit in that it addresses the two major barriers that lead to clinicians' limited use of prognostic indices (37). If a guide is other than extremely simple, clinicians will not remember the rule, and until recently that was sufficient to make it unfeasible. Hand-held computers and on-line programs ameliorate these problems, but a very simple rule that clinicians can retain in memory remains appealing. Second, unless the result of estimating prognosis is a change in clinical action, clinicians may wonder about the point. The guide that suggests that clinicians should administer H_2-receptor antagonists if patients are intubated or have a coagulopathy, and not intervene if these risk factors are absent, is as about as simple as they come and is closely linked to a nontrivial clinical action, the administration of prophylaxis. In making this link, one might say, we turned a prediction guide into a decision rule.

Post-test Probability Versus Relative Risks and Likelihood Ratios

A final point in presentation has to do with what information is captured in the prognostic index. If all items of history and physical are included, clinicians should be offered post-test probabilities. For instance, a prediction guide to differentiate between patients presenting with suspected deep venous thrombosis who do, or do not, have underlying clot focuses on history and physical examination (38). Thus, there is nothing that would allow an estimate of pretest probability independent of the guide. The same is true for the risk of bleeding in the ICU, and that is why we offered only post-test probabilities. It turns out that this situation characterizes most clinical prediction guides.

On the other hand, prognostic indexes may on occasion offer information that builds on prior estimates of probability that differ among patients. For instance, clinicians may use a variety of factors, including prevalence in the community, to estimate the likelihood that the patient is an alcoholic. They can then use answers to the questions in the CAGE (Cut down, Annoyed, Guilty, Eye-opener) prediction rule to generate LRs (e.g., for CAGE scores of 0/4, LR = 0.14; for scores of 1/4, LR = 1.5; for scores of 2/4, LR = 4.5; for scores of 3/4, LR = 13; and for scores of 4/4, LR = 100), and then apply these to the pre-test probability to generate a post test probability.

This final example brings us back to the conceptual point that provided the focus of an early part of this discussion: the overlap between issues of diagnosis and of prognosis.

REFERENCES

1. North American Symptomatic Carotid Endarterectomy Trial Collaborators. Beneficial effect of carotid endarterectomy in symptomatic patients with high grade carotid stenosis. *N Engl J Med* 1991;325:445–453.

2. Lindahl B, Toss H, Siegbahn A, et al. Markers of myocardial damage and inflammation in relation to long-term mortality in unstable coronary artery disease. *N Engl J Med* 2000;343:1139–1147.

3. The PIOPED investigators. Value of ventilation/perfusion scan in acute pulmonary embolism. Results of the prospective investigation of pulmonary embolism diagnosis (PIOPED). *JAMA* 1990;263:2753–2759.

4. Cook DJ, Fuller H, Guyatt GH, Canadian Critical Care Trials Group. Risk factors for gastrointestinal bleeding in critically ill patients. *N Engl J Med* 1994;330:377–381.

5. Cook DJ, Witt LG, Cook RJ, et al. Stress ulcer bleeding in the critically ill – a meta analysis. *Am J Med* 1991;91:519–527.

6. Recurrent renal calculi [editorial]. *BMJ* 1981;282:5.

7. Coe FL, Keck J, Norton ER. The natural history of calcium nephrolithiasis. *JAMA* 1977;239:1519–1523.

8. Ellenberg JH, Nelson KB. Sample selection and the natural history of disease. Studies of febrile seizures. *JAMA* 1980;243:1337–1340.

9. Sackett DL, Haynes RB, Guyatt GH, et al., eds. Making a prognosis. *Clinical epidemiology*, 2nd ed. Boston, MA: Little, Brown and Company, 1991:173–185.

10. Greenstein AJ, Sachar DB, Smith H, et al. Cancer in universal and left-sided ulcerative colitis: factors determining risk. *Gastroenterology* 1979;77:290–294.

11. Sackett DL, Whelan G. Cancer risk in ulcerative colitis: scientific requirements for the study of prognosis. *Gastroenterology* 1980;78:1632.

12. Stevenson R, Ranjadayalan K, Wilkinson P, et al. Short and long term prognosis of acute myocardial infarction since introduction of thrombolysis. *BMJ* 1993;307:349–353.

13. Knaus WA, Draper EA, Wagner DP, et al. APACHE II: a severity of disease classification system. *Crit Care Med* 1984;13:818–829.

14. Fleiss JL. Measuring agreement between two judges on the presence or absence of a trait. *Biometrics* 1975;30:651–659.

15. Donner A, Klar N. The statistical analysis of kappa statistics in multiple samples. *J Clin Epidemiol* 1996;9:1053–1058.

16. Cook RJ, Farewell VT. Conditional inference for subject-specific and marginal agreement: two families of agreement measures. *Can J Stat* 1995;23:333–344.

17. Meade MO, Cook RJ, Guyatt GH, et al. Interobserver variation in interpreting chest radiographs for the diagnosis of acute respiratory distress syndrome. *Am J Respir Crit Care Med* 2000;161:85–90.

18. McGinn T, Guyatt G, Cook R, et al. Measuring agreement beyond chance. In: Guyatt G, Rennie D, eds. *Users' guides to the medical literature: A manual for evidence-based clinical practice.* Chicago, IL: AMA Press, 2002.

19. Bhandari M, Guyatt GH, Sprague S, et al. Predictors of re-operation following operative management of fractures of the tibial shaft. *J Orthop Trauma* 2003;17(5):353–61.

20. Jollis JG, Ancukiewicz M, DeLong ER, et al. Discordance of databases designed for claims payment versus clinical information systems. Implications for outcomes research. *Ann Intern Med* 1993;119:844–850.

21. Green J, Wintfeld N. How accurate are hospital discharge data for evaluating effectiveness of care? *Med Care* 1993;31:719–731.

22. Rudy TE, Kubinski JA, Boston JR. Multivariate analysis and repeated measurements: a primer. *J Crit Care* 1992;7:30–41.

23. Cook EF, Goldman L. Empiric comparison of multivariate analytic techniques: advantages and disadvantages of recursive partitioning analysis. *J Chronic Dis* 1984;39:721–731.

24. Baxt WG. Application of artificial neural networks to clinical medicine. *Lancet* 1995;346: 1135–1138.

25. Guyatt GH, Rennie D, eds. *Users' guides to the medical literature: A manual for evidence-based clinical practice.* Chicago, IL: AMA Press, 2002:527.

26. Leigh JP. Assessing the importance of an independent variable in multiple regression: is stepwise unwise? *J Clin Epidemiol* 1988;41:669–677.

27. Cook DJ, Walter SD, Cook RJ, et al. Incidence of and risk factors for ventilator-associated pneumonia in critically ill patients. *Ann Intern Med* 1998;129:433–440.

28. Efron BE, Tibshirani RJ. *An introduction to the bootstrap.* New York: Chapman & Hall, 1993.

29. Cook D, Heyland D, Griffith L, et al. Risk factors for clinically important upper gastrointestinal bleeding in patients requiring mechanical ventilation. *Crit Care Med* 1999;27: 2812–2817.

30. Cook D, Guyatt GH, Rocker G, et al, Canadian Critical Care Trials Group. Cardiopulmonary resuscitation directives on admission to the intensive care unit. *Lancet* 2001;358:1941–1945.

31. Agresti A. *Categorical data analysis.* New York: John Wiley & Sons, 1990:306–346.

32. Guyatt G, Walter S, Cook D, et al. Regression and correlation. In: Guyatt G, Rennie D, eds. *Users' guides to the medical literature: A manual for evidence-based clinical practice.* Chicago, IL: AMA Press, 2002.

33. Hanley JA, McNeil BJ. A method of comparing the areas under receiver operating characteristic curves derived from the same cases. *Radiology* 1983;148:839–843.

34. Lemeshow S, Le Gall JR. Modeling the severity of illness of ICU patients: a systems update. *JAMA* 1994;272:1049–1055.

35. Hosmer DW, Lemeshow S. *Applied logistic regression.* New York: John Wiley & Sons, 1989.

36. McDonald CJ. Medical heuristics: the silent adjudicators of clinical practice. *Ann Intern Med* 1966;124:56–62.

37. Redelmeier DA, Lustig AJ. Prognostic indices in clinical practice. *JAMA* 2001;285: 3024–3025.

38. Wells PS, Hirsh J, Anderson DR, et al. Accuracy of clinical assessment of deep-venous thrombosis. *Lancet* 1995;345:1326–1330.

10

ASSESSING CLAIMS OF CAUSATION

Peter Tugwell and Brian Haynes

Chapter Outline

CLINICAL RESEARCH SCENARIO: CAUSE OR COINCIDENCE?

Do silicone breast implants *cause* rheumatologic diseases? Or if women with breast implants experience disorders such as rheumatoid arthritis, is this merely a *coincidence*? More than a million women have undergone surgical implantation of silicone breast implants. It is undisputed that the implants leak silicone into the surrounding tissues and cause local fibrosis. Several hundreds of breast-implant recipients have subsequently developed clinically significant symptoms of connective tissue diseases (CTDs), including Raynaud's phenomenon, fibromyalgia, and classic rheumatologic diseases such as scleroderma, lupus, and rheumatoid arthritis. Courts in the United States have awarded up to $14 million in damages to single cases.

Missing in these early legal decisions was systematic consideration of whether, in such a large population, these conditions would be expected to occur anyway, unrelated to silicone breast implants, that is, by coincidence. How does one assess whether silicone breast implants have caused an increase in these conditions?

After a number of these court decisions had been made in favor of the plaintiffs, a US federal court convened a National Science Panel, including one of us (Peter Tugwell) as a member (1). The panel was asked to assist in evaluating expert testimony and scientific evidence presented in lawsuits brought against silicone breast-implant manufacturers. We were to assess whether existing studies provide scientific evidence of an association between silicone breast implants and systemic classic/accepted CTD, atypical connective disease, and certain signs and symptoms identified by plaintiffs in the lawsuits. To do so, we performed a systematic review of published studies, using principles of causation to marshal the evidence for the court's decision.

As Peter Tugwell put it to the court in his deposition, "If we take rheumatoid arthritis, without implants the frequency in the population is 1% (1 woman in 100 women), so in 1 million women without implants, 10,000 (1% of 1 million) of these women will have rheumatoid arthritis ('expected number'). So the question we need to answer is: Were women with breast implants more likely to develop rheumatoid arthritis than women who had no implants?"

Studying whether one thing causes another is a challenging task. The best scientific test of this putative relationship would be a randomized controlled trial (RCT) in which women, initially free of connective tissue complaints, who consent to be part of this trial are randomly allocated to receive or not receive silicone breast implants, and then followed to assess the incidence of such complaints. A single RCT might settle such a matter if it were large enough to detect an important difference in the risk for CTDs, and if silicone breast implants were homogeneous enough in their nature to generalize from a single study. But both the difficulty and expense of mounting a convincing study and the diversity of medical devices (with different brands, construction, and continual changes) render definitive RCTs improbable. Further, as is often the case in causal questions, RCTs can be infeasible or unethical, especially if the potential cause is likely to be noxious, as for, say, smoking or asbestos or breast implants. If RCTs are not possible, more types of evidence are needed, although none by themselves will be close to compelling. To make matters worse, those who have a vested interest in avoiding a causal claim (e.g., that smoking is bad for health) frequently insist on "absolute truth," something that neither clinical epidemiology nor any other scientific approach can offer. Thus, we cannot provide in this chapter a recipe for a definitive study that you can conduct to assess a causal claim.

Nevertheless, principles and procedures for testing claims for causation have been widely accepted for more than half a century. These are based on the evidence accumulated from many investigations, each assessed for relative scientific merit and collectively weighed for the strength, consistency, and temporality of findings. We will explore these in this chapter and attempt to tie down a causal claim with several lines of evidence. We'll begin with the basic ground rules that have been established for studying causation before returning to the scenario and how it played out.

10.1 BASIC PRINCIPLES OF ASSESSING CAUSATION

Because multiple studies will be needed to assess a causal claim, and because each of these studies will have limitations of both method and execution, the general procedure for assessing causation will follow the principles set out in Chapter 2 for systematic reviews. We will begin with a review of these principles in light of assessing causation, and later in this chapter, after considering the special principles for *settling* questions of causation, we will return to this approach.

Although there are many variants of the principles for systematic reviews, those set out by Sir Austin Bradford Hill many decades ago are still both simple and powerful. These guides are summarized in Table 10-1 and can be used to organize the evidence that is to be retrieved and reviewed. It is important to bear in mind that these are not "criteria" or "rules" and that following the guides will lead to an assembly of evidence, usually with shades of gray, rather than a black-and-white conclusion. Thus, a decision about causation is best based on the weight of the evidence at the time of decision and, especially if the evidence is not strong, the decision may be later overthrown by better research. That said, weighing the evidence according to its strengths and weaknesses can often get us convincingly past the paralysis of insisting on absolute truth.

The best ("weightiest") evidence for causation comes from rigorous experiments in humans (i.e., RCTs). If experimental evidence is lacking, then

TABLE 10-1 Austin Bradford Hill's Guides for Assessing Causation (2), in Descending Order of Importance[a]

1. Experimental evidence: Is there evidence from true experiments in humans?
2. Strength of association: How strongly associated is the putative risk with the outcome of interest?
3. Consistency: Have the results been replicated by different studies, in different settings, by different investigators, and under different conditions?
4. Temporality: Did the exposure precede the disease?
5. Biological gradient: Are increasing exposures (i.e., dose and duration) associated with increasing risks of disease?
6. Coherence: Is the association consistent with the natural history and epidemiology of the disease?
7. Specificity: Is the exposure associated with a very specific disease rather than a wide range of diseases?
8. Plausibility: Is there a credible biological or physical mechanism that can explain the association?
9. Analogy: Is there a known relation between a similar putative cause and effect?

[a]In our view!

From Hill AB. *Principles of medical statistics*, 9th ed. London: Lancet, 1971, with permission.

TABLE 10-2   **Organization and Analysis of Evidence to Assess Claims of Causation**

Evidence from the hierarchy of research designs

- true experiments
- cohort studies
- case–control studies
- analytic surveys

Strength of association

Consistency–especially among studies of higher quality

Temporal sequence–from prospective studies

Gradient–by dose or duration of exposure

Sense–from epidemiology, biology, and analogy

---

strength of association from "lesser" studies becomes particularly important, and the quality of the studies pertaining to strength of association becomes paramount. Thus, prospective cohort studies with comparable controls and careful and independent (blinded) assessment of exposure and outcomes outweigh case–control studies and surveys, no matter how well the latter are done, provided the cohort study is competently done (e.g., successfully following a high proportion of its cohort).

This hierarchy of evidence is taken into account in the reorganization of Hill's guides shown in Table 10–2. In this, we have amalgamated the lesser guides into "sense."

10.2 EVIDENCE FROM TRUE EXPERIMENTS IN HUMANS

As we've mentioned, this is the most important guide in distinguishing between coincidence and causation. Optimally, this evidence will come from RCTs. In situations in which the potential cause is "internal" (e.g., high blood pressure) or "self-inflicted" (e.g., alcohol or drugs or smoking), "reverse trials" can be done. Trials of lipid lowering, blood pressure lowering, blood sugar lowering, smoking cessation, and so on convincingly contribute to our causal understanding of harmful factors in our internal environments, particularly when lowering the suspected culprit by many means–for example, drugs that work by different mechanisms–has the same effects on the outcomes of interest.

Some trials are clearly much harder to do than others. For example, a trial of blood pressure lowering is straightforward, but a trial of smoking cessation is not. Smokers could be allocated to be offered a special smoking cessation program or no intervention (often euphemistically called "usual care"), and both groups then followed to see whether harmful effects of smoking were less in the intervention group. Even if such an RCT were done, readers who recall Chapters 4 to 7 on testing treatments will appreciate the trouble in getting a "clean" answer from a study when at least two "Cs"–low compliance (with smoking cessation) in the intervention group and contamination (quitting smoking) in the control group– are likely to make a mess of the results.

In other situations, a trial of what proves to be a harmful substance can be done (or must be done!) because prior observational studies have suggested a benefit. For example, observational studies of combined estrogen–progestin hormonal replacement therapy (HRT) for postmenopausal women suggested a substantial cardiac benefit (5), but this was convincingly shown to be false by two RCTs (6,7). With the luxury of hindsight, follow-up re-evaluations of observational studies purported that these really showed the same result as RCTs after adjusting for differences in baseline features (8,9). It is self-evident that observational and experimental studies can produce results that are consistent with one another, but this is most likely to occur when observational studies take special measures to avoid biases that are inherently avoided in RCTs. Observational studies are usually done before RCTs and with fewer resources, so that their ability to reduce bias is limited, even if the investigators are aware of the possible biases. In addition, no amount of resources can eliminate unknown confounders in observational studies, whereas RCTs neutralize the effect of such biases by ensuring that they are randomly distributed to the groups being compared.

It is often claimed that observational studies are needed to look for rarer adverse effects of medications, but the sample sizes of "pivotal studies" required for approval are now increasing so that less common adverse effects can be detected. For example, pivotal studies of coxibs for pain and arthritis are now required to be large enough to detect adverse effect rates as low as 1% in RCTs (10). Where individual studies are too small, meta-analyses of RCTs should be considered. For example, a meta-analysis of RCTs showed the lack of efficacy of vitamin E for lowering the risk of cardiovascular events and a small increase in risk of death and cardiovascular events with use of β-carotene (11). Similarly, but less convincingly, Hemminki and McPherson's review of small hormone replacement trials (12) raised the possibility that hormone replacement therapy (HRT) was unlikely to lower cardiovascular risk long before the definitive trials confirmed that HRT was actually harmful.

Our key point is this: RCTs provide the best evidence for causation, so don't give up on the notion of doing an RCT to settle a causal issue just because it may be difficult or contentious to do. Many precedents exist where hoards of biased observational studies have been overthrown by a single, large, well-done RCT.

A brief statistical interlude: If we did an RCT of breast implants, or a reverse trial of removing them, to see if they cause musculoskeletal (MSK) complaints, Table 10–3 would be a good way to display the findings.

The results would then be calculated as the risk in exposed versus nonexposed. That is:

rate in exposed divided by rate in unexposed = a/(a + b) ÷ c/(c + d).

TABLE 10-3 Presenting the Results of a Randomized Controlled Trial of Silicone Breast Implants to Assess Their Effect on the Development of Musculoskeletal Disease

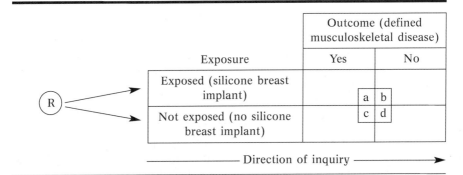

	Outcome (defined musculoskeletal disease)	
Exposure	Yes	No
Exposed (silicone breast implant)	a	b
Not exposed (no silicone breast implant)	c	d

——————— Direction of inquiry ———————➤

"R" refers to random allocation.

This is known as the "relative risk (RR)." We'll return to this shortly. Alas, in many situations an RCT is not possible for either ethical or, less often, logistical reasons.

In the case of silicone breast implants it would not be ethical to randomize women to receive them. It would be ethical to randomize willing participants for removal of the implants but perhaps unlikely that many would agree. Nevertheless, when we assemble the evidence, we will certainly want to look for any such trials.

10.3 COHORT STUDIES

Evidence from cohort studies (also known as cohort analytic studies) is the next most powerful method after the controlled trial. In cohort studies of silicone breast implants, at least two cohorts of patients would be identified and followed, one cohort of women who received the implants and the other cohort who did not. The women in these two cohorts should be similar in features other than the implants, for example, in age and sociodemographic status, so that "like is compared with like." Further, at the beginning of observation, the participants in both cohorts should be verified to be free of the outcome of interest–in this case rheumatologic disorders. These two groups are then followed by counting the rheumatologic outcomes that occur in each group. For the study to provide a convincing result, participants should not be lost during follow-up, and the study should be of adequate size to detect an association of a clinically important size.

Cohort studies are less rigorous than randomized trials for at least two reasons. First, the risk of bias is increased from potential differences in features between exposed participants and the controls. In a randomized trial, both known factors such as age, and unknown factors, are randomly distributed between the groups, a "bias free" basis for comparisons.

TABLE 10-4 Presenting the Results of a Cohort Study of Silicone Breast Implants to Assess Their Effect on the Development of Musculoskeletal Disease

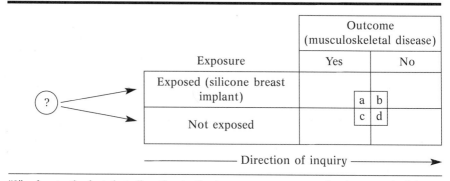

"?" refers to the fact that allocation to the two groups was not under the control of the investigator.

Second, there may be unequal searching for the endpoints in the two groups, with a less intense search in the control group. This was acknowledged as an issue in the breast-implant studies in December 1990, in a "Face to Face with Connie Chung" television program on the dangers of silicone breast implants, and attracted widespread attention. This was explicitly taken into account in two subsequent cohort studies (13,14) that restricted analysis of self-reported disease to 1990 or earlier to avoid bias from this intense media coverage. If we did a cohort analytic study of breast implants to see if the implants cause MSK complaints, Table 10-4 would be the way to display the findings.

The results would then be calculated as the risk in exposed versus nonexposed. That is:

rate in exposed divided by rate in unexposed = $a/(a + b) \div c/(c + d)$.

This is known as the "relative risk" again. We hope you are seeing a pattern. We'll return to this shortly.

10.4 CASE-CONTROL STUDIES

Case-control studies (sometimes known as case comparison studies or "trohoc"[1] research) are on the next step down the evolutionary ladder of evidence generation. Here "cases" are gathered, namely patients who already have the rheumatologic endpoint of interest. Controls, who definitely do not have the outcomes of interest, are then matched to cases, usually for age, gender, and any other important characteristic that might

[1]"Trohoc" is cohort spelled backwards, a term coined by Alvan Feinstein.

be related to the outcome of interest, except for exposure to the putative cause, that is, breast implants. Both groups are then questioned or examined for possible exposure or records are checked to ascertain whether they had received implants. Of importance, to avoid bias, ascertaining exposure should be done by someone who is unaware of whether the participants have, or do not have, the outcome(s) of interest.

This design is much easier and faster to implement than a cohort study because the bad outcomes have already appeared. However, a price must be paid for this ease of execution, and a large literature exists on examples of spurious associations found in case–control studies that were not borne out by subsequent cohort studies and/or randomized trials. But because of their simplicity, case–control studies can be a good place to start when generating and exploring causal hypothesis, especially for rare disorders. Traditional epidemiology texts provide detailed methods for doing such studies, and they are even described in some clinical epidemiology texts (15).

Alvan Feinstein provided a detailed analysis of the biases inherent in this study design and how to avoid many of them (16). Indeed, advocates of observational studies such as Feinstein claim that they can provide the same answers as RCTs about causal effects if their biases and other limitations are understood and, where possible, overcome. Table 10–5 lists some of the important principles for avoiding bias in case–control research. We agree that a badly done RCT can give incorrect answers and a well done observational study can give correct answers—but a well-designed and executed RCT trumps a well done observational study every time, because it is least susceptible to the many biases that can create false conclusions.

TABLE 10–5 Scientific Principles for Case–Control Studies[a]

1. Establish research hypothesis before the research is conducted
2. Define the exposure beforehand
3. Define inclusion and exclusion criteria for each person's baseline state
4. Exclude from the control group anyone with what could be the early signs of the outcome state or contraindications to exposure
5. Check and adjust for prognostic factors that differ between the comparison groups
6. Choose a selection process that eliminates or minimizes referral bias
7. Establish ways to eliminate or minimize recall bias
8. Establish ways to eliminate or minimize detection bias
9. Record unknown exposure as unknown, not absent
10. Manage participation bias

[a] From Feinstein AR. *The architecture of clinical research.* Philadelphia, PA: WB Saunders, 1985, with permission (16).

TABLE 10-6 Presenting the Results of a Case–Control Study of Silicone Breast Implants to Assess their Effect on the Development of Musculoskeletal Disease

	Outcome (musculoskeletal disease)	
Exposure	Yes	No
Exposed (silicone breast implant)	a	b
Not exposed	c	d

◄——————————— Direction of inquiry ———————————

If we did a case–control study of breast implants to see if they cause MSK complaints, Table 10-6 would be a way to display the findings.

Here the table looks the same as before, but the analysis is different. Because the study starts with people who have, or lack, the outcome of interest (MSK disease) and looks backwards in time to see if they were previously exposed or not exposed to the putative causal agent (silicone breast implants), we need to compare $a/(a + c)$ with $b/(b + d)$. This is called the "relative odds." Typically, in such studies, the relative frequencies of "a" compared with "c," and "b" compared with "d," are very low. Thus, the equation can be simplified as $a/c \div b/d$, which becomes ad/bc. This provides an estimate of RR. So statistically the estimate of association is basically the same as for an RCT or a cohort study.

10.5 ANALYTIC SURVEYS

Analytic surveys are on the bottom rung of the evidence ladder. In these, a survey is conducted in which individuals are assessed for whether they have the condition of interest or the exposure of interest, and the correlation of the findings for these two assessments is determined. For example, for silicone breast implants, a surveyor could stand on a street corner and ask women passing by whether they had any connective tissue complaints and noting whether they had breast implants. Clearly, any association found could be due to any number of known or unknown confounders. Lack of association could also be misleading. Although some of the potential biases can be anticipated and minimized (e.g., through random sampling techniques, training interviewers, and avoiding leading questions), other biases cannot be anticipated and minimized with this approach.

If we did an analytic survey of breast implants to see if they cause MSK complaints, Table 10-7 would be an appropriate way to display the findings.

Here the appropriate analysis would be the same as for a cohort study or RCT.

TABLE 10-7   **Presenting the Results of an Analytic Survey of Silicone Breast Implants to Assess Their Effect on the Development of Musculoskeletal Disease**

Exposure	Outcome (musculoskeletal disease)	
	Yes	No
Exposed (silicone breast implant)	a	b
Not exposed	c	d

Direction of inquiry ⬉

By now, you no doubt have discerned a pattern: we're making much of the importance of various study design options for obtaining valid conclusions about possible causal relations, but the results can come out looking the same in tables and statistics. That's precisely why we are emphasizing research methods and not statistics. Statistics can brew any type of data and concoct P values and confidence intervals. But there is a world of difference in how nourishing the results will be that depends on the ingredients and how they are prepared. So we repeat our previous advice: Learn how to conduct sound research and be sure to have a statistician along with you so that the results are properly analyzed.

10.6 STRENGTH OF ASSOCIATION

The magnitude of the association between the exposure and the outcome is known as the "strength of the association." In controlled trials it is often expressed as the "absolute risk reduction" [or risk difference (RD)] or relative risk reduction (RRR), as we've shown for Tables 10-3, 10-4, 10-6, and 10-7. The relative merits of these trials are discussed in Chapters 5 and 6 on therapeutic trials. For cohort studies the RR is usually employed, that is, how many more times the outcome of interest is found in patients exposed versus unexposed. For case–control studies instead of using a ratio of risks (RR), we use a ratio of odds [odds ratio (OR)]: the odds of a case patient being exposed, divided by the odds of a control patient being exposed.

Table 10-8 shows the range of RRs for a number of conditions positively associated with smoking. Note that the RR with lung cancer is 15 whereas that of ischemic heart disease is only 1.6. To appreciate the impact, it is also necessary to look at the baseline prevalence rate. For lung cancer this is 14 per 100,000/year in contrast to ischemic heart disease, which is 572 per 100,000/year. Thus, despite a much lower RR for ischemic heart disease than for lung cancer, smoking causes many more deaths per 100,000/year from ischemic heart disease than from lung cancer (320 versus 195).

TABLE 10-8 Fatal Diseases Associated with Smoking—Based on a Study of Male British Doctors (17)

	Standardized Mortality per 100,000/year				
	Life-long Nonsmoker (a)	Current Cigarette Smoker (b)	Relative Risk (b/a)	Absolute Excess Risk Per 100,000 Man/year (b–a)	Attributable Proportion[a] (%)
Cancer of lung	14	209	15.0	195	31
Ischemic heart disease	572	892	1.6	320	15

[a]Attributable proportion: Proportion of cases explained by "current smoking."
From Doll R, Peto R, Wheatley K, et al. Mortality in relation to smoking: 40 years' observations on male British doctors. *BMJ* 1994;309(6959):901–911, with permission.

It is more challenging to show that no association exists because the ability to rule out an increase in RR of a specified size is limited by the number of participants you can assemble and the event rate expected among them. Those who will tolerate no increase in risk will then never be satisfied. The best you can do is to specify in advance the level of RR increase that is "acceptable" (or at least, detectable with available resources) and then carry out the analysis to see if the result is either well below this level or clearly above it. All the issues and procedures for determining the power of a study apply here, as detailed in Chapter 6 and elsewhere.

10.7 CONSISTENCY

The repetitive demonstration of an association by different investigators, using different research designs in different settings, constitutes consistency. Typically, in a meta-analysis, if the confidence intervals for the outcomes of the individual studies overlap, and statistical tests for heterogeneity are negative (see Chapter 2), then consistency has been shown. If a meta-analysis has not been done, especially if the available studies are too disparate to allow quantitative summary of the findings across studies, then consistency can be in the "eyes of the beholder" and subject to considerable disagreement among observers, depending on their point of view. A "vote counting" approach to consistency (i.e., counting the number of studies with positive findings, compared with the total number of studies) is far from satisfactory (Table 2–3), especially if the preponderance of studies are negative, because negative study results are often found when the individual studies are too small to detect even a sizable increase in risk. These smaller studies can also be a nuisance when many of them are alongside a few large studies. A case can be made in this situation for sorting the studies based on size and quality, then looking for consistency among the larger, higher quality studies. Obviously, this will be more convincing if the procedure for doing this is set out in advance, before the findings of individual studies are considered.

10.8 TEMPORAL SEQUENCE

A consistent sequence of events of exposure to the putative cause, followed by the occurrence of the outcome of interest, is required for a positive test of temporality. In the case–control and retrospective cohort studies (for example, a retrospective review of charts to go back to identify women who had the implants and then compare their subsequent complaints) it can be difficult to ascertain whether the first appearance of symptoms was before or after the implant. A prospective cohort would exclude women who had prior complaints, thus ensuring that temporality could be assessed.

10.9 GRADIENT

The demonstration of an increasing risk or severity of the outcome in association with an increased "dose" or duration of exposure satisfies this rule. For example, the association between homocysteine and coronary heart disease in Table 10–9 shows a gradient.

10.10 SENSE

The first element of "sense" is satisfied when the evidence is in agreement with our current understanding of the distributions of causes and outcomes in humans ("ecologic sense"). For example, suicide rates fell in the United Kingdom after establishment of a Good Samaritans help line. These studies are very easy to do, with figures typically drawn from publicly available sources. They are also very hard to believe as causal evidence because they do not guarantee any connection between one phenomenon

TABLE 10–9 Odds Ratios for Death from Coronary Heart Disease for Quartiles of Homocysteine Levels in Men[a][b] (18)

Homocysteine Levels	Mean Homocysteine Level	Odds Ratio (95% CI)
<10.25 μmol/L	8.77 μmol/L	1.00 (0.73 to 1.38)
10.25 to 12.32 μmol/L	11.26 μmol/L	1.43 (1.07 to 1.92)
12.33 to 15.16 μmol/L	13.56 μmol/L	1.46 (1.08 to 1.97)
≥15.17 μmol/L	19.13 μmol/L	2.90 (2.04 to 4.12)

[a]Adjusted for apolipoprotein B levels and systolic blood pressure.
[b]Reproduced with permission of the American College of Physicians.
From Wald NJ, Watt HC, Law MR, et al. Homocysteine and ischemic heart disease: results of prospective study with implications regarding prevention. *Arch Intern Med* 1998;158:862–867; High homocysteine levels were associated with increased CHD in men, Abstract of *ACP J Club* 1998;129:51, with permission.

(suicide) and the other (Samaritan help lines). That is because in ecologic studies, the data concerning the two phenomena are derived from different sources. In this particular case, the causal link was challenged when it was noted that that the decline in suicide rates also coincided with a more plausible cause, changing the cooking gas supply from deadly coal gas to sleepy North Sea gas (19). Thus, the ecologic study is even below the lowly analytic survey that we disparaged earlier in this chapter. An example of ecologic sense for breast implants and connective tissue disorder would be if we were to observe an increase in sales of breast implants followed by an increase in medical insurance charges for connective tissue disorders. Even if this were true, it would be impossible to establish a direct connection without doing a more sophisticated study, higher in the feeding chain of Table 10–2.

The second element of "sense" inquires whether the results of the article are in harmony with our current understanding of the responses of cells, tissues, organs, and organisms to stimuli ("biologic sense"). For example, the relationship between homocysteine and coronary heart disease has been known for some time from animal studies that show that hyperhomocysteinemia causes platelet and vascular damage that can lead to atherosclerosis. Similarly, studies in humans that show elevated serum levels of homocysteine through inborn errors of metabolism and nutritional deficiencies, especially of folate, are associated with vascular damage (20). This kind of sense is remarkably easy to find, given the vast amount of biologic research that has been done and the infinite capability of the human mind to conceive of plausible connections among phenomena.

The third element of "sense," the limitation of the association to a single putative cause and single effect can be useful, as seen with thalidomide and phocomelia. This concept is called "specificity," and it is helpful when present but is exceedingly rare.

Finally, causal arguments can proceed by "analogy" or by similarity to a known cause. This test for causation would be satisfied, for example, if silicone was similar in chemical structure to an agent that was known to cause chronic inflammatory responses in human connective tissues.

The implant case provided an interesting example of an attempt to make the case for a causative link by establishing a new disease labeled systemic silicone-related disorder (SSRD). The executive committee of the Silicone-Related Disorders Research Group proposed a preliminary set of operational criteria for SSRD: a current or past silicone gel–filled breast implant currently or in the past plus the presence of three major criteria or two major criteria and four minor criteria or one major criterion and seven minor criteria (21).

The National Science Panel concluded that they do not yet support the inclusion of SSRD in the list of accepted diseases, for four reasons. First, the requirement of the inclusion of the putative cause (silicone exposure) as one of the criteria does not allow the criteria set to be tested objectively without knowledge of the presence of implants, thus incurring incorporation bias (22). Second, there are few objective signs. Third, the constellation proposed is not unique, that is, the majority of components in the proposed SSRD criteria are already included in the signs and symptoms of other accepted diseases (e.g., scleroderma, Sjögren syndrome, systemic lupus erythematosis, fibromyalgia, and chronic fatigue syndrome), with the only differentiating feature being exposure to a silicone breast implant. Finally, there is no established association of the criteria set with the putative cause (exposure to silicone gel and/or silica) through well-controlled studies.

10.11 ASSEMBLING THE EVIDENCE CONCERNING A CAUSAL CLAIM

Following this consideration of the relationship of various types of evidence to causal claims, it is now time to assemble the evidence regarding the question of breast implants and CTD in a systematic fashion. Briefly, in protocols for studies or systematic reviews of causation, you should describe the features of the investigation that are noted here.

✓ **Research question.** Describe the research question (or questions) that defines which of Bradford Hill's criteria for causation will be addressed, along with the exposures (breast implants, in this case) and outcomes (CTDs, in this case).

✓ **Literature search.** Outline the methods you will use to do a comprehensive literature search for both original articles and review articles.

✓ **Study selection.** Include criteria for selection and methods of reducing bias in this assessment.

✓ **Data extraction and assessment of study merit.** Detail the procedure for extracting the details of the purpose, study participants, exposure, controls, blinding, and clinical outcomes for each eligible study and the methods of assessing their merit.

✓ **Analysis.** Indicate the approach you will use to summarize and present the findings of studies, including statistical issues and interpretation.

✓ **Results.** These should directly address the research question.

✓ *Research question.*

In women of all ages, are those who have a silicone breast implant more likely than those who do not have an implant to have specified signs/symptoms of CTDs or a diagnosis of classical/accepted CTDs during the time the implant is in place?

As for other research areas, the question needs to include the five PICOT components specifying the patient population, intervention/exposure, comparison group, outcomes, and time.

✓ *Literature search.*

We identified potentially relevant studies through a computerized search of bibliographic databases and a review of references cited in retrieved articles. We developed a prespecified list of search terms (detailed in Appendix 10.1) to identify different subsets of rheumatologic/autoimmune disease in women with implants in the following bibliographic databases: MEDLINE, Current Contents, HealthStar, Biological Abstracts, EMBASE, Toxline, and Dissertation Abstracts. The results of these searches were compared with the 3,615 articles submitted by legal counsels from both sides to identify additional relevant studies not captured in the computerized searches. We were unaware of which counsel provided the studies that we reviewed.

Note that this comprehensive searching approach is necessary for researchers who need to be exhaustive (or to convince a court of law!). PubMed Clinical Queries (*http://web.ncbi.nlm.nih.gov/entrez/query/static/ clinical.shtml*) has both sensitive and specific search strategies for etiology evidence to get you started.

✓ *Study selection.*

Two reviewers screened articles and abstracts independently and judged them to be eligible or ineligible according to predetermined inclusion criteria, as follows: human studies, total number of participants fewer than 10, and appropriate control group of either healthy or women who were not exposed who fulfilled the requirements of the study. Case–control studies had to include controls with no history of the disease in question, and cross-sectional studies had to include populations not selected on the basis of either exposure or disease. When we encountered multiple publications of the same data, we included in the review only the publications that were most complete, published studies over unpublished dissertations, and the most recent publications over otherwise similar reports. We included abstracts and imposed no language restrictions. We found 21 eligible studies through the literature search and 3 additional ones from the material submitted by the legal counsels.

This process is very similar to the one detailed in Chapter 2, so we recommend that you review that chapter if you need more procedural detail.

✓ Data extraction and assessment of study merit.

Two independent reviewers used a standard form to collect information on study participants, exposure, controls, blinding, and clinical outcomes from the selected manuscripts. Discrepancies in data extraction were discussed and resolved through consensus.

In collaboration with David Henry in Newcastle, Australia, George Wells and our group (23) developed the Newcastle-Ottawa Scale for assessing the quality of cohort and case–control studies. We applied this to 21 of the 24 included studies, including 10 cohort studies and 11 case–control studies, omitting this assessment for the three cross-sectional studies. The details of the criteria are listed in Appendix 10.2 and illustrated for cohort studies in Table 10–10.

✓ Analysis.

Sample size: We didn't make formal power calculations. However, a large number of patients were assessed in the ten cohort and three cross-sectional studies (cohorts studies: 22,862 patients exposed, 113,849 not exposed; cross-sectional studies: 11,061 patients exposed, 388,882 not exposed). Also, 11 case–control studies were conducted, with the number of cases varying from 35 to 532 and the number of controls varying from 35 to 2,507 across the various outcomes of interest. Given the number of patients assessed and the number of studies conducted, the power of finding any association was high.

Data synthesis and statistical methods: For non-randomized studies, it is important to adjust for the effects of potential confounding factors in estimating measures of association. We reported adjusted RRs or ORs, corrected for the effects of confounding factors if they were provided in the published study; otherwise we calculated and reported unadjusted RRs and ORs.

The nonoccurrence of the outcome of interest (i.e., no outcome events) for cohort studies and nonoccurrence of exposure for case–control studies presents arithmetic problems in calculating these measures of association, resulting in indeterminate values. For cohort studies, if no outcomes occurred for both study groups, we did not calculate the RRs, and if no outcomes occurred in only one group, a risk difference (RD) (i.e., the difference between the rates) was calculated. For case–control studies, if no exposures occurred in either the case or control groups, no OR calculation was made. In addition to the point estimate, 95% CI estimates were used. These define a range within which the true value for the association between exposure and outcome is most likely to be found.

TABLE 10–10 Quality Assessment of Cohort Studies of Breast Implants and Connective Tissue Disorders

Study	Selection				Comparability	Outcome		
	Representativeness of Exposed Cohort	Selection of Nonexposed Cohort	Ascertainment of Exposure	Demonstration Outcome of Interest Not Present at Start of Study	Comparability of Cohorts on the Basis of Design or Analysis	Ascertainment of Outcome	Adequate Length of Follow-up	Adequacy of Follow-up
Edworthy 1998	*	*	*	*	**	*	*	
Friis 1997	*	*	*	*		*	*	*
Gabriel 1994	*	*	*	*	**	*	*	*
Giltay 1994	*	*	*		**	*	*	*
Nyren 1998a	*	*	*	*	**	*	*	*
Nyren 1998b	*	*	*	*	**	*	*	*
Park 1998	*	*	*		*	*	*	
Sanchez 1995		*	*	*	**	*	*	*
Wells 1994		*	*		**			
Winther 1998	*	*	*			*	*	*

*Study has fulfilled the criteria for the item listed at the top of each column. A blank cell indicates that the criteria have not been met. See Appendix 10.2 for an explanation of criteria.

**Signifies that study groups were comparable for age as well as one or more additional unspecified variables.

As shown in Tables 10–4 and 10–7, the magnitude of the association between an exposure to an intervention and an outcome of interest is expressed as a RR for cohort and cross-sectional studies; an OR is most appropriate for case–control studies (Table 10–6) and is preferred by many statisticians for prospective studies as well. The RR is a ratio of the risk of the outcome of interest in the group exposed to the intervention to the risk of the outcome in the group not exposed. For the OR, the ratio of the odds of experiencing the outcome to not experiencing the outcome in the exposed group is compared to the odds in the group not exposed to the intervention. An RR or OR of 1.0 indicates no observed association between the exposure and the outcome.

✓ Results.

1. Evidence from true experiments: no RCTs were found.
2. Strength of Association: As can be seen in Tables 10–11 and 10–12, in the 10 cohort and 14 case–control studies, no association was found between breast implants and rheumatologic diseases. In our silicone breast implant systematic review, we were able to say that no study found a statistically significant association with the MSK diseases of interest, that is, no association was evident between breast implants and any of the individual established or atypical connective tissue disorders. Thus, the strength of association is nil.
3. Consistency: The breast-implant studies were conducted by 24 different groups in 24 different settings, showing consistency in the absence of an effect across both case–control and cohort studies. The results in Table 10–11 are consistent in that all of the classic/accepted diagnoses reported had a risk estimate whose confidence interval included 1, in the case of ORs or RRs, or 0, in the case of RD. There was, however, some inconsistency in the results reported for the symptom groupings: arthralgias, lymphadenopathy, myalgias, sicca, skin changes, and stiffness. For each of these categories, there was a single study in which the risk estimate(s) had a 95% CI that did not include 1, yet in every instance, there were other studies that did not confirm this association. None of these symptoms, therefore, met the Hill criterion for consistency (2).
4. Temporal sequence. From prospective studies, seven cohort studies stated that they excluded individuals with previous symptoms and provided estimates, which excluded participants who had disease-predating implants. None of these showed an association of connective tissue disorders with breast implants.
5. Gradient: In the implant studies, there was no evidence of increased frequency of rheumatologic disorders with the duration of exposure to the implant—by dose or duration of exposure.
6. Sense—from epidemiology, biology, and analogy: In the breast-implant case, the lawyers presented large amounts of information on the effects of silicone polymers and their products on the histology and laboratory tests of immune function, including slides of silicone that had migrated to distal tissues from the implant.

Table 10–11 Association Between Silicone Breast Implants and Classical/Accepted Connective Tissue Diseases

End point	Author, Year	Frequencies[a]		RR/OR (95% CI)[b]	Risk difference (%)	D[c]	E[d]	A[e]
Ankylosing spondylitis	Friis et al., 1997	0/2,570	NR	NA	NA	E		
	Gabriel et al., 1994	0/749	3/1,498		−0.20 (−0.43, 0.03)	E	C	+
	Nyren et al., 1998	1/7,442	0/3,353		0.01 (−0.01, 0.04)	E	C	
Arthritis associated with inflammatory bowel disease	Gabriel et al., 1994	1/749			0.13 (−0.13, 0.40)	E	C	+
Chronic fatigue syndrome	MacDonald et al., 1996	1/35	2/35	0.49 (0.01, 9.84)		D	C	+
Fibromyalgia	Nyren et al., 1998	9/7,442	5/3,353	1.10 (0.3, 3.0)		E	R	+
	Wolfe and Anderson, 1999	3/505	3/764	1.52 (0.31, 7.56)		D	R	+
Giant cell (temporal) arteritis	Friis et al, 1997	3/2,570	10/11,023	1.29 (0.35, 4.67)		E	C	
	Nyren et al., 1998	1/7,442	0/3,353		0.01 (−0.01, 0.04)	E	C	
Hashimoto thyroiditis	Friis et al., 1997	0/2,570	NR	NA	NA	E		
	Gabriel et al., 1994	10/749	21/1,498	1.00 (0.47, 2.13)		E	R	+
Localized or discoid lupus	Friis et al., 1997	0/2,570	NR	NA	NA	E		
	Nyren et al., 1998	1/7,442	0/3,353	1.35 (0.06, 33.18)		B	C	
Mixed connective tissue disease	Goldman et al., 1995	0/150	49/4,079	0.00 (0.00, 2.68)		B	R	+
	Sanchez-Guerrero et al., 1995	0/1,183	0/86,318	NA	NA	E		
	Teel, 1997	0/3	24/1,577			D	C	+
Multiple sclerosis	Nyren et al., 1998	3/7,429	4/3,351	0.5 (0.2, 0.9)		E	R	+
	Winther et al., 1998	2/1,135	2/7,071	6.23 (0.88, 44.18)		E	C	
Myasthenia gravis	Winther et al., 1998	0/1,135	1/7,071		−0.01 (−0.04, 0.01)	E	C	
Polyarteritis nodosa	Friis et al., 1997	0/2,570	NR	NA	NA	E		
	Nyren et al., 1998	0/7,442	0/3,353	NA	NA	E		

(continued)

Table 10-11 Continued

End point	Author, Year	Frequencies[a]		RR/OR (95% CI)[b]	Risk difference (%)	D[c]	E[d]	A[e]
Polychondritis	Gabriel et al., 1994	1/749	0/1,498		0.13 (−0.12, 0.40)	E	C	+
Polymyalgia rheumatica	Gabriel et al., 1994	2/749	1/1,498	4.00 (0.36, 44.04)		E	C	+
	Friis et al., 1997[f]	3/2,570	10/11,023	1.29 (0.35, 4.67)		E	C	
	Nyren et al., 1998	5/7,442	0/3,353		0.07 (0.01, 0.13)	E	C	
Polymyositis/ dermatomyositis	Friis et al., 1997	0/2,570	2/11,023		−0.02 (−0.04, 0.01)	E	C	
	Goldman et al., 1995	0/150	36/4,079	0.00 (0.00, 3.71)		B	R	+
	Hennekens et al., 1996	20/10,830	727/384,713	1.52 (0.79, 2.37)		B	R	+
	Nyren et al., 1998	1/7,442	0/3,353		0.01 (−0.01, 0.04)	E	C	+
	Sanchez-Guerrero et al., 1995	0/1,183	12/186,318		−0.01 (−0.02, −0.01)	E	C	
	Teel, 1997	0/17	24/1,577			d	c	+
Psoriatic arthritis	Friis et al., 1997	0/2,570	NR	NA	NA	E	C	
	Gabriel et al., 1994	0/749	1/1,498		−0.07 (−0.20, 0.06)	E	C	+
	Nyren et al., 1998	0/7,442	2/3,353		−0.06 (−0.14, 0.02)	E	C	
Raynauds disease/ phenomenon	Collado Delfa et al., 1998	0/81	1/72		−1.39 (−4.09, 1.31)	E	C	
	Giltay et al., 1994	12/235	7/210	1.53 (0.61, 3.82)		E	C	
	Park et al., 1998 (cosmetic)	1/110	3/128	0.39 (0.04, 3.68)		E	C	+
	Park et al., 1998 (breast cancer)	7/207	5/88	0.60 (0.19, 1.82)		E	C	
	Wells et al., 1994	1%	0%	0.49 (0.02, 2.80)[g]		E	R	+
Rheumatoid arthritis	Dugowson et al., 1992	1/300	12/1,456	0.41 (0.05, 3.13)		D	R	+
	Edworthy et al., 1998	11/1,112	6/727	1.44 (0.50, 4.15)		E	R	+
	Friis et al., 1997	7/2,570	16/11,023	1.88 (0.77, 4.56)		E	C	
	Gabriel et al., 1994	0/749	2/1,498		−0.13 (−0.32, 0.05)	E	C	+
	Goldman et al., 1995	5/146	383/4,079	0.35 (0.14, 0.85)		B	C	

(continued)

Table 10-11 Continued

End point	Author, Year	Frequencies[a]		RR/OR (95% CI)[b]	Risk difference (%)	D[c]	E[d]	A[e]
	Hennekens et al., 1996	107/10,830	6,322/384,713	1.18 (0.97, 1.43)		B	R	+
	Nyren et al., 1998	11/7,442	5/3,353	1.3 (0.7, 2.5)		E	R	+
	Park et al., 1998 (breast cancer)	1/207	1/88	0.43 (0.03, 6.72)		E	C	+
	Sanchez-Guerrero et al., 1995	3/1,183	392/86,318	0.90 (0.30, 2.60)		E	R	+
	Wolfe and Anderson, 1999	3/464	3/764	1.66 (0.33, 8.23)		D	R	+
Sarcoidosis	Friis et al., 1997	0/2,570	NR	NA	NA	E		
	Gabriel et al., 1994	0/749	2/1,498		−0.13 (−0.32, 0.05)	E	R	+
	Nyren et al., 1998	2/7,442	2/3,353	0.45 (0.06, 3.20)		E	C	+
Scleroderma	Burns et al., 1996	2/274	14/1,184	0.95 (0.21, 4.36)		D	R	+
	Edworthy et al., 1998	0/1,112	3/727			E	C	+
	Englert et al., 1996	3/286	4/253	0.52 (0.11, 2.41)	−0.41 (−0.88, 0.05)	D	R	+
	Friis et al., 1997	1/2,570	1/11,023	4.29 (0.27, 68.55)		E	C	+
	Gabriel et al., 1994	0/749	0/1,498	NA	NA	E		+
	Goldman et al., 1995	0/150	64/4,079	0.00 (0.00, 2.05)		B	R	+
	Hennekens et al., 1996	10/10,830	314/384,713	1.84 (0.98, 3.46)		B	R	+
	Hochberg et al., 1996	11/837	31/2,507	1.11 (0.55, 2.24)		D	R	+
	Lacey et al., 1997	2/189	13/1,043	1.48 (0.34, 6.93)		D	R	+
	Nyren et al., 1998	0/7,442	3/3,353		−0.09 (−0.19, 0.01)	E	C	
	Sanchez-Guerrero et al., 1995	0/1,183	14/86,318		−0.02 (−0.02, 0.01)	E	C	
	Teel, 1997	0/55	24/1,577			D	C	+
	Wells et al., 1994	0%	0%	NA	NA	E		
Sjögren syndrome	Edworthy et al., 1998	5/1,112	4/727	0.99 (0.17, 5.94)		E	R	+
	Friis et al., 1997	1/2,570	1/11,023	4.29 (0.27, 68.55)		E	C	
	Gabriel et al., 1994	1/749	0/1,498		0.13 (−0.13, 0.40)	E	C	+

(continued)

Table 10–11 Continued

End point	Author, Year	Frequencies[a]	RR/OR (95% CI)[b]	Risk difference (%)	D[c]	E[d]	A[e]
	Goldman et al., 1995	1/149	47/4,079	0.58 (0.08, 4.19)		B	C	
	Hennekens et al., 1996	22/10,830	752/384,713	1.49 (0.97, 2.28)		B	R	+
	Nyren et al., 1998	1/7,442	0/3,353		0.01 (−0.01, 0.04)	E	C	
	Sanchez-Guerrero et al., 1995	0/1,183	2/86,318		0.00 (−0.01, 0.00)	E	C	
	Teel, 1997	4/161	24/1,577	1.60 (0.50, 4.70)		D	R	+
Systemic lupus erythematosus	Edworthy et al., 1998	3/1,112	3/727	0.94 (0.17, 5.23)		E	R	+
	Friis et al., 1997	1/2,570	5/11,023	0.86 (0.10, 7.34)		E	C	
	Goldman et al., 1995	0/150	179/4,079		−4.39 (−5.02, −3.76)	B	C	
	Hennekens et al., 1996	32/10,830	1,561/384,713	1.15 (0.81, 1.63)		B	R	+
	Nyren et al., 1998	3/7,442	3/3,353	0.70 (0.30, 1.60)		E	R	+
	Sanchez-Guerrero et al., 1995	0/1,183	96/86,318		−0.11 (−0.13, −0.09)	E	C	
	Strom et al., 1994	1/133	0/100	2.28 (0.09, 56.45)		D	C	+
	Teel, 1997	2/191	24/1,577	0.8 (0.2, 3.4)		D	R	+
	Wells et al., 1994	0%	0%	NA	NA	E		

For full references, refer to article (24).

[a]Frequencies for cohort/cross-sectional studies are the number of cases/number exposed and the number of cases/number not exposed. Frequencies for case–control studies are the number exposed/number of cases and the number exposed/number of controls. A few frequencies were reported as percentages, as shown. NR, not reported.

[b]For case–control studies, the odds ratio (OR) is used. For cohort/cross-sectional studies [with the exception of Wells et al. 1994, and the estimates reported in Goldman et al. 1995 the relative risk (RR) is used. 95% CI, 95% confidence interval; NA, not available.

[c]Study design: E, subjects selected based on exposure (cohort study); D, subjects selected based on disease (case–control study); B, subjects selected based on both exposure and disease (cross-sectional study).

[d]Estimate: R, odds ratio/relative risk reported by authors; C, odds ratio/relative risk calculated by reviewers.

[e]Adjusted: +, study controlled for ≥1 factor in the design or in the analysis.

[f]Giant cell (temporal) arteritis and polymyalgia rheumatica combined.

[g]Estimate possibly reported incorrectly in article.

From Tugwell P, Wells G, Peterson J, et al. Do silicone breast implants cause rheumatologic disorders? A systematic review for a court-appointed national science panel. *Arthritis Rheum* 2001;44:2477–2484, with permission.

TABLE 10–12 **Summary of Associations Between Classical/Accepted Connective Diseases and Silicone Breast Implants (24)**

No Data Reported	No Evidence of Appreciable Risk (all confidence intervals cross 1)	Disagreement (confidence intervals for 1 or more diagnoses cross 1)	Agreement on Appreciable Risk (no confidence interval crosses 1)
Morphea	Ankylosing spondylitis Arthritis associated with inflammatory bowel disease Chronic fatigue syndrome Dermatomyositis/polymyositis Fibromyalgia Hashimoto thyroiditis Localized or discoid lupus Mixed connective tissue disease Multiple sclerosis Myasthenia gravis Polyarteritis nodosa Polychondritis Polymyalgia rheumatica Psoriatic arthritis Raynaud syndrome Rheumatoid arthritis Sarcoidosis Scleroderma Sjögren syndrome Systemic lupus erythematosus Temporal arteritis Vasculitis Wegener granulomatosis	None	None

From Tugwell P, Wells G, Peterson J, et al. Do silicone breast implants cause rheumatologic disorders? A systematic review for a court-appointed national science panel. *Arthritis Rheum* 2001;44:2477–2484, with permission.

Systematic reviews such as this are observational studies themselves and biases can creep in. The principle of consistency of different original study types for causation can and should be applied to reviews as well. The results presented here are consistent with those of other published reviews. For example, an independent review group established by the Minister of Health in the United Kingdom concluded that there was no epidemiologic evidence for any link between silicone gel breast implants and any established CTDs (25). The report also concluded that there was no good evidence for the existence of atypical CTDs. A subsequent published report from the Institute of Medicine on the safety of silicone breast implants reached two conclusions relevant to the results reported here (26). First, the report confirms that there does not appear to be any evidence of a novel syndrome in women with breast implants. Second, the report concurs with the interpretation that epidemiologic evidence shows that CTDs are not more common in women with breast implants than in women without breast implants.

This conclusion of the absence of an association has resulted in such claims now being unacceptable in court. For example, in the state of Oregon, no lawyers can use expert witnesses or testimony to claim a general causal link between silicone gel breast implants and any systemic illness or syndrome.

The process of weighing in on breast implants in a legal setting raised several key ethical issues. The first relates to the ethics of making recommendations unless the scientific basis is strong. It is a matter of opinion, but the four of us on the US National Science Panel were convinced that we had not found evidence for an association, let alone a clinically important effect (27). We were concerned that the rules of evidence might be very different in a court of law but were reassured by the following summary of the way in which research evidence can be assessed in a court of law (28). To help the judge evaluate the soundness of the methodology and overall "reliability" of scientific theory advocated by an expert, the US federal court directed district courts to consider the following factors (which the federal court labeled as its "general observations"): (a) falsifiability of the theory, (b) peer review and publication of the theory, (c) known or potential rate of error and the existence of standards controlling the research on which the theory is based, and (d) general acceptance of the methodology underlying the theory in the scientific community [a remnant of the *Frye v. United States* test, from a case involving polygraph evidence (3,4)]. The *Daubert v. Merrell Dow Pharmaceuticals* opinion (4) specifically explained that the words "scientific" and "knowledge" in the Federal Rule 702 imply that the testimony must be grounded "in the methods and procedures of science," be more than "subjective belief or unsupported speculation," and be supported by appropriate validation "based on what is known." The court explained that the distinction between "validity" and "reliability," that is, between a scientific test or principle and its application in the particular case, approximates the methodology/conclusion distinction. The requirement that an expert's testimony relate to "scientific knowledge" is one of evidentiary reliability, and in the determinations as to whether the expert's testimony relates to "scientific knowledge," the trial judge must focus "solely on principles and methodology, not on the conclusions that they generate."

Another major ethical issue is the independence of scientists who are asked for their opinion. In this instance and likely in most others, it proved very difficult to find scientists who were knowledgeable yet had not been an advocate for the patients or the manufacturers. Many scientists refrain from testifying as expert witnesses because they are concerned about the potential for bias and loss of credibility and want to protect their reputations for scientific integrity. Indeed, our experience confirmed this; despite open disclosure of industry support and acceptance thereof by the lawyers for both sides, only after the recommendations became known did the lawyers for the plaintiffs claim conflict of interest with a carefully orchestrated media campaign (Peter Tugwell was one of the targets). Furthermore, during the videotaped depositions, a lawyer was admitted to the courtroom who, although not a member of either legal team, was allowed to cross-examine one panel member (not PT) and mount an *ad hominem* attack on the member's character and qualifications. We also felt it unethical that, without due warning, panel members were required to release files, telephone records, meeting notes, handwritten notes on published articles, and early drafts of the report. Thus, many working documents were made available to the lawyers and were used for legal maneuvering during the subsequent depositions and used by counsel in an effort to discredit panel members during subsequent testimony. A legitimate question is whether court-appointed neutral experts should have to hand over such materials and, if so, which types.

Our exhaustive review of research evidence for causal claims also brought the feasibility of such reviews into sharp focus. Systematic reviews of evidence for causal claims can have important effects both medically and legally, but the price to be paid for getting involved in them can be very high, especially if conducted for legal purposes. The breast-implant review proved to be a much, much larger project than any of us involved ever predicted! Our background (with Cochrane reviews and the credibility it gave us in court, even though the studies in this case were not controlled trials) proved to be invaluable. Although small in comparison with the monetary claims in the breast-implant litigation, the costs incurred by the court, as well as our panel and legal advisors were substantial (several million dollars), largely because the work took much longer than predicted. Our recommendations (27) should help subsequent panels function more efficiently. In addition, the costs incurred by selection panels will be substantially reduced if the members of scientific panels are selected from registries such as those recently established by Duke University Law School's Private Adjudication Center and the American Association for the Advancement of Science (29).

REFERENCES

1. Diamond BA, Hulka BS, Kerkvliet NL, et al. *Silicone breast implants in relation to connective tissue diseases and immunoloic dysfunction: a report by a National Science Panel to the Honorable Sam C. Pointer, Jr., coordinating judge for the federal breast implant multi-district litigation.* Birmingham: Federal Judicial Center, November 1998.

2. Hill AB. *Principles of medical statistics*, 9th ed. London: Lancet, 1971.

3. Frye v. United States. 54 App. D.C. 46, 293 F. 1013. 1923.

4. Daubert, et al. v. Merrell Dow Pharmaceuticals. 92–102 June 28 1993, 113 S Ct 2768.

5. Stampfer MJ, Colditz GA. Estrogen replacement therapy and coronary heart disease: a quantitative assessment of the epidemiologic evidence. *Prev Med* 1991;20(1):47–63.

6. Rossouw JE, Anderson GL, Prentice RL, et al. Risks and benefits of estrogen plus progestin in healthy postmenopausal women: principal results from the women's health initiative randomized controlled trial. *JAMA* 2002;288(3):321–333.

7. Hulley S, Grady D, Bush T, et al. Heart and Estrogen/Progestin Replacement Study (HERS) Research Group. Randomized trial of estrogen plus progestin for secondary prevention of coronary heart disease in postmenopausal women. *JAMA* 1998;280(7): 605–613.

8. Nelson HD, Humphrey LL, Nygren P, et al. Postmenopausal hormone replacement therapy: scientific review. *JAMA* 2002;288:872–881.

9. Humphrey LL, Chan BK, Sox HC. Postmenopausal hormone replacement therapy and the primary prevention of cardiovascular disease. *Ann Intern Med* 2002;137(4):273–284.

10. Bombardier C, Laine L, Reicin A, et al. VIGOR Study Group. Comparison of upper gastrointestinal toxicity of rofecoxib and naproxen in patients with rheumatoid arthritis. *N Engl J Med* 2000;343(21):1520–1528.

11. Vivekananthan DP, Penn MS, Sapp SK, et al. Use of antioxidant vitamins for the prevention of cardiovascular disease: meta-analysis of randomised trials. *Lancet* 2003; 361(9374):2017–2023.

12. Hemminki E, McPherson K. Impact of postmenopausal hormone therapy on cardiovascular events and cancer: pooled data from clinical trials. *BMJ* 1997;315:149–153.

13. Sanchez-Guerrero J, Colditz GA, Karlson EW, et al. Silicone breast implants and the risk of connective-tissue diseases and symptoms. *N Engl J Med* 1995;332(25):1666–1670.

14. Hennekens CH, Lee IM, Cook NR, et al. Self-reported breast implants and connective-tissue diseases in female health professionals. A retrospective cohort study. *JAMA* 1996;275(8): 616–621.

15. Hulley SB, Cummings SR, Browner WS, et al. *Designing clinical research. An epidemiologic approach*, 2nd ed. Philadelphia, PA: Lippincott Williams & Wilkins, 2001.

16. Feinstein AR. *The architecture of clinical research*. Philadelphia, PA: WB Saunders, 1985.

17. Doll R, Peto R, Wheatley K, et al. Mortality in relation to smoking: 40 years' observations on male British doctors. *BMJ* 1994;309(6959):901–911.

18. Wald NJ, Watt HC, Law MR, et al. Homocysteine and ischemic heart disease: results of prospective study with implications regarding prevention. *Arch Intern Med* 1998;158: 862–867; High homocysteine levels were associated with increased CHD in men, Abstract of *ACP J Club* 1998;129:51.

19. Fox R. The suicide drop—why? *R Soc Health J* 1975;95:9–13, 20.

20. McCully KS. Vascular pathology of homocysteinemia: implications for the pathogenesis of arteriosclerosis. *Am J Pathol* 1969;56(1):111–128.

21. Silverman S, Borenstein D, Solomon G, et al. Preliminary operational criteria for systemic silicone related disease (SSRD). *Arthritis Rheum* 1996;39(Suppl. 9):S51.

22. Sackett DK. Bias in analytic research. *J Chronic Dis* 1979;32:51–63.

23. The Newcastle-Ottawa Scale (NOS). Assessing the quality of non-randomized studies in meta-analysis. Presented to: The 3rd Symposium on Systematic Reviews: Beyond the Basics-Improving Quality and Impact, St. Catherine's College, Oxford, Jul. 2000.

24. Tugwell P, Wells G, Peterson J, et al. Do silicone breast implants cause rheumatologic disorders? A systematic review for a court-appointed national science panel. *Arthritis Rheum* 2001;44:2477–2484.

25. Sturrock RD, Batchelor JR, Harpwood V, et al. *Silicone gel breast implants: the report of the independent review group*. Cambridge, MA: Jill Rogers Associates, 1998.

26. Bondurant S, Ernster V, Herdman R, eds. *Safety of silicone breast implants*. Washington, DC: National Academy Press, 1999.

27. Hulka BS, Kerkvliet NL, Tugwell P. Experience of a scientific panel formed to advise the federal judiciary on silicone breast implants. *N Engl J Med* 2000;342(11):812–815.

28. Berger MA. Procedural paradigms for applying the Daubert test. *Minn Law Rev* 1994;78: 1345–1348.

29. Kaiser J. Project offers judges neutral science advice. *Science* 1999;284:1600.

APPENDIX 10.1 SILICONE BREAST-IMPLANT LITERATURE SEARCH STRATEGY

The following search strategies were used for searching the silicone breast-implant literature in MEDLINE for connective tissues diseases, including Raynaud's phenomenon, fibromyalgia, and classic rheumatologic diseases such as scleroderma, lupus, and rheumatoid arthritis. These strategies were then translated for searching in the following other databases: Current Contents, Health STAR, Biological Abstracts, CINAHL and Embase.

Set   Search 1:

1	breast implants/ or breast implantation/
2	(breast adj3 implant$).tw.
3	(breast adj3 (augmentation or reconstruction)).tw.
4	(breast adj3 prosthes#s).tw.
5	or/1-4
6	breast/
7	breast$.tw.
8	"prosthesis and implants"/
9	exp silicones/ or silicone$.tw,hw.
10	or/7-9
11	(5 or 6) and 10
12	exp mammaplasty/ or mammaplasty.tw.
13	surgery, plastic/
14	breast/su
15	or/12-14
16	(augment$ or implast$).tw.
17	(reconstruct$ or cosmetic or prosthes#s).tw.
18	15 and (16 or 17)
19	5 or 11 or 18
20	exp arthritis, rheumatoid/
21	(felty$ adj2 syndrome).tw.
22	(caplan$ adj2 syndrome).tw.
23	(rheumatoid nodule).tw.
24	(sjogren$ adj2 syndrome).tw.
25	(sicca adj2 syndrome).tw.
26	(still$ disease).tw.
27	(spondylitis adj2 ankylosing).tw.
28	(bechterew$ disease).tw.
29	(arthritis adj2 rheumat$).tw.
30	scleroderma, circumscribed/
31	((scleroderma adj localized) or progressive or diffuse or systemic),tw,
32	exp scleroderma, systemic/
33	((crest or crst) adj syndrome).tw.
34	morphea.tw,sh. or dermatosclerosis.tw.
35	sclerodacty$.tw.

36	exp calcinosis/ or calcinosis.tw.
37	exp esophageal motility disorders/
38	esophag$.tw.
39	ataxia telangiectasia/
40	telangiectasia, hereditary hemorrhagic/
41	telangiectasia.tw.
42	osler-rendu.tw.
43	louis-bar.tw.
44	raynaud's disease/ or raynaud$.tw.
45	exp lupus erythematosus, systemic/
46	(lupus adj (nephritis or erythematosus or disseminatus)).tw.
47	libman-sacks.tw.
48	antiphospholipid syndrome/
49	antiphospholipid.tw.
50	dermatomyositis/ or dermatomyositis.tw.
51	polymyositis/
52	myositis.tw,sh. or polymyositis.tw.
53	arthritis, psoriatic/
54	(psoriatic adj2 (arthrit$ or arthropathica)).tw.
55	exp vasculitis/
56	angiitis.tw.
57	vasculitis, allergic cutaneous/
58	vasculitis.tw,sh.
59	arteritis.tw.
60	(thrombophlebitis or phlebitis).tw.
61	thromboangiitis.tw.
62	(behcet$ or churg-strauss).tw.
63	wegener$.tw.
64	(mucocutaneous lymph).tw.
65	exp inflammatory bowel diseases/
66	ulcerative colitis.tw.
67	crohn$.tw.
68	(colitis or ileitis or enteritis).tw.
69	(rectocolitis or proctocolitis).tw.
70	inflammatory bowel.tw.
71	polychondritis, relapsing/
72	polychondritis.tw.
73	fibromyalgia/
74	(fibromyalgia or fibrositis).tw.
75	muscular rheumatism.tw.
76	fatigue syndrome, chronic/
77	(chronic fatigue).tw.
78	myalg$.tw.
79	encephalomyelitis.tw.
80	encephalomyelitis.tw.
81	or/20–80
82	81 and 19

Set   Search 2

1   breast implants/ or breast implantation/
2   (breast adj3 implant$).tw.
3   (breast adj3 (augmentation or reconstruction)).tw.
4   (breast adj3 prosthes#s).tw.
5   or/1-4
6   breast/
7   breast$.tw.
8   "prosthesis and implants"/
9   exp silicones/ or silicone$.tw,hw.
10   or/7-9
11   (5 or 6) and 10
12   exp mammaplasty/ or mammaplasty.tw.
13   surgery, plastic/
14   breast/su
15   or/12-14
16   (augment$ or implast$).tw.
17   (reconstruct$ or cosmetic or prosthes#s).tw.
18   15 and (16 or 17)
19   5 or 11 or 18
20   connective tissue diseases/
21   exp cartilage diseases/
22   cellulitis/
23   exp collagen diseases/
24   cutis laxa/
25   dupuytren's contracture/
26   homocystinuria/
27   marfan syndrome/
28   mixed connective tissue disease/
29   exp mucinoses/
30   neoplasms, connective tissue/
31   noonan syndrome/
32   osteopoikilosis/
33   exp panniculitis/
34   pseudoxanthoma elasticum/
35   mctd.tw.
36   (sharp syndrome).tw.
37   (human adjuvant).tw.
38   (mixed connective tissue).tw.
39   sclerosis-like.tw.
40   (fibrous banding).tw.
41   (skin thickening).tw.
42   arthralgia/
43   (arthralgia or polyarthralgia).tw.
44   or/20-43
45   19 and 44

Set   Search 3

1   breast implants/ or breast implantation/
2   (breast adj3 implant$).tw.
3   (breast adj3 (augmentation or reconstruction)).tw.
4   (breast adj3 prosthes#s).tw.
5   or/1–4
6   breast/
7   breast$.tw.
8   "prosthesis and implants"/
9   exp silicones/ or silicone$.tw,hw.
10   or/7–9
11   (5 or 6) and 10
12   exp mammaplasty/ or mammaplasty.tw.
13   surgery, plastic/
14   breast/su
15   or/12–14
16   (augment$ or implast$).tw.
17   (reconstruct$ or cosmetic or prosthes#s).tw.
18   15 and (16 or 17)
19   5 or 11 or 18
20   randomized controlled trial.pt.
21   controlled clinical trial.pt.
22   controlled clinical trials/
23   exp cross-sectional studies/
24   cross-sectional.tw.
25   prospective.tw.
26   retrospective.tw.
27   exp cohort studies/
28   exp case-control studies/
31   control$.tw. or random$.tw.
32   or/20–31
33   19 and 31
34   limit 33 to human

The following search strategies were used for searching the silicone breast-implant literature in the Toxline and Dissertation Abstracts databases.

Toxline Search

1   (breast implant$ or breast) and silicone$
2   exclude medline

Dissertation Abstracts

1   (breast implant$ or breast).tw.
2   silicone$.tw.
3   1 and 2

APPENDIX 10.2 GRADING OF OBSERVATIONAL STUDIES—NEWCASTLE-OTTAWA SCALE (23)

Case–Control Studies

Note: A study can be awarded a maximum of one star (signified by an asterisk) for each numbered item within the Selection and Exposure categories. A maximum of two stars can be given for Comparability.

Selection

1. Is the case definition adequate?
   a. yes, with independent validation *
   b. yes, e.g., record linkage or based on self reports
   c. no description
2. Representativeness of the cases
   a. consecutive or obviously representative series of cases *
   b. potential for selection biases or not stated
3. Selection of Controls
   a. community controls *
   b. hospital controls
   c. no description
4. Definition of Controls
   a. no history of connective tissue disease *
   b. no description of source

Comparability

1. Comparability of cases and controls on the basis of the design or analysis
   a. study controls for age *
   b. study controls for any additional factor *

Exposure

1. Ascertainment of exposure to breast implants
   a. secure record e.g., surgical records *
   b. structured interview where blind to case/control status *
   c. interview not blinded to case/control status
   d. written self report or medical record only
   e. no description
2. Same method of ascertainment of implants for cases and controls
   a. yes *
   b. no
3. Non-response rate
   a. same rate for both groups *
   b. non respondents described
   c. rate different and no designation

Cohort studies

Note: A study can be awarded a maximum of one star for each numbered item within the Selection and Outcome categories. A maximum of two stars can be given for Comparability

Selection

1. Representativeness of the exposed cohort
   a. truly representative of average women with implants in the community *
   b. somewhat representative of average women with implants in the community *
   c. selected group of users e.g., nurses, volunteers
   d. no description of the derivation of the cohort
2. Selection of the non exposed cohort
   a. drawn from the same community as the exposed cohort *
   b. drawn from a different source
   c. no description of the derivation of the non exposed cohort
3. Ascertainment of exposure to implants
   a. secure record e.g., surgical records *
   b. structured interview *
   c. written self report
   d. no description
4. Demonstration that outcome of interest was not present at start of study
   a. yes *
   b. no

Comparability

1. Comparability of cohorts on the basis of the design or analysis
   a. study controls for age *
   b. study controls for any additional factor *

Outcome

1. Assessment of outcome
   a. independent blind assessment *
   b. record linkage *
   c. self report
   d. no description
2. Was follow-up long enough for outcomes to occur?
   a. yes (5 + yrs) *
   b. no
3. Adequacy of follow up of cohorts
   a. complete follow-up—all subjects accounted for *
   b. subjects lost to follow-up unlikely to introduce bias (small number lost– >80% follow up or description of those lost) *
   c. follow-up rate <80% and no description of those lost
   d. no statement

GENERATING OUTCOME MEASUREMENTS, ESPECIALLY FOR QUALITY OF LIFE

Peter Tugwell and Gordon Guyatt

Chapter Outline

11.1 Measuring mortality
11.2 Laboratory measures
11.3 Health-related quality of life
11.4 Selecting measurement instruments

CLINICAL RESEARCH SCENARIO

The idea for OMERACT (the Outcome Measures in RheumAtology Clinical Trials) was conceived in 1989 when one of the authors (Peter Tugwell) and a colleague, Maarten Boers, were discussing what endpoints should be included in trials for rheumatoid arthritis. We concluded that, despite several conferences and meetings held from 1980 on the endpoints employed in rheumatology, clinical trials remained problematic.

Rheumatoid arthritis and other musculoskeletal disorders (such as osteoarthritis, osteoporosis, and lupus) have many clinical features, such as pain, swelling, and deformities of joints, but none of these individual features makes for a clear picture of the patient's clinical state. More than 30 clinical and laboratory measurements, such as erythrocyte sedimentation rate (ESR), had been used as "major endpoints" in published trials for rheumatoid arthritis, with a similar situation for osteoarthritis, lupus, and osteoporosis. Nevertheless, when we looked closely, the measures selected were often not comprehensive and yet showed considerable overlap, and many were insensitive to what otherwise appeared to be important changes in the clinical state of the patient. Opinions on the solution varied widely, with a "transatlantic" divide between the European and North American camps. The stalemate was impeding progress and hampering the development and testing of new treatments.

We decided to bring together the experts in the field from around the world, both clinicians and methodologists. We met in Maastricht, the Netherlands, under the auspices of appropriate international organizations in the area. The objective was to forge a consensus on the following: how to establish a minimum core set of measurements, the utility of pooling endpoints, and minimum important differences based on the available literature.

MACTAR PET (McMaster–Toronto Patient Elicitation Technique) was a product of this quest for better measures for rheumatologic disorders. Conventional generic and disease-specific health-related quality of life (HRQoL) questionnaires usually ask a standard set of questions that may or may not apply to a particular patient—some areas may be irrelevant and some relevant areas may not be included. Irrelevant questions create unwanted noise in the responses to such questionnaires and lack of questions in relevant areas have the potential to reduce responsiveness—the ability to detect all the important changes, even if they are small. Furthermore, identifying the most relevant concerns of the patient is important to reflect real-life clinical decision making, which focuses on issues that patients judge most important. These considerations stimulated Peter Tugwell and his colleague, Claire Bombardier, to develop and test a patient preference questionnaire for assessing disability in clinical trials by focusing only on those activities that the patient feels are both important and directly affected by the disease."

It is a truism that a study is only as good as its outcome. We deal with selection of measurements and the use of surrogate measurements extensively in other chapters, especially Chapter 5 (therapy) and Chapter 8 (diagnostic tests). We'll briefly review some of the same issues here, but only to set the stage for the main focus of this chapter, measures of "health-related quality of life."

11.1 MEASURING MORTALITY

Mortality is a legitimate outcome in studies in which it is the dominant concern (e.g., in septic shock). Measuring mortality is seldom a problem unless you lose patients to follow-up, which should not happen if you have designed and executed your study well. However, unless the mortality rate is high (such as in an intensive care unit or with certain cancers), only the largest trials have the option of using mortality as the primary outcome measure.

The intended outcome of most studies is the improvement of health, ideally to a state of optimal physical, mental, and social well-being (1). Further, in industrialized countries, only one third of the burden from disease is due to mortality and two thirds is due to physical, mental, and social disability (2). Although the inverse is true in low- and middle-income countries, a third of the burden of disease in these domains is still due to the impact on well-being. Thus, we require appropriate outcome measures for those medical interventions that are designed to improve well-being in addition to, or instead of, extending the duration of the patient's life. This is certainly true for musculoskeletal disease trials described in the opening scenario for this chapter.

11.2 LABORATORY MEASURES

Laboratory changes that predict benefit or harm are often used as "surrogate endpoints" to substitute for clinical endpoints when too large a sample size or too long a patient follow-up is needed to assess treatment effects on mortality or morbidity. Benefit can be determined by an increase in levels of biomarkers such as CD4 cell count for AIDS morbidity and mortality, or by a decrease, for example, in blood cholesterol for cardiovascular disease or in blood pressure for stroke.

A necessary but not sufficient requirement for using a surrogate measure is that its values are known to be strongly related to a clinical outcome of interest. Bone mineral density (BMD) is often used in trials of osteoporosis prevention. However, although it is reasonably accurate in predicting the risk of subsequent fracture in the absence of therapy, the increase in BMD seen with therapy does not translate well into fracture reduction with efficacious agents such as bisphosphonates. Indeed, with fluoride, despite an increase in BMD, the fracture risk is actually increased! In fact, changes in bone density bear essentially no relation to the magnitude of reductions in the risk of non-vertebral fractures with antiosteoporosis therapy (3). Because of such problems, the number of surrogate endpoints accepted by regulatory agencies for drug approval has been increasingly restricted. In the United States, at the time of writing, surrogates were limited to blood pressure, low-density lipoprotein (LDL) cholesterol, and hemoglobin A_{1c}.

Investigators may over-interpret and pharmaceutical companies may inappropriately market changes in surrogate outcomes, targeting clinicians whose training emphasizes "mechanisms," and by omitting health outcomes as the criterion for assessing the effects of interventions (4,5,6). Surrogate biomarkers are also commonly used for assessing harm, for example, serum transaminases for liver toxicity, serum creatinine for renal toxicity, electrocardiographs for cardiotoxicity. The justification for including these biomarkers is that many trials are powered only for detecting a relatively frequent beneficial outcome, and the resulting sample size is much too small to detect side effects whose frequency is expected to be lower than the event rate for the outcomes assessing benefit.

A salutary lesson of the dangers of surrogate outcomes to assess harm was provided by the use of endoscopic ulcers as a surrogate for clinically important gastrointestinal (GI) events in pivotal trials of nonsteroidal antiinflammatory drugs (NSAIDs). For more than 30 years endoscopic ulcers were routinely used as the surrogate outcome for clinically serious events. A landmark study in the 1990s showed that the proportion of endoscopic ulcers that ever became clinically symptomatic is as low as 15% (7).

This issue of surrogate outcomes is a complex area that we will not address comprehensively here. If you wish to decide whether it is justifiable to use surrogate outcomes, look for a systematic review of observational studies of the relation between the surrogate outcome and the target clinical outcome, along with a review of randomized trials that have evaluated the impact upon both the surrogate and the clinical outcome. Our view is that surrogates should not be used in the absence of sound evidence of a strong relation between a putative surrogate and a clinically important outcome. Without such evidence, changes in surrogate outcomes should be viewed as "hypothesis-generating signals" for further formal testing (8). See also the section on surrogate markers in Chapter 5, on therapy.

11.3 HEALTH-RELATED QUALITY OF LIFE

Of the many measurement options available to clinical researchers, well-being is perhaps closest to the mark for what is important to patients. Because well-being is a complex concept or attribute, its definition has been the subject of great debate (9–13). It is variably interpreted as HRQoL or function. Fitzpatrick and colleagues distinguish "global definitions" from "component definitions" (14). Global definitions express well-being in general terms such as global judgments of health or satisfaction with life, whereas component definitions break the concept into specific parts or dimensions (14). They have proposed the following classification of components: physical function, symptoms, psychological well-being, social well-being, cognitive functioning, role activities, personal constructs (i.e., life satisfaction, stigmata, and spirituality), and satisfaction with care. Investigators have suggested different subsets based on the general public's views, consensus conferences, content, and factor analysis.

Measurement of well-being poses challenges that are not found in other areas of measurement. One of these challenges arises because quite different instruments may be needed for measuring differences between individuals at a point in time versus changes within individuals over time. The latter is required for clinical trials. The first type of instrument asks questions such as: who, at this point, has better quality of life, and whose quality of life is not so good? The technical term for such measures is "discriminative instruments." The second type of instruments asks: who has improved more, who has improved less, and who has deteriorated? The technical term for these measures is "evaluative instruments."

Consider a possible item on a questionnaire concerning quality of life: are you physically and mentally able to work outside the home? Such a question is central to discriminating between those with superior and those with inferior quality of life. However, if you are designing an instrument as an outcome measure for use in trials of rehabilitation for chronic disease, the question is liable to be useless. The reason is that, for many rehabilitation programs, the goals are more modest, and few, if any, patients ever return to work. Thus, this item would be critical for a discriminative instrument but readily rejected for an evaluative measure.

11.4 SELECTING MEASUREMENT INSTRUMENTS

"Measurement instrument" is a commonly used term that originated in clinical medicine and originally referred to physical measuring devices such as the stethoscope and sphygmomanometer. Nowadays, measurement instruments include questionnaires as well, calibrated to predict or detect diagnosis, prognosis, or clinical responsiveness.

Although it is always tempting to "build a better mousetrap" and design your own outcome instrument (15), this makes it difficult to compare results with other studies or clinical practice and challenging to use meta-analytic techniques to pool across studies that rely on a variety of instruments. Thus, groups such as OMERACT urge investigators to use a common set of "core" measures to facilitate comparison (and, if appropriate, pooling) across studies. These core measures can, of course, be supplemented by the additional measures favored by the investigators in a specific study.

Whether you use an existing measure or plan to develop a new one, your protocol should address nine questions in its section describing your study's outcome instrument(s):

1. What is the research question?
2. What methods of searching for studies of relevance were used?
3. Are all relevant dimensions of the morbidity or mortality outcome included?
4. Was the method of selecting individual items for inclusion appropriate?
5. Are the items measured in a sensible way?
6. Is the measurement responsive enough to detect clinically important changes or new events?
7. Does your measurement approach include a search for adverse effects?
8. Is the format appropriate for your study (i.e., type of administration and time)?
9. Are the results interpretable by clinicians, patients, and policymakers?

What Is the Research Question?

For our studies of rheumatoid arthritis, we needed to address the following question:

> Which outcome measures should be included as a core set in trials of interventions for patients with rheumatoid arthritis when testing a new monotherapy or a combination of disease-modifying agents.

What Methods of Searching for Original Articles Were Used?

> In 1989, when planning the initial OMERACT conference, we spent considerable time retrieving and reviewing published articles in the rheumatology literature that addressed outcomes used in clinical trials of interventions in patients with rheumatoid arthritis. At that time,

good search strategies for outcomes had not been developed, and details of many of the outcome instruments were found in the references in the reports of the clinical trials. We also contacted investigators in the field and did unsystematic searches in databases such as MEDLINE. We identified 33 outcome measures (see Table 11–1).

TABLE 11–1 OMERACT Outcome Measurements[a]

AIMS–overall assessment
AIMS–physical function scale
AIMS–psychological status scale
American Rheumatism Association (ARA) Remission
Arthritis Impact Measurement Scales (AIMS)–Pain scale
C-reactive protein (European)
Disease Activity Score (DAS)
Erythrocyte sedimentation rate
Grip strength
Haataja
Health Activity Questionnaire (HAQ) (disability)
Hemoglobin
Lansbury
Lee
Mallya
McMaster–Toronto Patient Preference Function Questionnaire (MACTAR)
Morning stiffness
Pain (Visual Analog Scale)
Patient global
Paulus
Physician global
Platelets
Pooled
Proximal Inter Phalangeal joint (PIP) circumference
Riel
Ritchie Score
Scott
Stoke
Swollen joint count
Swollen joint score
Tender joint count
Tender joint score
Walk time

[a]Readers interested in the details of these and current measures should consult the OMERACT Web site at *http://www.jrheum.com/omeract/1-5toc.html.*

TABLE 11-2 Search Strategy for Retrieving Studies of Quality-of-life Measurement Instruments from MEDLINE[a]

1. (health assessment question$ or HAQ).tw.
2. (medical outcomes study).tw.
3. (health utilit$ index).tw.
4. (health adj2 quality life).tw.
5. Quality of Life/
6. (quality life or value life).tw.
7. 5 or 6
8. (scale or scales or question$ or outcome or measur$ or instrument$).tw.
9. Questionnaires/
10. 8 or 9
11. 7 and 10
12. or /1-4
13. 11 or 12
14. exp rheumatoid arthritis/
15. 14 and 15

[a]The terms with a backslash (/) are Medical Subject Heading (MeSH) terms. MeSH is the indexing system used by MEDLINE. The terms with .tw. after them are textwords. The textword function searches the title (TI) and abstract (AB) fields. This is done when a MeSH term is not available or to be more thorough in the searching. When searching for textwords where prefix, suffix or other such variations need to be taken into account, you may truncate the term you are searching by adding the truncation symbol ($) to the end of the word (i.e., question$ will also search for question, questions, questionnaire, questionnaires etc.).

In 1989, we knew most of the researchers in the field and searched by using the references in articles we had accumulated in our personal collections. The standards for systematic reviews have improved a great deal since then. If we were to do this again, we would use the MEDLINE search strategy suggested by our librarian colleague Jessie McGowan (see Table 11-2).

If we had done this search, we would have found that the following additional endpoints had been published in Index Medicus cited journals before 1989: Sickness Impact Profile (16), Index of Well-being (17), Functional Status index (18), Convery Polyarticular Disability Index (19), and Toronto Questionnaire (20).

Are All Relevant Dimensions of the Morbidity or Mortality Outcome Included (Comprehensiveness/Content Validity)?

Investigators must identify the spectrum of intended and unintended outcomes they need to monitor. Different subsets of these have been advocated based upon elicitation of the views on dimensionality of the general public, consensus conferences, content, and factor analysis.

OMERACT had to address the fact that when we started in 1989 the Food and Drug Administration (FDA) in the United States relied on joint counts (tender and swollen joints), sedimentation rate, and physicians' global assessments in pivotal trials of new drugs in rheumatic diseases and did not accept the inclusion of patient-based outcomes. For OMERACT, background papers reviewing the dimensions were developed and circulated beforehand. At the first OMERACT meeting, voting was conducted as to which dimensions should constitute a minimal core set of outcomes. Participants registered their preferences using voting pads. In addition to the expected physical signs and laboratory tests, in contrast to their exclusion from the regulator's criteria the following 'patient reported outcomes' [PRO's] were given high rankings: physical disability, pain, and patient global assessment. Table 11–3 shows the rank order of the votes.

TABLE 11–3 Summary of Voting on Efficacy Endpoints (21)

Endpoints Vote		
Final (after nominal group process)	First (at the beginning of the conference)	Measure
9.1	8.9	Swollen joints
9.0	8.5	Physical disability (patient report)
8.6	8.2	Pain
8.2	8.3	Tender joints
8.1	5.8	Radiographs
8.0	7.7	Patient global
7.3	6.8	Acute-phase reactants
4.3	5.9	Physician global
3.3	5.5	Psychosocial (patient report)
2.9	4.9	Patient preference
2.0	3.9	Grip strength
2.0	3.3	Extraarticular disease
1.2	1.7	Synovial tissue
0.7	4.2	Morning stiffness

From Tugwell P, Boers M, OMERACT Committee. Developing consensus on preliminary core efficacy endpoints for rheumatoid arthritis clinical trials. *J Rheumatol* 1993;20: 555–556, with permission.

At the sixth and seventh OMERACT meetings we included a patient group for the first time (22). They reviewed the dimensions in the current core set and identified fatigue and sleep as important omissions.

The OMERACT example has so far focused upon detecting benefits of interventions. In selecting outcomes, equal attention needs to be paid to detecting adverse effects. Where the intervention is known to cause side effects, or if the intervention is designed to reduce the side effects of another agent (e.g., misoprostol to protect against the GI inflammation and ulceration caused by NSAIDs that are commonly prescribed for pain relief for patients with arthritis), then investigators must include these domains in the designated outcome measures.

It is also important to look for unexpected adverse outcomes. The occurrence of unexpected side effects is quite common and we must continue to look for methods that would better identify unexpected events such as thalidomide phocomelia, benoxyprofen hepatorenal disease, ACE-inhibitor angioneurotic edema, indomethacin dementia, indomethacin hip, remicade infections, etanercept demyelinating disease, ibuprofen aseptic meningitis, mycophenolate mofetil gout, and increased cardiovascular events with rofecoxib.

The current approach for detecting adverse drug reactions (ADRs) is rudimentary. Regulatory agencies endorse a number of standardized instruments for assessing ADRs in clinical trials of pharmacological and biological agents (e.g., the COSTART system developed by the US FDA; *http://www.ntis.gov/search/product.asp?ABBR=PB95269023&starDB= GRAHIST*). These ensure that both expected and unexpected effects are recorded, but as we will discuss in the section on responsiveness in the subsequent text, most studies are grossly underpowered to document low-frequency but important ADRs.

Was the Method of Selecting Items for Inclusion Appropriate?

In the mid 1980s, while planning new studies in rheumatoid arthritis, we found that the item selection for existing instruments was based on a variety of statistical approaches; these often reflected the frequency of the occurrence of a reduction in physical, social, and emotional functioning but did not explicitly address the importance to the individual patient. We therefore interviewed 50 patients with rheumatoid arthritis. We did this in groups of 10 patients until we obtained no new information. As is shown in Table 11–4, those items most important to patients showed substantial variation across patients.

Many of these items important to patients were not included in the most commonly used questionnaires. We then developed a standardized approach based on goal attainment scaling (24), resulting in the MACTAR (M[A]Cmaster Toronto ARrthritis) Patient Preference Function questionnaire, and a subsequent version, the MACTAR Problem Elicitation Technique (PET). The questionnaire asks patients to describe the specific ways in which the arthritis affects their daily life and then to rank them in order and, in the PET version, to also rate on a visual analog scale (VAS) the importance of each item. These rankings and VAS results are used to weight the disability scores.

TABLE 11-4 **Activities Affected by Arthritis According to Patients (23)**

Disability	Ranking of Importance				
	Ranked First	Ranked 1-2	Ranked 1-3	Ranked 1-5	Not Ranked Among First Five Activities
Walking	14	18	20	29	21
Housework	6	8	11	12	38
Cooking	5	6	9	12	38
Sewing	1	2	7	10	40
Gardening	0	1	3	8	42
Working	3	3	4	6	44
Going to church	0	1	2	6	44
Golfing	2	4	5	6	44
Driving	2	2	4	6	44
Climbing stairs	1	4	4	6	44

From Tugwell P, Bombardier C, Buchanan WW, et al. The MACTAR patient preference disability questionnaire–an individualized functional priority approach for assessing improvement in physical disability in clinical trials in rheumatoid arthritis. *J Rheumatol* 1987;14:446-451, with permission.

GG used a similar approach in a study examining HRQoL in patients recruited from a secondary-care respiratory clinic. Following a literature review, 100 patients identified which of 123 preselected items were problems for them and indicated how important those items were (25). When we found that the activities associated with problematic dyspnea were extremely diverse, we chose an "individualized question" approach to measuring day-to-day dyspnea. The questionnaire emerging from the item reduction process asks patients to identify five important activities in which they experience dyspnea and then monitors the extent of their shortness of breath while performing these five activities (26).

Conventional questionnaires ask a standard set of questions that may or may not apply to a particular patient. Where items are irrelevant, this creates unwanted noise in the responses; where items that assess important areas are missing, this reduces responsiveness and the ability to discriminate between patients. Outcome measures and their component items should reflect areas that are important to patients suffering from the disease of interest. For morbidity, this should be derived from what patients say about how the illness affects their lives. For example, for a patient who is a carpenter, manual strength and dexterity are essential for livelihood; although these attributes would be important to anyone, mild impairment could pose much less difficulty for someone involved in sales or teaching.

Having individual items differ between patients needn't cause problems in analysis and interpretation as long as you are measuring the same underlying construct in each patient and your goal is to measure changes within people over time (called "evaluation" in the technical terms we have introduced). As it happens, we are never measuring exactly the same thing for every patient in quality-of-life measures. For instance, if we ask about dyspnea climbing stairs, each patient is thinking about a different set of stairs. If we ask about difficulty doing housework, patients have different burdens of housework about which they are thinking. So as long as we are measuring the same construct (shortness of breath in daily living, for instance) in each patient over time (say, before and after an intervention), it matters little that the individual items differ from patient to patient.

If your goal is measuring differences between individuals at one point in time (called "discrimination" in the technical language we've introduced), the situation is more problematic. MACTAR and the dyspnea domain of the Chronic Respiratory Questionnaire (CRQ) were designed for evaluative and not for discriminative purposes. A chapter in the Users' Guides to the Medical Literature, and the references cited there, provide a more detailed discussion of the properties needed for discriminative and evaluative instruments (27).

If the item selection instrument yields many more items than can be included in the final questionnaire, it is necessary to select a subset. Again, there are many statistical techniques for this, including sophisticated ones such as principal component analysis (*http://www.epa.gov/bioindicators/primer/pca.html*), but we would argue that the approach should at least incorporate the number of patients who listed the item as a problem (item frequency), the importance attached to the items by the patients, and (if your primary purpose is measuring within-person change over time) the potential responsiveness of the items (the ability to detect change if it is present).

We have concentrated on "disease-specific" questionnaires that focus on patients with musculoskeletal and respiratory conditions. Where it is important to be able to compare results across conditions, you need to include a "generic" questionnaire. By definition, generic questionnaires include a broad array of items that will detect overall change in health. We commonly include both a disease-specific and a generic questionnaire to be sure to detect minimally important changes in items specific to the disease with the former and overall changes in the latter. The most widely used generic instrument is the Short-Form-36 Health Survey (SF 36), which despite its title has performed remarkably well in clinical trials (28–32). The items were drawn from an original 245-item questionnaire used in a study by the Rand Corporation in the 1970s to compare the impact of alternative health insurance systems on health status and utilization. The conceptual approach covers both mental and physical concepts, including behavioral functioning, perceived well-being, social and role disability, and personal evaluations in general. The last item is intended to capture the impact of health problems not directly included in the other questions. Scoring is complex and requires automated software. This includes presenting the results of the set of eight scales (Physical Functioning, Role Limitations–Physical, Role Limitations–Emotional, Pain, Social Functioning, Mental Health, Vitality, and General Health Perceptions) or two component scores (Physical and Mental), leading to a score between 0 and 100 with perfect health being 100. The SF 36 has been extensively validated in many populations with many conditions and in different languages; it has been shown to be responsive in a number of musculoskeletal conditions (19). The SF 36 can be self-administered or used in personal or telephone interviews.

The SF 36 has many variants, including a number of shorter instruments such as the SF 20 and SF 12, that reduce the load on the respondent. These tend to become too narrow in focus and have not been shown to perform as well, so we would recommend using the 36-item version.

Are the Items Measured in a Sensible Way?

The key elements that need to be considered that affect whether the items selected for an instrument are "sensible" include how well items are worded for patients, how specific the items are, how simple or complex they are, the time span they cover, the type of scale, and how they are scored.

The credibility or face validity of the measure should be assessed by obtaining a copy of the measure/questionnaire and by reviewing it carefully to assess the following. First, if patients are to be asked to respond, is the item phrased in "plain language" so that the patient will understand? A small sample of patients of different ages and education levels should be interviewed to determine if the item meets this requirement.

Second, how specific are the questions? Does the questionnaire ask only general questions at a dimension level (such as limitation in physical function) or at a subdimensional level (such as limitation in self-care or a particular component such as limitation in dressing, or does it detail individual behavioral activity within a component such as difficulty in buttoning shirts)? It is important to note that an individual can have difficulty in specific behavioral activities (e.g., doing buttons) but have no limitations in her ability to dress because of aids, adaptation, or modified clothing.

Third, how complex are the questions? "Doing up buttons" is a question on the commonly used Health Assessment Questionnaire that focuses on fine movements of the hands; compare this with "difficulty in dressing," which includes many more movements (33).

Fourth, does each question refer to a specific period appropriate for the particular intervention? Without reminders describing the baseline state, 1 to 2 weeks is as long as most people can be expected to recall for most quality-of-life measures. In our 6-month cyclosporine studies using the MACTAR, we reminded patients of what they said at baseline and asked them if their difficulty with each specific important function had improved, stayed the same, or worsened. This still implies that they could remember their state 6 months ago well enough to be able to judge whether they had improved or deteriorated, an assumption that one could question (34).

Fifth, is the scale appropriate in the type and number of the response categories? The detail in scaling of a question is an important predictor of its responsiveness/sensitivity to change. A dichotomous response [yes/no] is likely to be less responsive than a more detailed scale such as a Visual Analogue Scale or multiple categories such as (a) No difficulty, (b) Some difficulty, (c) Much difficulty, (d) Cannot do. The reason for this is that patients can reliably discriminate change in smaller "chunks" than four categories, although probably not beyond seven categories (35). Indeed, seven categories is a popular choice of number, with some empirical support (36).

Sixth, are the responses to individual questions aggregated into a summary score? The combination of items into a global score or index is a subject of much controversy. Some authors simply add up the scores for individual questions, whereas others have designed systems of weighting individual questions before adding them up. Some use Guttman scaling, which implies unidimensional scales, whereas others use factor analysis, principal component analysis, or discriminant analysis. For the American College of Rheumatology (ACR) composite endpoint that was derived from the OMERACT core set (joint counts, pain, ESR, disability, patient global, clinician global), it was decided to combine the items into a single score to avoid the problem of multiple major outcomes and also to allow the clinician to understand the calculation of the score (37).

Using the above core set of outcome measures for RA trials (the reduced set of most preferred measures, derived from the initial candidates in Table 11–1), 40 different definitions of improvement were tested, using a three-step process. First, we performed a survey of rheumatologists, using actual patient cases from trials, to evaluate which definitions corresponded best to rheumatologists' impressions of improvement, eliminating most candidate definitions of improvement. Second, we tested 20 remaining definitions to determine which maximally discriminated effective treatment from placebo treatment and also minimized placebo response rates. With eight candidate definitions of improvement remaining, we tested to see which were easiest to use and were best in accord with rheumatologists' impressions of improvement. The following definition of improvement was selected: 20% improvement in tender and swollen joint counts and 20% improvement in three of the five remaining ACR core set measures: patient and physician global assessments, pain, disability, and an acute-phase reactant. Additional validation of this definition was carried out in a comparative trial, and the results suggested that the definition is statistically powerful and does not identify a large percentage of placebo-treated patients as having improved.

Is the Measurement Responsive Enough to Detect Clinically Important Changes or New Events?

For the OMERACT core set, responsiveness was assessed in three ways. To begin, a consensus exercise was performed at the first OMERACT conference using a Latin square design (38). We presented different small groups, each with a cross-sectional representation of the different disciplines attending the OMERACT conference, with different magnitudes of relative change in each of the measures in the proposed core set and asked them to assess which ones were important in the context of a new therapy for patients with rheumatoid arthritis. The resulting estimates of important relative change were 19% for tender joint counts, 15% for swollen joint counts, 21% for pain, 18% for disability, and 25% for ESR.

Second, a large dataset of the National Institutes of Health–funded Collaborative Studies consortium was analyzed using a series of different cut-points for the individual components to identify what difference best discriminated between active drug and placebo (37). The best discrimination was achieved with a 20% improvement in each of these items.

Third, the approach developed by Redelmeier was applied (39). Each of 40 patients with different levels of severity of rheumatoid arthritis was assessed using the preliminary core set. Then, the patients were asked to discuss their arthritis with three other patients for 5 minutes each. At the end of each discussion the patient was asked to decide if their severity was greater, the same, or worse than the patient with whom they had just been talking. This again gave estimates close to 20% for important relative differences in the preliminary core set.

Although a 20% change in someone with minimal problems is a smaller absolute change than in someone with severe problems, these estimates of approximately 20% were remarkably stable in this study across different levels of severity and in further testing of the relative efficiencies of each of the components and the core set to confirm the responsiveness of both (24,40–42).

This summary score, that is, percentage of patients who achieve an overall relative score increase of 20%, is the same adopted by the ACR and is commonly referred to as the ACR20. On the basis of this the US FDA guidelines now require the ACR20 to be assessed as a major outcome in pivotal trials of new agents for rheumatoid arthritis.

The ACR20 assesses the minimum important difference. Some clinicians are also interested in "major" improvement, and data on responsiveness and sample size is also available now for larger changes such as the ACR50 and ACR70. ACR20, 50, and 70 findings are usually presented as the proportion of patients who responded in the experimental group, compared with the proportion who responded in the control group (CG), for example, 55% of the intervention group (IG) and 27% of the CG achieved an ACR20 response (i.e., a 20 percentage point response in 5 of the 7 components of the ACR Score), whereas 22% of the IG and 9% of the CG showed an ACR50 response.

Typically, clinicians' enthusiasm for intervening decreases progressively as they see results presented in terms of relative risk reduction, absolute risk reduction, or the number needed to treat (NNT), the inverse of absolute risk reduction) (43). The importance of identifying the minimally important difference (MID) and the achievement of a minimal disease activity state in absolute terms, and a research plan to estimate this, was endorsed at the OMERACT 6 meeting in 2002 (44). Reporting absolute change, the number needed to treat (NNT), and number needed to harm (NNH) are being encouraged in presenting the clinical results of Cochrane Reviews in musculoskeletal disease (45).

The usefulness of an outcome measure depends on its responsiveness, that is, its ability to detect important changes even if the changes are small. Responsiveness is proportional to the change in score that constitutes an important difference (the "signal" that the instrument is trying to detect) and is inversely proportional to the variability in score in stable patients (this is the noise, which makes the signal difficult to detect). The ratio of the MID (or if that is unavailable, the change produced by a treatment of known benefit) to the within-subject variability in stable patients is directly related to sample size requirements and is one of the most useful indexes of the responsiveness of an outcome measure (46).

It is possible to check out how the responsiveness of the instrument chosen ranks against other published instruments. One of us (Gordon Guyatt) worked as part of a team that conducted a systematic review evaluating the relative responsiveness of generic- and disease-specific questionnaires by pooling effect sizes across studies (47). Although there were instances in which generic instruments appeared as responsive as specific ones, in the overall analysis the disease/condition-specific questionnaires proved more responsive than general or generic questionnaires.

Other ways of establishing the MID include:

1. Relate changes in outcome measures to better known existing measures of function (e.g., for cardiorespiratory problems, the New York Heart Association classification) or clinical diagnosis (such as the change in score needed to move individuals in or out of the diagnostic category of depression) (48).

2. Relate changes in outcome measures to patients' global ratings of the magnitude of change they have experienced (49); we have used this approach for the MACTAR, too (23).

3. Use an approach based on item response theory that essentially describes the status of individuals with a particular score according to their likely status on a number of easily interpreted questionnaire items (50).

Does Your Measurement Approach Include a Search for Adverse Effects?

Although pharmacoepidemiology has long assessed adverse consequences of interventions by increased mortality, the responsiveness of outcome measures designed to detect important increases in adverse effects has not received the same attention as those outcomes intended to assess benefit.

The statistical planning of clinical trials is usually aimed at investigating efficacy rather than safety because the intention is to develop beneficial therapies. The mechanism of action of a drug, or adverse reactions seen among similar drugs ("class effect"), may guide the monitoring of adverse events in a trial, and common adverse effects will often be detected during early phase clinical trials. However, it is difficult to plan for unexpected events, especially ones that are rare and difficult to detect.

The VIGOR (VIOXX GI Clinical Outcomes Research) study (51) has provided some insights into this issue. This was a patient- and clinician-blinded randomized controlled trial in which 8,076 patients with rheumatoid arthritis were enrolled. The study was designed to assess whether rofecoxib resulted in fewer clinically important upper gastrointestinal (GI) adverse events than a NSAID, naproxen. An important difference in NNH was found for the primary outcome of symptomatic upper GI ulcers and the secondary outcome of ulcer complications (*Perforations, *Pyloric *Obstruction, clinical *Bleeds–known as POBs) in favor of rofecoxib. Unexpectedly, it was discovered that the incidence of myocardial infarction (MI) in the VIGOR study was much higher in the rofecoxib group. Initially it was unclear whether this was due to an increased rate from the new drug, rofecoxib, or due to a cardio-protective effect of the comparator drug, naproxen. The drug was subsequently withdrawn by the company in 2004 after they found that further placebo-controlled trials confirmed this cardiovascular toxicity 'signal.' However, following a public outcry from the 'pain epidemic' resulting from its withdrawal, in 2005 first the FDA in the US, and shortly afterwards Canada's Federal Ministry of Health, held public hearings that pointed out that the 83% increase in the relative risk over the baseline risk 1.2 per 100 per year in low-risk adults over 65 only translated to an absolute increase of mostly non-fatal myocardial infarctions of 1 per 100 per year (*http://decisionaid.ohri.ca/nsaid.html*). This led to both agencies recommending the reintroduction of rofecoxib with a 'black box warning' of the cardiovascular risk.

Current regulatory guidelines are not designed to capture unexpected side effects. Assessment of adverse events in these "coxib" trials again follows a parallel logic of focusing primarily on the known GI adverse events of NSAIDs; indeed a reduction in these is the major putative advantage of the coxibs. At one time, endoscopy was used widely as the surrogate outcome for clinically serious events such as bleeding. The Misoprostol Ulcer Complication Outcomes Safety Assessment (MUCOSA) study showed, however, how inaccurate the computed estimates of clinical GI events were when based upon endoscopic ulcers (7). This resulted in a loss of credibility for the perforation, ulcer, and bleeding (PUB) index because this largely reflected the endoscopic ulcer frequency that grossly overestimates the clinical impact.

The finding of an unexpected increase in cardiovascular events in the rofecoxib arm of the VIGOR study (51,52) has some troubling implications. First, should all future coxib studies be powered to detect cardiovascular differences? Table 11–5 shows that sample sizes of 20,000 to 80,000 would be needed to show this in populations without high-risk

TABLE 11–5   Number of Patients Needed to Detect a 50% Relative Increase in the Proportion of Patients Experiencing the Outcome of Interest (53)

Endpoint	Control Rate (%)	Sample Size for a 50% Relative Difference
Benefit		
ACR20	29	171
GI Toxicity		
GI events	3.15	2,400
Ulcers (U)	3.0	2,500
Bleeds (B)	0.9	9,000
Perforations (P)	0.1	78,000
Obstructions (O)	0.0	—
PUB (P + U + B) (VIGOR study)	4.0	1,900
PUB (P + U + B) (CLASS study)	1.8	4,000
POB (P + O + B) (VIGOR study)	1.0	8,000
POB (P + O + B) (CLASS study)	0.55	14,000
CV events		
CV (patients not on aspirin)	0.4	20,000
Myocardial infarction only	0.1	80,000
Hypertension	0.8	10,000
Composite outcome		
(P + O + B + CV + Hypertension)	2.1	3,000

GI, gastrointestinal; CV, cardiovascular.

From Tugwell P, Judd M, Fries J, et al. Powering our way to the elusive effect: proposal to include a "basket" of predefined designated endpoints in each organ system in all controlled trials. *J Clin Epidemiol (in press)*, with permission.

groups. Is this a "wake-up call" that argues strongly for including endpoints that will detect such an increase in unexpected events in any of the major organ systems? This magnifies the sample size requirements even further. We need to think seriously about options that will substantially improve the likelihood that such increases will be detected.

Vital information concerning rare, serious adverse events will be obtained only after a large number of exposures to the drug. A reasonable chance of detecting these side effects will often not arise within a study of drug efficacy but in postmarketing surveillance studies, or Phase IV clinical trials that are simpler in design and that involve more patients. Further, prospective cohort studies, in which investigators follow a number of patients over time and those taking the drug are compared to those not taking the drug, are beginning to be required by regulatory agencies for new classes of interventions, for example, for anti–tumor necrosis factor (anti-TNF) biological agents. Although not a clinical trial, one may have to rely on such datasets to provide a reasonable chance for rare serious events to be detected if they arise. Sophisticated analysis is needed to control for potential confounding variables that may be associated with the decision of the patient to take the medication. Such techniques, of course, can only go so far; residual confounding will remain a possibility.

Using Table 11–5, let's look at how further expanding composite outcomes could help increase the responsiveness of outcome assessment for both expected and unexpected adverse effects (54,55). By virtue of increasing the event rate by combining events, fewer patients are required to detect a specified relative treatment effect (say 50%). A doubling of the base rate requires one third to one fourth as many patients (Furburg C. Personal communication, 2001.). The POB index is one such composite outcome using one organ system. Composite outcomes have also included more diverse content including: mortality and morbidity (MI, stroke, and death) (56); invasive breast cancer, coronary heart disease, stroke, and pulmonary embolism (57); cancer recurrence or death (58,59); and various presentations in different organ systems of thrombosis, bleeding, and anaphylaxis (60). So one option for coxib studies would be to combine thromboembolic complications such as acute MI, unstable angina, sudden death, thrombotic strokes, and pulmonary embolism, because they are all vascular events, in a composite endpoint with POB.

The greater the variability in underlying pathogenesis, however, the more questionable the composite. A composite limited to arterial atheroembolic events, and another to events in the venous circulation, would have greater internal cohesion. The OMERACT ACR core set (tender and swollen joint counts, patient and physician global assessments, pain, functional assessment, and a measure of acute-phase reactant) combines different outcomes for efficacy (61), although the purpose is not to increase the number of events but to capture all aspects of a construct (disease severity/functional consequences) that clinicians believe strongly are so biologically related they are ready to call them aspects of the same thing.

As can be seen in Table 11–5 if we combine cardiovascular endpoints such as MI, angina, heart failure, and hypertension in a composite outcome with POB, the sample size reduces dramatically to well within the study sample size. In view of the importance of detecting unforeseen important effects, this could logically be taken further to designate serious endpoints in each organ system and to agree on an inclusion frequency criterion such as 1% greater in the experimental group than in the CG. If the nominal P value is not adjusted for multiple comparisons, the sensitivity increases, as does the number of false positives. Thus, it should be used as a secondary rather than a primary outcome, that is, to raise hypotheses rather than to test them. Indeed, there are several limitations to creating composite endpoints to detect adverse effects (including the possibility that sample size might be increased rather than decreased and that the approach will generate many false positives), as we will return to in the discussion about Figure 11–1A and B in the subsequent text.

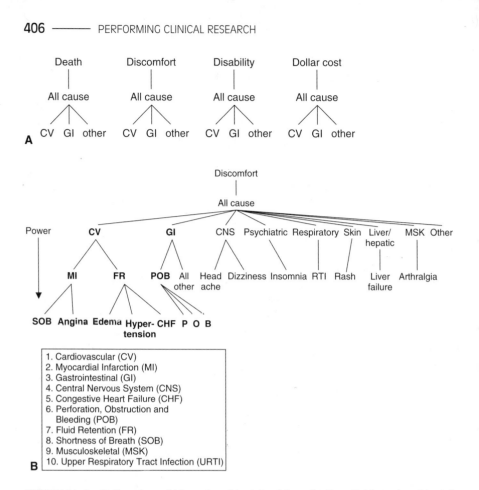

FIGURE 11–1 A: Overview of hierarchy of toxicity data collection; **B:** hierarchy of toxicity data collection for discomfort (53). (From Tugwell P, Judd M, Fries J, et al. Powering our way to the elusive effect: proposal to include a "basket" of predefined designated endpoints in each organ system in all controlled trials. *J Clin Epidemiol (in press)*, with permission.)

The "basket" depicted in Figure 11–1 presents a hierarchical approach to presenting safety information in a way that is meaningful to the decision making of physicians or patients. First, it provides an overall evaluation of the basket (Figure 11–1A), providing a general indicator of what is happening. Second, the endpoints in the basket would then be assessed using appropriate descriptive statistics for the frequency of their occurrence according to a hierarchical scheme (Figure 11–1B). Here we have very high power for the top levels and decreasing but reasonable power for the middle levels, and, finally, use descriptive statistics for the lowest levels. Third, an estimate of the probability of the occurrence of the various endpoints would eventually be determined through the analysis of large databases so that the estimates can be based on large number of patients from a wide population group.

We need to be very careful in how we construct our basket of side effects in organs. POB works because all three are complications of NSAID ulcers. If we add gastroenteritis and appendicitis, we do not gain power just because we have a larger basket. With cardiovascular events, we might look at a full index, but if there is no effect on arrhythmias or aneurysms, then including them will not increase our power to detect cardiovascular events. Indeed, the sample size will rise because of the extra "noise" created by including the noncontributing elements of arrhythmias and aneurysms. In the coxib area, a cluster of MI-related events such as MI death, nonfatal MI, and angina can increase power while maintaining a particular mechanism—that of thrombosis. Another cluster, which combines fatal and non-fatal events, might be edema, hypertension, and congestive heart failure; this would speak to a fluid retention effect. Thus, we need the all-cause and all-single-organ-cause "alarm" systems for the unexpected, but we need groupings of problems with putatively common mechanisms to preserve some power.

There are several disadvantages to composite outcomes, including: if the endpoints are not related, then statistical noise is added that may obscure the real outcome differences; if patients can experience several endpoints, it is important to properly and fully use all the information; if the endpoints are not equally important, too small a sample size may result for the more important but rarer endpoints; differences in importance of endpoints also raises problems with the interpretation of any differences found; it is still not possible to detect statistical significance of individual endpoints; and the composite outcome could be the same in each group but with important differences in different endpoints. Concerns have also been raised that use of composite outcomes tempts investigators to extend the range of fishing that is inevitable in looking at adverse events, creating multiple constellations of events that, without adjustment for multiple comparisons, result in lots of spurious associations (62,63).

Is the Format Appropriate for Your Study?

Feasibility needs to be the final check when deciding which outcomes to include. Patient questionnaires requiring more than 1 hour to complete often need to be broken into more than one session. Once selected, the outcome instrument needs to be pre-tested. Investigators should pay careful attention to incomplete responses in this test phase to identify difficulties with comprehension, layout, method of delivery, cultural or sensitive personal issues, and so on (8).

Are the Results Interpretable by Clinicians, Patients, and Policymakers?

Note that the OMERACT approach assesses the improvement in proportions of individual patients, that is, as discrete measures. Commonly, results of outcomes are presented as means of all patients, that is, as continuous measures. Means are potentially misleading for specifying MIDs in interventions because they hide the distribution of responses—clinicians who assume that each individual who experiences the mean effect are liable to make flawed clinical decisions. Depending on the distribution of the individual differences, the same mean difference can have very different implications. For example, if the MID for disability is 20% and a study showed a mean improvement of 15%, this might mean that all the patients improved by approximately 15%, so that none of them achieved the minimum important difference. It could also mean that half the patients improved by a much larger amount—for example, 30%—and the other half didn't improve at all. If this were the case, clinicians would find the important improvement in half the patients of vital interest. We therefore suggest for individual-based therapies that the MID be established as described in preceding text. Investigators conducting clinical trials should then calculate the proportion of patients who achieved this MID (64,65).

It is being increasingly appreciated that although this is the best approach for individual-focused care, a complementary strategy may aid in communicating the magnitude of an effect of a population-focused intervention to those responsible for making decisions on community interventions (e.g., public health clinicians and health policy makers). For example, a change in mean blood pressure in a population of a magnitude that would be trivial in an individual (e.g., 2 mm Hg) would translate into a large reduction in the number of strokes in a population. In this case, you are classifying patients into risk groups within a population and the clinical significance requires an estimate of the change in risk across the population to which the individual belongs, with the caveat that there must be appropriate checking that reducing the risk does indeed translate into the amplified reduction in clinical events. Again, the principle is the same as for the NNT approach: a naïve interpretation of the mean difference may lead to an underestimation of the impact of the intervention because a proportion of individuals may be much more responsive.

CONCLUSION

Given that the development and validation of measures for well-being are complex and challenging, why should we bother? What matters to patients should count foremost in our studies, especially when their afflictions cause nonfatal miseries and incapacities. Although we have guided you through many details of the process for rheumatoid arthritis, we haven't taken you through all the details of doing original research to develop and validate outcome measures (although we've cited many good examples of such research along the way). We've cautioned against contributing to the profusion of HRQoL instruments by developing another; if it's absolutely necessary, you'll need to consult other texts to complement what we've presented here.

We conclude with this admonition from Lord Kelvin (of Kelvin thermometer fame) (66): "I often say that when you can measure what you are speaking about and express it in numbers you know something about it; but when you cannot measure it, when you cannot express it in numbers, your knowledge is of a meager and unsatisfactory kind: it may be the beginning of knowledge, but you have scarcely, in your thoughts, advanced to the stage of science, whatever the matter may be." In other words, if you can't measure it, you can't study it–a mantra of quantitative methods. The authors of this book are quantitative researchers–you will note that a limitation is the absence of a chapter on qualitative research–and so pay ready deference to this mantra. When you are contemplating doing your own research and have formulated a question, an excellent next step is to determine whether there are valid and feasible methods for measuring the outcomes in which you are interested. If you suspect not, think at least twice–with the large number of quality-of-life instruments now available, you may well be able to find a satisfactory, if not perfect, measure. If after due consideration you still conclude that a satisfactory measurement instrument is not available, then you have two choices: scale back your question based on available outcome measures or develop and validate your own outcome measures before you begin the study. The latter will set back your schedule for testing interventions in the short-term–but it is essential to progress. One way to proceed is to test the intervention with available outcome measures and also include in the study a validation component for some measures that you have reason to believe will capture the outcomes you most wanted to measure. With good planning, that approach won't greatly increase the cost of your project and will put you in a better position for your next investigation.

REFERENCES

1. Preamble to the Constitution of the World Health Organization as adopted by the International Health Conference, New York, 19–22 June, 1946; signed on 22 July 1946 by the representatives of 61 States (Official records of the World Health Organization, no. 2, p. 100) and entered into force on 7 April 1948. New York: 1948.

2. Murray C, Lopez A. The Global Burden of Disease A comprehensive assessment of mortality and disability from diseases, injuries, and risk factors in 1990 and projected to 2020. Boston, MA: World Health Organization, Harvard School of Public Health, World Bank, 1996.

3. Guyatt GH, Cranney A, Griffith L, et al. Summary of meta-analyses of therapies for postmenopausal osteoporosis and the relationship between bone density and fractures. *Endocrinol Metab Clin North Am* 2002;31:659–679.

4. Furberg CD, Herrington DM, Psaty BM. Are drugs within a class interchangeable? *Lancet* 1999;354:1202–1204.

5. Sobel BE, Furberg CD. Surrogates, semantics, and sensible public policy. *Circulation* 1997;95:1661–1663.

6. Psaty BM, Weiss NS, Furberg CD, et al. Surrogate end points, health outcomes, and the drug-approval process for the treatment of risk factors for cardiovascular disease. *JAMA* 1999;282:786–790.

7. Silverstein FE, Graham DY, Senior JR, et al. Misoprostol reduces serious gastrointestinal complications in patients with rheumatoid arthritis receiving nonsteroidal anti-inflammatory drugs. A randomized, double-blind, placebo-controlled trial. *Ann Intern Med* 1995;123:241–249.

8. Bucher H, Guyatt G, Cook D, et al. Surrogate outcomes. In: Guyatt G, Rennie D, eds. *Users' guides to the medical literature: A manual for evidence-based clinical practice.* Chicago, IL: AMA Press, 2002.

9. Spitzer WO. State of science 1986: quality of life and functional status as target variables for research. *J Chronic Dis* 1987;40:465–471.

10. Bergner M. Quality of life, health status, and clinical research. *Med Care* 1989; 27(Suppl. 3):S148–S156.

11. Patrick DL, Erickson P. Assessing health-related quality of life for clinical decision-making. In: Walker SR, Rosser R, eds. *Quality of life assessment*, Key issues in the 1990's. Dordrecht: Kluwer Academic Publishers, 1993:11–63.

12. McDaniel RW, Bach CA. Quality of life: a concept analysis. Rehabilitation. *Nursing Research* 1994;3:18–22.

13. McDowell I, Newell C. *Measuring Health: a guide to rating scales and questionnaires*, 2nd ed. New York: Oxford University Press, 1996.

14. Fitzpatrick R, Davey C, Buxton MJ, et al. Evaluating patient-based outcome measures for use in clinical trials. *Health Technol Assess* 1998:2:i–iv, 1–74.

15. Liang MH, Cullen K, Larson M. In search of a more perfect mousetrap (health status or quality of life instrument). *J Rheumatol* 1982;9:775–779.

16. Bergner M, Bobbitt RA, Pollard WE, et al. The sickness impact profile: validation of a health status measure. *Med Care* 1976;14:57–67.

17. Fanshel S, Bush JW. A health status index and its application to health services outcome. *Operation Research* 1970;18:1021–1066.

18. Jette AM. Functional Status Index: Reliability of a chronic disease evaluation instrument. *Archives of Physical Medicine and Rehabilitation* 1980;61:395–401.

19. Convery FR, Minteer MA, Amiel D, et al. Polyarticular disability: a functional assessment. *Arch Phys Med Rehabil* 1977;58:494–499.

20. Helewa A, Goldsmith CH, Smythe HA. Independent measurement of functional capacity in rheumatoid arthritis. *J Rheumatol* 1982;9:794–797.

21. Tugwell P, Boers M, OMERACT Committee. Developing consensus on preliminary core efficacy endpoints for rheumatoid arthritis clinical trials. *J Rheumatol* 1993;20:555–556.

22. Kirwan J, Heiberg T, Hewlett S, et al. Outcomes from the patient perspective workshop at OMERACT 6. *J Rheumatol* 2003;30:868–872.

23. Tugwell P, Bombardier C, Buchanan WW, et al. The MACTAR patient preference disability questionnaire—an individualized functional priority approach for assessing improvement in physical disability in clinical trials in rheumatoid arthritis. *J Rheumatol* 1987;14:446–451.

24. Buchbinder R, Bombardier C, Yeung M, et al. Which outcome measures should be used in rheumatoid arthritis clinical trials? Clinical and quality-of-life measures' responsiveness to treatment in a randomized controlled trial. *Arthritis Rheum* 1995;38:1568–1580.

25. Guyatt GH, Townsend M, Berman LB, et al. Quality of life in patients with chronic airflow limitation. *Br J Dis Chest* 1987;81:45–54.

26. Guyatt GH, Berman LB, Townsend M, et al. A measure of quality of life for clinical trials in chronic lung disease. *Thorax* 1987;42:773–778.

27. Guyatt GH, Naylor CD, Juniper EL, et al. Quality of Life. *JAMA* 1997;277:1232–1237; Guyatt G, Rennie D. *Users' guides to the medical literature: A manual for evidence-based clinical practice.* Chicago, IL: AMA Press, 2002.

28. Ware JE, Sherbourne CD Jr. The MOS 36-item short-form health survey (SF-36). I. Conceptual framework and item selection. *Med Care* 1992;30:473–483.

29. Katz JN, Larson MG, Phillips CB, et al. Comparative measurement sensitivity of short and longer health status instruments. *Med Care* 1992;30:917–925.

30. Jenkinson C, Coulter A, Wright L. Short form 36 (SF 36) health survey questionnaire: normative data for adults of working age. *BMJ* 1993;306:1437–1440.

31. Jenkinson C, Wright L, Coulter A. *Quality of life measurement in health care: a review of measures and population norms for the UK SF-36.* Oxford: Health Services Research Unit, University of Oxford, 1993.

32. Ware JE, Jr., Kosinski M, Keller SD. *SF-36 physical and mental health summary scores: a user's manual.* Boston, MA: The Health Institute, New England Medical Center, 1994.

33. Fries JF. Toward an understanding of patient outcome measurement. *Arthritis Rheum* 1983;26:697–704.

34. Guyatt GH, Norman GR, Juniper EF, et al. A critical look at transition ratings. *J Clin Epidemiol* 2002;55:900–908.

35. Streiner DL, Norman GR. *Health measurement scales: a practical guide to their development and use,* 3rd ed. New York: Oxford University Press, 2003.

36. Jaeschke R, Singer J, Guyatt GH. A comparison of seven-point and visual analogue scales: data from a randomized trial. *Controlled Clinical Trials* 1990;11:43–51.

37. Felson DT, Anderson JJ, Boers M et al, American College of Rheumatology. Preliminary definition of improvement in rheumatoid arthritis. *Arthritis Rheum* 1995; 38:727–735.

38. Box GEP, Hunter WG, Hunter SJ. *Statistics for experimenters.* New York: John Wiley & Sons, Inc, 1978.

39. Redelmeier DA, Goldstein RS, Guyatt GH. Assessing the minimal important difference in symptoms: a comparison of two techniques. *J Clin Epid* 1996;49:1215–1219.

40. Wells G, Boers M, Shea B et al, International League of Associations for Rheumatology. Sensitivity to change of generic quality of life instruments in patients with rheumatoid arthritis: preliminary findings in the generic health OMERACT study. OMERACT/ILAR Task Force on Generic Quality of Life. Life Outcome Measures in Rheumatology. *J Rheumatol* 1999;26:217–221.

41. Tugwell P, Wells G, Strand V et al, Leflunomide Rheumatoid Arthritis Investigators Group. Clinical improvement as reflected in measures of function and health-related quality of life following treatment with leflunomide compared with methotrexate in patients with rheumatoid arthritis: sensitivity and relative efficiency to detect a treatment effect in a twelve-month, placebo-controlled trial. *Arthritis Rheum* 2000;43:506–514.

42. Ortiz Z, Shea B, Garcia DM, et al. The responsiveness of generic quality of life instruments in rheumatic diseases. A systematic review of randomized controlled trials. *J Rheumatol* 1999;26:210–216.

43. Jaeschke R, Guyatt G, Barratt A, et al. Measures of Association. In: Guyatt G, Rennie D, eds. *User's guides to the medical literature: A manual for evidence-based clinical practice.* Chicago, IL: AMA Press, 2002.

44. Wells G, Anderson J, Boers M, et al. MCID/Low Disease Activity State Workshop: summary, recommendations, and research agenda. *J Rheumatol* 2003;30(5):1115–1118.

45. Osiri M, Suarez-Almazor ME, Wells GA, et al. Number needed to treat (NNT): implication in rheumatology clinical practice. *Ann Rheum Dis* 2003;62:316–321.

46. Guyatt G, Walter S, Norman G. Measuring change over time: assessing the usefulness of evaluative instruments. *J Chronic Dis* 1987;40(2):171–178.

47. Wiebe S, Guyatt G, Weaver B, et al. Comparative responsiveness of generic and specific quality-of-life instruments. *J Clin Epidemiol* 2003;56(1):52–60.

48. Testa MA, Simonson DC. Assessment of quality-of-life outcomes. *N Engl J Med* 1996;334:835–840.

49. Juniper EF, Guyatt GH, Willan A, et al. Determining a minimal important change in a disease-specific quality of life questionnaire. *J Clin Epidemiol* 1994;47(1):81–87.

50. Valderas JM, Alonso J, Prieto L, et al. Content-based interpretation aids for health-related quality of life measures in clinical practice. An example for the visual function index (VF-14). *Qual Life Res* 2004;13(1):35–44.

51. Bombardier C, Laine L, Reicin A et al. VIGOR Study Group. Comparison of upper gastrointestinal toxicity of rofecoxib and naproxen in patients with rheumatoid arthritis. *N Engl J Med* 2000;343(21):1520–1528.

52. Boers M. NSAIDS and selective COX-2 inhibitors: competition between gastroprotection and cardioprotection. *Lancet* 2001;357:1222–1223.

53. Tugwell P, Judd M, Fries J, et al. Powering our way to the elusive effect: proposal to include a "basket" of predefined designated endpoints in each organ system in all controlled trials. *J Clin Epidemiol (in press)*.

54. Cannon CP. Clinical perspectives on the use of composite endpoints. *Control Clin Trials* 1997;18(6):517–529.

55. Cannon CP, Sharis PJ, Schweiger MJ, et al. Prospective validation of a composite end point in thrombolytic trials of acute myocardial infarction (TIMI 4 and 5). Thrombosis in myocardial infarction. *Am J Cardiol* 1997;80:696–699.

56. Cook NR, Hebert PR, Manson JE, et al. Self-selected posttrial aspirin use and subsequent cardiovascular disease and mortality in the physicians' health study. *Arch Intern Med* 2000;160:921–928.

57. Writing Group for the Women's Health Initiative Investigators. Risks and benefits of estrogen plus progestin in healthy postmenopausal women principal results from the women's health initiative randomized controlled trial. *JAMA* 2002;288(3):321–333.

58. Beck RW, Chandler DL, Cole SR, et al. Interferon beta-1a for early multiple sclerosis: CHAMPS trial subgroup analyses. *Ann Neurol* 2002;51:481–490.

59. Blute ML, Bostwick DG, Seay TM, et al. Pathologic classification of prostate carcinoma: the impact of margin status. *Cancer* 1998;82:902–908.

60. Cannon CP, Sharis PJ, Schweiger MJ, et al. Prospective validation of a composite end point in thrombolytic trials of acute myocardial infarction (TIMI 4 and 5). Thrombosis In Myocardial Infarction. *Am J Cardiol* 1997;80:696–699.

61. Felson DT, Anderson JJ, Boers M, et al, The Committee on Outcome Measures in Rheumatoid Arthritis Clinical Trials. The American College of Rheumatology preliminary core set of disease activity measures for rheumatoid arthritis clinical trials. *Arthritis Rheum* 1993;36:729–740.

62. Freemantle N, Calvert M, Wood J, et al. Composite outcomes in randomized trials: greater precision but with greater uncertainty? *JAMA* 2003;289(19):2554–2559.

63. Montori VM, Permanyer-Miralda G, Ferreira-Gonzalez I, et al. Validity of composite end points in clinical trials. *BMJ*. 2005 Mar 12;330(7491):594–6.

64. Guyatt GH, Juniper EF, Walter SD, et al. Interpreting treatment effects in randomised trials. *BMJ* 1998;316:690–693.

65. Guyatt GH, Osoba D, Wu AW, et al. Methods to explain the clinical significance of health status measures. *Mayo Clin Proc* 2002;77:371–383.

66. Lord Kelvin. Electrical units of measurement, 1883 viewed August 20, 2004 at *http://www.rasch.org/rmt/rmt143c.htm*.

Becoming a Clinical Researcher

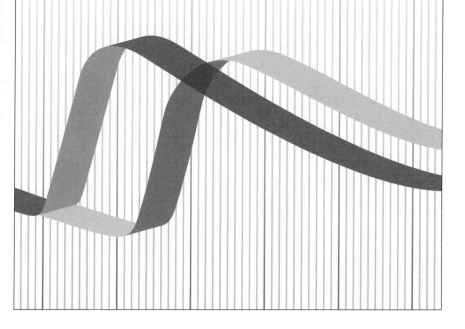

BECOMING A SUCCESSFUL CLINICIAN-INVESTIGATOR

Dave Sackett

I wrote this section with both the mentors and the mentored in mind. However, my primary target is the reader who is being mentored, whom I will call "you." I hope it will also help mentors (whom I will call "they") identify their duties and evaluate their effectiveness.

I think that the determinants of your "academic success" as a clinician–investigator (defined in terms of principal investigatorship, lead authorship, promotion, tenure, career awards, honors, power, and reputation) are not "academic" (defined in terms of intelligence, theoretic understanding, mastery of a body of knowledge, and teaching skills) (1,2). Some clinician–investigators fail because they are crazy. Others fail because they lack minds that are "prepared" to generate important questions based on their clinical observations. However, the range of their intelligence is so compressed at the top of the scale that, even if it were an important determinant, attempts to correlate it with success are doomed. Furthermore, academic failure is common to both those who do and those who don't understand the theory and know the facts, and among those who are and aren't excellent teachers. The ability to generate novel, imaginative hypotheses does play a role in the academic success of basic researchers. However, this rarely applies in patient-based and clinical-practice (3) research (where the hypotheses are usually common knowledge and often originate with patients). Finally, I'm confident that none of you will seriously argue that being a nice person is a prerequisite for academic success.

What, then, are the determinants of your academic success as a clinician–investigator? I've concluded that they are three: mentoring, creating periodic priority lists, and time management. However, the evidence supporting my conclusions is of shaky validity. Most of it is based on a Level 4 case-series (4) of young academics I've mentored and to whom I've taught priority lists and time management. I've also repeated Level 2b cohort observations of individuals who did and didn't receive mentoring or employ time management. In addition, I've made several Level 3b case–control observations of academics who clearly were and were not successful.

A literature search provided some confirmation for my conclusions, but no higher levels of evidence. Applying the Medical Subject Headings

(MeSH) terms MENTORS (510 hits) and TIME MANAGEMENT (901 hits) didn't turn up any Level 1 evidence, but the Level 2 to 4 evidence I encountered there (5–13) supports my thesis. I also found important evidence on the experiences and perceptions of women in medicine (14,15). A final note of caution: most of the clinician scientists I've mentored and observed in the United States, Canada, and the United Kingdom have been hospital-based internists. If you and your mentor are from another health discipline, you will have to decide whether and where the conclusions and recommendations I make in this section apply to you.

12.1 MENTORING

Mentoring is vital to your success as an academic clinician. For example, graduates of US-style primary care internal medicine research fellowship programs were five times more likely to publish at least one paper and were three times more likely to be principal investigators (PIs) on a funded research grant if they had an "influential mentor" during their fellowship (16). Effective mentoring is of two sorts, depending on whether you are a newcomer or an established academic. For newcomers (such as graduate students or new faculty), mentoring provides four advantages. First, it provides *resources* without obligations. Second, it provides *opportunities* without demands. Third, it provides *protection*. Fourth, it provides *advice* without coercion. I hope it's already obvious (and I'll reinforce this point later) that it requires an already successful and secure academic to provide this sort of mentoring.

By *resources*, I mean that a really good mentor would provide you with:

- space to work
- productivity-enhancing equipment
- free photocopy, e-mail, and Internet
- occasional secretarial support
- money to attend courses and meetings
- salary supplements if your fellowship doesn't provide for necessities and simple graces and
- bridge funding your research until you get your first grant.

In some departments, all or most of these resources are provided by the chair, and in others, none. In either setting, your mentor should "wheel and deal" until the resources are in place. You should be spared both the time and the humiliation of begging for these resources on your own.

By *opportunities* at the beginner's level, I mean the systematic examination of everything that crosses your mentor's desk for its potential contribution to your scientific development and academic advancement:

1. The opportunity to join one of your mentor's ongoing research projects. This can provide more than just "hands-on" practical experience in the application of your graduate course content. You can also learn how to create and function as a member of a collaborative team and to develop skills in research management.

Taking on a piece of your mentor's project to run, analyze, present, and publish is a two-edged sword. On the one hand, it provides an excellent opportunity to go beyond the classroom and develop your practical skills in data management and analysis. Moreover, it gives you the opportunity to start to learn how to combine "science and showbiz" in presenting your results and writing for publication, and your CV will benefit.

On the other hand, being given a project by your mentor can be harmful. The greatest risk here is that your mentor might "give" you a predesigned substudy or research project and encourage you to use it as your major (e.g., thesis) learning focus. Although often done with the best intention, accepting this "gift" is bad for you because taking on a predesigned project robs you of the opportunity to develop your most important research skills. First, you'll lose the opportunity to learn how to recognize and define a problem in human biology or clinical care. Second, you'll lose the opportunity to learn how to convert that problem recognition into a question that is both important and answerable. Third, you'll lose the opportunity to learn how to select the most appropriate study architecture to answer your question. Fourth, you'll lose the opportunity to identify and overcome the dozens of "threats to validity" that occur in any study. These four skills are central to your development as an independent investigator. Without these skills, you'll master only the methods that are required for your "given" project. Like the kid who received a shiny new birthday hammer, you'll risk spending the rest of your career looking at ever less important nails to pound with your same old limited set of skills.

2. The opportunity to carry out duplicate, blind (and, of course, confidential) refereeing of manuscripts and grants. The comparison of these critiques not only sharpens your critical appraisal skills but also permits you to see your mentor's refereeing style and forces you to develop your own.

3. The opportunity to accompany your mentor to meetings of ethics and grant-review committees to learn firsthand how these groups function.

4. The opportunity, as soon as your competency permits, to join your mentor in responding to invitations from prominent, refereed journals to write editorials, commentaries, or essays. Not only will the joint review and synthesis of the relevant evidence be highly educational but it will also provide you the opportunity to learn how to write with clarity and style (see Chapter 16, on preparing reports for publication.). Finally, it will add an important publication to your CV. As soon as your contribution warrants, you should become the lead author of such pieces. The ultimate objective is for you to become the sole author (all the sooner if your mentor casts a wide shadow).

One note of caution about invited chapters for books: unless the book is a very prestigious one, its authorship adds little or no weight to your CV.

5. The opportunity to take over some of your mentor's invitations and to learn how to give "boilerplate" lectures (especially at nice venues and for generous honoraria).

6. Your inclusion in the social as well as academic events that comprise the visit of colleagues from other institutions.

7. The opportunity to go as part of a group to scientific meetings, especially annual gatherings of the research clan. This has several advantages. First, it gives you the chance to meet and hear the old farts in your field. Second, it allows you to meet and debate with the other newcomers who will become your future colleagues. Third, you can compare your impressions and new ideas with your mentor while they are fresh, in a relaxed and congenial atmosphere.

   Another note of caution: spending time going to meetings carries risks as well as benefits, as I'll describe under time-management at the end of this section.

8. The opportunity to observe, model, and discuss teaching strategies and tactics in both clinical and classroom situations. When you are invited to join your mentor's clinical team, you can study how they employ different teaching strategies and tactics as they move from the post-take/morning report, to the daily review round, to the clinical skills session, to grand rounds. With time, you should take over these sessions and receive feedback about your performance. The same sequence should be followed in teaching courses and leading seminars in research methods.

As you become an independent investigator, your opportunities mature and incorporate two additional areas. First, your mentor should start nominating you to more advanced opportunities for increasing your academic experience, networking, and recognition. Examples here include scientific committees (e.g., grant-review committees), task forces (e.g., for the development of methodological standards or evidence-based guidelines), and symposia (especially those that can result in first-authored publications). Second, your mentor should start nominating you for academic posts, writing letters of support, and counseling you as you negotiate space, support staff, rank, and salary. Finally, your mentor should continue to be available for discussions of your triumphs and troubles and for letters of support as you proceed through the various stages of academic development, promotion, and tenure.

It is important that these opportunities are offered without coercion and are accepted without resentment. Crucially, they must never involve the off-loading of odious tasks with little or no academic content from overburdened mentors to the beholden mentored.

By *advice*, I mean providing frequent, unhurried, and safe opportunities for you to think your way through both your academic and social development. Topics here include your choices of graduate courses, the methodological challenges in your research projects, the pros and cons of working with a particular set of collaborators, and how to balance your career with the rest of your life. For example, some mentors refuse to discuss academic issues at such sessions until they have gone through a checklist of items encompassing personal and family health, relationships, finances, and the like. Their advice should take the form of "active listening," should focus on your development as an independent thinker, and should eschew commands and authoritarian pronouncements.

As long as gender-based inequalities exist in running households and raising children, mentors must be knowledgeable and effective in addressing and advising about the special problems that women face in academic careers (17). Although in one study only 20% of female academics stated that it was important to have a mentor of the same gender (14), it is imperative that all women pursuing academic careers have easy access to discussing and receiving informed, empathic advice about issues such as timing their pregnancies, parental leave, time-out, part-time appointments, sharing and delegating household tasks, and the like. When the principal mentor is a man, these needs are often best met by specific additional mentoring around these issues from a woman.

I'll discuss your mentor's role in helping you evaluate your "priority list" and time management strategies later in this chapter.

When listening to you sort through a job offer, it is important for your mentor to help you recognize the crucial difference between "wanting to be wanted for" and "wanting to do" a prestigious academic post. You'd be crazy not to feel elated at "being wanted for" any prestigious job, regardless of whether it matched your career objectives and academic strengths. However, an "actively listening" mentor can help you decide whether you really "want to do" the work involved in that post. It is here that they may help you realize that a post is ill matched to your interests, priorities, career stage, competencies, or temperament.

By *protection*, I mean insulating you from needless academic buffeting and from the bad behavior of other academics. Because science advances through the vigorous debate of ideas, designs, data, and conclusions, you should get used to having yours subjected to keen and critical scrutiny. For the same reason, you needn't be tossed in at the deep end. Thus, for example, you should rehearse formal presentations of your research in front of your mentor (and whoever else is around). They can challenge your every statement and slide in a relaxed and supportive setting. As a result (especially in these days of PowerPoint), you can revise your presentation and rehearse your responses to the likely questions that will be asked about it. The objective here is to face the toughest, most critical questions about your work for the first time at a rehearsal among friends, not following its formal presentation among rivals and strangers.

Similarly, your mentor can help you recognize the real objectives of the critical letters to the editor that follow your first publication of your work. Most of them are attempts to show off (the "peacock phenomenon"), to protect turf, and to win at rhetoric, rather than to promote understanding. When serious scientists have questions about a paper, they write to its authors, not to the editor. Your mentors also can help you learn how to write responses that repeat your main message, answer substantive questions (if any), and ignore the tawdry slurs that your detractors attempt to pass off as harmless wit.

Finally, disputes between senior investigators often are fought over the corpses of their graduate students. This means you. Your mentor must intervene swiftly and decisively whenever they detect such attacks on you, especially those related to your sex, race, gender, or sexual orientation. The intention of your tutor's rapid retaliation needn't be to overcome your attacker's underlying prejudice or jealousy. It should merely make the repercussions of picking on you so unpleasant for him that he never tries it again. If it wasn't already part of your core training, a study of the classic paper on "how to swim with sharks" should be part of this exercise (18).

I don't believe that academics ever outgrow their need for mentoring. As you become an established investigator, you'll require gentle confrontation about whether you are becoming a recognized "expert" and taking on the bad habits that inevitably accompany that state (19). Moreover, given the huge number of highly prestigious but simply awful chairs and deanships that are pressed upon even unsuccessful academics, these offers need the dispassionate (even cynical) eye of a mentor who can help you distinguish the golden opportunities from the black holes. Finally, mentors can help senior academics find the courage to seize opportunities for radical but fulfilling and even useful changes in the directions of their careers. For example, I am ever indebted to my then mentor Bill Spaulding, who helped me confirm the sense, and then find the courage, to repeat my internal medicine residency shortly before my fiftieth birthday.

What should you look for when picking a mentor (or in sizing up the one to whom you've been assigned)? I think your mentor should possess six crucial prerequisites:

1. Your mentor has to be a competent scientist. Although most mentors will be clinicians as well, this needn't be the case. Some of the most successful academic clinicians I know (including me) were mentored by biostatisticians.

2. Your mentor must not only have achieved academic success themselves, but must also treat you accordingly. That is, your mentor must feel secure enough about their own academic success that they are not only comfortable taking a back seat to you in matters of authorship and recognition. They must actively pursue this secondary role. Everything fails if your mentor competes with you for recognition. Unfortunately, such competition is common, and you should seek help from your chair or program director if this happens to you (I devote lots of time to trying to resolve such conflicts before they destroy friendships and damage careers).

3. Your mentor should not directly control your academic appointment or base salary. Such controls interfere with the free and open exchange of ideas, priorities, aspirations, and criticisms. For example,

you may find it difficult to turn down an irrelevant, time-consuming task offered by your mentor if they also control your salary.

4. Your mentor must like mentoring and must be willing to devote the time and energy required to do it well. This includes a willingness to explore and solve both the routine and the extraordinary scientific and personal challenges that arise when they take on this responsibility.

5. Some institutions still lack policies for stopping the tenure clock for childbirth and caring for a young child, or for "re-entry" rights and discounted "resume gaps." Your mentor should be informed about these, and she should fight for these rights when they are lacking.

6. Finally, your mentor must periodically seek feedback from you about how well they are performing. They must periodically evaluate their own performance, decide whether they remain the best person to mentor you, and identify ways to improve their mentoring skills.

Do the benefits of mentoring flow just one way, or do mentors benefit as well? A qualitative study of Faculty Advisors in Maryland identified several benefits of being a mentor (20):

- An enhanced academic reputation from spotting and developing highly talented young people.
- The development of a dependable junior colleague.
- The satisfaction of repaying a past debt owed to their own mentors.
- The thrill and pride of seeing a protégé succeed.
- The enjoyment and excitement of taking partial credit for the protégé's success.

12.2 MAKING AND UPDATING YOUR "PRIORITY LIST"

You should start making and updating your "priority list" as soon as you gain the smallest degree of control over your day-to-day activities and destiny. This control might start the day you take up your first faculty appointment, or maybe after your successful thesis defence. Updating, discussing, and acting on this list will be central to your academic success throughout the rest of your career. You should review and update this list at least every 6 months, and more often if needed. Discussion of this list is a key element of the mentoring process. For established academics, your mentor need no longer be a senior colleague; indeed, the most effective mentoring I'm receiving in the twilight of my career comes from younger colleagues.

Making, updating, and following your priority list is trivially simple in format, dreadfully difficult in execution, and vital to both your academic success and happiness. The list has four elements:

List 1: Things you're doing now that you want to *quit.*

List 1a: Things you've just been asked to do that you want to *refuse* to do.

List 2: Things you're not doing that you want to *start* doing.

List 3: Things you're doing that you want to *keep doing*.

List 4: Strategies for *improving the balance* within your lists by shortening List 1 (*want to quit*) and by lengthening List 2 (*want to start*) over the next 6 months.

Note that the entries on this list are about *doing* (things like research, clinical practice, teaching, and writing). They are not about *having* (things like space, titles, rank, or income). Note, too, that there are no "cop-out" entries for "things you *have* to do." These "have-to-do" entries must be thought through until they can be allocated to either List 1 (*want to quit or refuse*) or List 3 (*want to keep doing*).

You can generate Lists 1 (*want to quit or refuse*) and 3 (*want to keep doing*) by reviewing your diary for the period since your last update. List 1a (*want to refuse*) comes from your mail and from recalled conversations with bosses or colleagues who were attempting to transform their problems into your problems.

List 2 (*want to start*) is more exciting. It comes from multiple sources:

- the next research question that logically follows the answer to your last one
- ideas that arise from successes and failures with your patients
- brainstorms that occur while reading, or during conversations with colleagues
- ideas that are formed during trips to meetings or other research centers
- inspirations that arise in reading other people's research in depth and with a critical eye
- long-held aspirations that are now within reach
- job offers
- changes in life goals or personal relationships
- and so on.

Contemplating the length and content of List 3 (*want to keep doing*) enables self-diagnosis and insight. If it's long, is it comfortable but complacent, stifling further growth? Worse yet, is it the list of an expert, comprising the tasks required to protect and extend your personal "turf" in ways that are leading you to commit the "sins of expertness?" (19)

The next, crucial step is to titrate Lists 2 (*want to start*) and 3 (*want to keep doing*) against List 1 (*want to quit or refuse*). Academic and personal disaster results from a dislocation between what you are doing and what is expected of you. This dislocation is inevitable when you fail to stop doing enough old things on List 1 (*want to quit or refuse*) to make it possible to pursue List 2 (*want to start*) while keeping up with List 3 (*want to continue*).

Dislocation and its sequelae are not new, and their causes have been acknowledged for decades. The special vulnerability of clinicians was reported over 20 years ago when they were already experiencing the constant pressure of trying to provide more and better patient care with resources that had already begun to diminish (21).

For "time-imbalanced" clinician–scientists, there are two outcomes. First, you can work day and night, keep up, and trade your family, friends, and emotional well-being for a reputation as a "world-class" academician. Second, regardless of whether you work day and night, you can fall behind and gain a reputation as a "nonfinisher." Either way, you increase your risk of slipping into emotional exhaustion, cynicism, feeling clinically ineffective, and developing a sense of depersonalization in dealing with patients, colleagues, and family (22). The term "burnout" has been applied to the resulting deterioration of values, dignity, spirit, and will. This process can start early in your career (even during your training), can take years to become full-blown, but by then has a poor prognosis in terms of ever gaining career satisfaction or personal well-being.

Making and updating lists has two goals, then. One is the prevention of burnout. The other is the realization of a set of research, teaching, and clinical activities that would make it fun to go to work.

All the foregoing leads to List 4, a tactical plan for *improving the balance* within your lists by terminating entries in Lists 1 (*want to quit or refuse*) and having more time for Lists 2 (*want to start*) and 3 (*want to continue*). You will add greatly to your academic reputation when your List 4 (*improving the balance*) advocates gradual and orderly change through evolution, such as giving 6-months notice on List 1 (*want to quit*) entries and helping find and train your successor. Along the way, you can gain administrative skills by sorting out which of the tasks on List 1 (*want to quit or refuse*) can be delegated to your assistants, with what degrees of supervision and independence. By the same token, it will greatly damage your academic reputation if your List 4 (*improving the balance*) calls for revolution, resignation, or running away.

My colleagues in psychiatry taught me that troubled families achieve about 80% of the benefits of family therapy before they ever sit down with a therapist. The explanation is that they have already acknowledged their problem and have resolved to seek help in solving it. I likewise suggest that most of your benefits from the periodic priority list will occur before it is presented and discussed with your mentor. Nonetheless, additional insights can come with presenting your lists to someone else. Moreover, additional List 4 strategies for *improving the balance*, such as learning how to say "no" constructively, can arise in these discussions.

Aspiring clinician–investigators, especially women, often face their greatest academic demands during the period of greatest physical and emotional dependency of their children and partners. The ability to discuss gender-specific conflicts in balancing priorities with an informed, empathic mentor is essential.

The strategies in List 4 for *improving the* balance that emerge from these discussions often focus on the effective and efficient use of time, which leads us to the third determinant of academic success: time management.

12.3 TIME MANAGEMENT

The most important element of time management for academic success is setting aside and ruthlessly protecting time that is spent *writing for publication*. I've encountered several successful academics whose only control over their schedule has been protected writing time. Conversely, I've met very few academics who have succeeded without protecting their writing time, regardless of how well they controlled the other elements of their schedules. For some academics, this protected writing time occurs outside "normal" working hours, but the price of such nocturnal and week-end toil is often paid by family and friends, and is a setup for burnout. The prototypically successful academic sets aside 1 day per week (except during periods of intensive clinical responsibilities; *vide infra*) for this activity and clearly means it by telling everyone that they aren't available for chats, phone calls, committees, classes, or departmental meetings that day.

I've never admired the publications of any academics who told me that writing was easy for them; those whose work I admire tell me that they find it very difficult to write (although many find it nonetheless enormously enjoyable and gratifying). Given the difficulty of writing well, no wonder so many academics find other things to do when they should be writing for publication. The great enemy here is procrastination, and rigorous self-imposed rules are needed for this protected writing time:

- it is *not* for writing grants
- *not* for refereeing manuscripts from other academics (aren't they already ahead of you with their writing?)
- *not* for answering electronic or snail mail
- *not* for keeping up with the literature
- *not* for responding to nonemergencies that can wait until day's end
- *not* for making lists of what should be written about in the future
- *not* for merely outlining a paper and
- *not* for coffee breaks with colleagues.

Early on, self-imposed daily quotas of intelligible prose may be necessary, and these should be set at realistic and achievable levels (as small as 300 coherent words for beginners).

It is imperative that no interruptions occur on writing days. Unless you are protected by a ruthless secretary and respected by garrulous colleagues, this often can best be achieved by creating a "writing room" away from the office; whether this is elsewhere in the building or at home depends on distractions (and family obligations) at these other sites (for a time, I simply traded offices with a colleague who wrote the same day as I). Writing in a separate, designated room permits you to create stacks of drafts, references, and the other organized litter that accompanies writing for publication. It also avoids your unanswered mail, unrefereed manuscripts, undictated patient charts, and the other distracting, disorganized litter of a principal office. Moreover, if e-mail is disabled in the computer in your writing office, a major cause for procrastination is avoided.

Mondays hold three distinct advantages as writing days. First, the things that "can't wait" are much more likely to arise on Fridays, and very few things that arise over the weekend cannot wait until Monday night or Tuesday. Second, a draft that gets off to a good start on Monday often can be completed during brief bits of free time over the next 4 days and sent out for comments by the week's end. Third, the comforting knowledge on a Sunday night that Monday will be protected for writing can go far in improving and maintaining your mental health, family function, and satisfaction as an aspiring academic. And, of course, the more of your colleagues who write on the same day each week, the greater the opportunity for trading offices and the fewer the conflicts in scheduling meetings on other days in the week.

The second important element of time management requires you to schedule clinical activities with great care. On the one hand, you want to maximize the delivery of high-quality care and high-quality clinical teaching. On the other hand, you want to avoid, or at least minimize, conflicts with the other elements of your academic career. Of course, your clinical work should complement your research. Indeed, your clinical observations, frustrations, and failures should be a major source of the questions you pose in your research. But both teaching and research require your full attention. Having to switch back and forth between them several times a week is a recipe for frustration and failure.

I reckon this conflict is best resolved in inpatient disciplines by devoting specific blocks (of, say, 1 month) of "on-service" time to nothing but clinical service and teaching. When on service, your total attention is paid to the needs of patients and clinical learners. No time is spent writing, traveling, attending meetings, or teaching nonclinical topics. This total devotion to clinical activities often will permit you to take on more night call and a greater number of patients and clinical learners (on my medical inpatient service at Oxford, I was on call every third day, with my clinical team of up to 16 learners and visitors, and I admitted 230 patients per month; and in addition to our individual daily bedside rounds my Fellows and I provided 13 hours of extra clinical teaching each week).

When "off-service," your time and attention should shift as completely as possible to research and nonclinical teaching. Ideally, you should have no night call when you are off service. Moreover, you should not routinely see every admitted patient at a post-hospital outpatient follow-up visit (again on my service, postadmission and predischarge telephone conversations with the patients' GPs reduced outpatient follow-up to <5% of my admissions).

If you are worried about getting rusty or out of date between your months on service, precede them by shadowing a colleague for a week just before reassuming command (I alternated between the coronary care and intensive care units for my "warm-up" weeks). Like so many other elements of your academic success, this sort of time management is fostered by the development of a team of like-minded individuals who spell one another in providing excellent clinical care. A survey of physicians in their second decade of clinical practice suggested that there needs to be at least three like-minded clinicians to make this strategy work (23).

Clinicians in other fields (e.g., intensive care and many of the surgical specialties) sometimes find it preferable to allocate time to clinical practice in units of 1 week. Another variant of scheduling is practiced by two of my former residents whose current incomes are derived solely from private practice. They devote 3 weeks of each month to intensive clinical practice in order to free up the fourth for their highly successful applied research programs.

This still leaves you with the outpatient dilemma. Academic clinicians usually accept ambulatory referrals to their general or subspecialty clinics one or two half-days every week. In addition to the time you spend during the clinic session itself, you have to spend several hours during the following 2 to 3 days chasing down lab results, talking with referring clinicians, and dictating notes. This additional time conflicts with your research, teaching, and travel to meetings and other centers, diminishing your research and writing productivity, peace of mind, and fun.

Moreover, I think that this pattern of weekly clinics lowers the quality of patient care. What happens when you are 1,000 km away when one of your outpatients gets sick during the diagnostic tests you've ordered or has an adverse reaction after starting a new treatment regimen?

A solution you should at least consider is to stop holding your outpatient sessions every week and concentrate them into back-to-back-to-back clinics just once a month. By staying in town for the few days following this outpatient "blitz," you can tie up the loose ends of four clinic sessions all at once (especially if you can delegate chasing down lab results), and the rest of your month is free for academic activities.

One of the sadder realities of pursuing an academic career is to be forced to consider your teaching commitments under the heading of time management. Of course, the opportunities and requests for teaching are endless, and the worthiness and fun of teaching are huge. That's why some universities have started to recruit and support clinician–scientists who focus on education research. However, unless you're an education-researcher, most universities offer tiny (or even negative) rewards for your teaching efforts and accomplishments. Your promotion and tenure remain dominated by first-authored publications in high-impact journals. Put quite simply, the time you spend teaching is time taken away from performing and (especially) from publishing your research. No wonder, then, that so many clinical research institutes boast that their recruits need not do any teaching. And no wonder that those who oversee your career investigator award will caution you against spending "too much time" teaching.

The following advice is for academic clinicians at the start of their careers:

1. Examine your university's teaching requirements (if any) for promotion and tenure and be sure you meet them. But focus your teaching so that it helps, not hinders, your career development, and be sure to keep a record of your teaching.

2. During your months on the inpatient clinical service (when you're not writing anyway), spend huge amounts of time teaching clinical

skills/therapeutics/clinical physiology/evidence-based medicine (EBM) at the bedside, and earn a reputation as an outstanding clinical teacher. But don't go on service when there are no students and housestaff to teach, and don't do clinical teaching when you're off service.

3. If your university runs a graduate program in your field, become a junior co-tutor with the best teacher you can find. You will not only earn teaching credits while consolidating your own methodological learning but you will also pick up useful teaching strategies and tactics from a seasoned senior colleague. However, you should avoid the energy-sink of taking responsibility for organizing or running an entire course.

4. Consider joining the best graduate teacher in your field as a junior co-supervisor of a graduate student. Again, you will earn teaching credits while you improve your methodological skills and learn how to supervise the next generation of graduate students. In doing so, you'll need to walk a thin line. On the one hand, you could benefit from becoming a co-investigator and co-author of the work that emerges from this supervision. On the other, you must avoid "muscling in" on the graduate student's project and diminishing the credit (such as lead authorships) they receive. If you take on this co-supervision, it would be important to agree at the start, preferably in writing, about everyone's role, responsibilities, and rules for authorship.

5. Never teach on your writing day.

6. Once you are an established, tenured academic, reverse your role. Teach a lot, organize courses, protect the next generation from excessive teaching demands, and invite new faculty colleagues to join you as co-tutors and co-supervisors.

My final advice about time management concerns taking time to go to annual scientific and clinical meetings. Such meetings are usually fun and relaxing. They also can be highly educational (especially, as noted earlier, when you attend with your mentor), and sometimes offer the chance to meet or at least observe the ephemeral experts in the field. However, you have to pay the opportunity costs of attending meetings. You have taken time away from your teaching and patients, and especially from your writing. I know lots of world-renowned clinician scientists who seldom or never go to annual meetings (which should show you that attending them is not a prerequisite for academic success).

You might want to set up and follow some rules about annual meetings. I close with the set I give my fellows:

1. Never go to an annual meeting for the *first* time unless you have submitted an abstract that will get published in a journal (thus inaugurating your CV).

2. Never go to that meeting a *second* time until you have a full paper based on that earlier abstract in print or in press (thus making a major contribution to your CV and academic recognition).

3. *Thereafter*, only go to that meeting if *both* Rule 2 has been met *and* this year's abstract has been selected for oral presentation (or if you have been invited to give the keynote lecture).

REFERENCES

1. Sackett DL. On the determinants of academic success as a clinician-scientist. *Clin Invest Med*; 2001;24:94–100.

2. Murdoch C. Academic medicine. Academic medicine is still hospital based. *BMJ* 2002; 324:1275.

3. Sackett DL. The fall of "clinical research" and the rise of "clinical-practice" research. *Clin Invest Med* 2000;23:331–333.

4. Centre for Evidence-Based Medicine at the University of Oxford: Levels of Evidence. Accessed at *http://cebm.jr2.ox.ac.uk/docs/levels.html*.

5. Verrier ED. Getting started in academic cardiothoracic surgery. *J Thorac Cardiovasc Surg* 2000;119(Part 2):S1–S10.

6. Morzinski JA, Diehr S, Bower DJ, et al. A descriptive, cross-sectional study of formal mentoring for faculty. *Fam Med* 1996;28:434–438.

7. Goldman L. Blueprint for a research career in general internal medicine. *J Gen Intern Med* 1991;6:341–344.

8. Rogers JC, Holloway RL, Miller SM. Academic mentoring and family medicine's research productivity. *Fam Med* 1990;22:186–190.

9. Applegate WB. Career development in academic medicine. *Am J Med* 1990;88:263–267.

10. Stange KC, Heckelman FP. Mentoring needs and family medicine faculty. *Fam Med* 1990;22:183–185.

11. Williams R, Blackburn RT. Mentoring and junior faculty productivity. *J Nurs Educ* 1988;27:204–209.

12. Eisenberg JM. Cultivating a new field: development of a research program in general internal medicine. *J Gen Intern Med* 1986;1:S8–S18.

13. Bland CJ, Schmitz CC. Characteristics of the successful researcher and implications for faculty development. *J Med Ed* 1986;61:22–31.

14. Palepu A, Friedman RH, Barnett RC, et al. Junior faculty members' mentoring relationships and their professional development in US medical schools. *Acad Med* 1998; 73:318–323.

15. Levinson W, Kaufman K, Clark B, et al. Mentors and role models for women in academic medicine. *West J Med* 1991;154:423–426.

16. Steiner JF, Lanphear BP, Curtis P, et al. Indicators of early research productivity among primary care fellows. *J Gen Intern Med* 2002;17:845–851.

17. Mason MA, Goulden M. Do babies matter: the effect of family formation on the life long careers of women. *Academe* 2002;88(6):21–27.

18. Johns RJ. How to swim with sharks: the advanced course. *Trans Assoc Am Physicians* 1975;88:44–54.

19. Sackett DL. The sins of expertness and a proposal for redemption. *BMJ* 2000;320:1283.

20. Romberg E. Mentoring the individual student: qualities the distinguish between effective and ineffective advisors. *J Dent Ed* 1993;57:287–290.

21. McCue JD. The effects of stress on physicians and their medical practice. *N Engl J Med* 1982;306:458–463.

22. Maslach C, Leither MP. *The truth about burn-out*. San Francisco: Josey-Bass, 1997:13–15.

23. Spears BW. A time management system for preventing physician impairment. *J Fam Pract* 1981;13:75–80.

13

PREPARING A RESEARCH PROTOCOL TO IMPROVE ITS CHANCES FOR SUCCESS

Gordon Guyatt

Readers will note the lack of evidence supporting the suggestions I make in this chapter. Evidence for the entire corpus is based on unsystematic personal experience and observations. So, the strength of inference is limited. The accompanying checklist summarizes the suggestions.

Tips for a successful research proposal checklist:

✓ Ask the right question.
✓ Know your granting agency/agencies.
✓ Ensure optimal collaboration and advice.
✓ Ensure your proposal is well presented.
✓ Discuss your prior work.
✓ Consider a feasibility study.
✓ Go early to your Institutional Review Board.
✓ Ensure you will get credit for what you do.

✓ Ask the right question.

You can follow each of the steps I outline below, but if you have started with the wrong question, you are doomed. What are the characteristics of the right question? Aside from the PICOT format described in Chapter 1 and elsewhere in this book, there are several key considerations.

First, you must find the question compelling. Taking the protocol through numerous iterations, securing feedback that will often be helpful (and sometimes not), and responding to that feedback require enormous time and energy. Tailoring your grant to the granting agency (see subsequent text) and dealing with the shocking administrative hassle associated with grant preparation also consume plenty of time and energy and are considerably less fun. Passionate interest in your question is a prerequisite for maintaining enthusiasm through this arduous process.

Second, the question must be important and the target agency and the reviewers must view it as important. There are a number of components to consider when pondering the importance of your question.

Is There Sufficient Doubt About the Answer?

Research hypotheses that are very unlikely to be correct, or are almost certainly correct, will not be a good choice for the expenditure of scarce research dollars.

What Is the Burden of Illness?

Is the population relevant to your grant large or small? Is the problem you are addressing associated with appreciable mortality, morbidity, or suffering? Consult Chapter 3 for the steps to documenting the burden of illness.

Does the Relevant Clinical Community Think There Is a Problem?

Carotid endarterectomy for atherosclerotic disease of the carotid arteries was a major industry long before anyone conducted a randomized trial to test its effectiveness. However, it was not until the negative results of a randomized trial examining the impact of extracranial to intracranial artery anastomosis that vascular surgeons accepted that there was a problem that needed addressing. One way of documenting the clinical community's interest is by conducting a survey. If you do it well, you will be able to publish the results.

What Is the Potential Economic Impact of Answering Your Question?

If somewhere not too far down the road is a health care innovation that could reduce resource expenditure, granting agencies are likely to find your question more attractive. As I will note later, if costs are an important issue, involvement of a health economist is crucial.

What Are the Costs of Conducting the Research Relative to the Potential Health and Economic Benefits?

A junior colleague of mine is passionately interested in predictors of knee injury in young athletes. Knowing the predictors may lead to interventions that reduce injury incidence, although one might be skeptical about the likelihood of effective interventions arising from the results. This would clearly be a great question if $50,000 would provide the answer. To do the study properly, however, would require $500,000, an amount that I, and other colleagues with whom the graduate student consulted, thought that a granting agency would likely consider disproportionate to the importance of the question. Although my colleague has not given up, the question has moved from the top of her research agenda.

Is Your Question in Fashion (with Someone or Other)?

Health issues relevant to older white men in heavily industrialized countries have generally found great favor among funders. If you are interested in investigating the impact of a new (or even old) product produced by the pharmaceutical industry, it will increase your chance of funding. HIV, women's health issues, and aboriginal health issues have had, and continue to have, their particular markets. If there is no funding source that finds your question appealing, you will have more trouble securing dollars to conduct your work.

My colleagues and I are currently very interested in ensuring that patients' values and preferences are appropriately considered in health care decision making. Many of our physician colleagues do not currently consider this issue important, limiting our chances of funding. At the time of writing, we are in the process of recruiting nurse co-investigators and are planning to target some of our funding requests to agencies that fund nursing research and whose reviewers will certainly consider our questions important. This example provides one illustration of the exigencies of searching for funds to carry out work that you consider important.

Is Your Question Not Only Not (Definitively) Answered, but Also the Logical Next Step?

To nail down the answer to this question, you must begin with a systematic review. As detailed in Chapter 2, and worth emphasizing here, all research must build on what has gone before. One can easily argue that unless investigators have an optimal understanding of prior research, they cannot properly justify or design the project that represents the next step. Furthermore, that optimal understanding should involve a systematic review of the existing literature; a less-than-systematic approach runs a serious risk of bias and presents a misleading picture of the existing state of affairs. The extreme of this argument, with which I have much sympathy, is that it is unethical to undertake a new piece of research without a systematic review of what investigators have already accomplished.

For instance, before submitting for funding for our randomized trial of alternative ways of nailing tibial fractures, we conducted and published a systematic review of the impact of reamed versus unreamed nailing on nonunion for lower-extremity long-bone fractures (1). As it turned out, we found a very large beneficial effect of reamed nailing in decreasing rates of nonunion (relative risk 0.33; 95% CI, 0.16–0.68, $P = 0.004$). The randomized trials that generated this estimate were, however, of limited quality. Problems included lack of concealment, lack of blinding in adjudication of outcomes, lack of standardized management protocols, and violation of the intention to treat principle.

When we considered fracture sites separately, we found that the apparent benefit of reamed nailing was appreciably larger with femoral (relative risk, 0.24; 95% CI, 0.07–0.82) than with tibial (relative risk, 0.44; 95% CI, 0.21–0.93) fractures. Although these results are consistent with the same underlying effect for both femur and tibia, the inference is weaker for tibial fractures, with the upper boundary of the confidence interval approaching no effect.

We went on to conduct a second meta-analysis examining the evidence regarding the treatment of open tibial shaft fractures (2). In the two studies that we identified, which compared reamed and unreamed nails in open tibial fractures, the wide confidence intervals around the point estimates in the risk of re-operation (0.75; 95% CI, 0.43–1.32) and the risk of nonunion (0.70; 95% CI, 0.24–1.67) reflect their small sample size (total $n = 132$). Again, the results are not inconsistent with a common underlying treatment effect, but the weaker effect generates additional doubt about the relative merit of reamed and unreamed nailing of tibial fractures.

These results and informal conversations with orthopedic trauma surgeons persuaded us that although there was limited doubt about the benefits of reamed nailing in femoral fractures, the optimal approach in tibial fractures remained unsettled. The results of a systematic survey of orthopedic trauma surgeons, demonstrating variation in both opinion and practice, further strengthened this inference (3). This formal survey found near consensus regarding the benefits of the reamed approach in femoral fractures but considerable disagreement for tibial fractures. Putting together the magnitude of the apparent effects, the methodological limitations of the studies, and the prevailing opinion, we decided to consider the femoral fracture issue settled, but the best management of tibial fractures was unresolved. Granting agencies agreed with the assessment, and, at the time of writing, the trial has enrolled more than 1,200 patients of a target sample size of 1,300 patients.

Conducting a systematic review has another merit (assuming of course, that someone else has not recently completed such a review and done a good job of it)–you are likely to be able to publish the result right away, and long before you ever publish the results of your study. This not only provides a step forward in your academic career but also enhances your credibility in your investigational field. Your systematic review can figure prominently when you present your work to date (see the following text). Further, citation counts are higher for systematic reviews than for nonsystematic reviews and often higher than for original articles.

✓ *Know your granting agency/agencies.*

There is no doubt that knowing your agencies is critical. It is knowledge that is also difficult to fully integrate as a neophyte investigator. I speak in the following text about how critical it is to have a good mentor–a person to help you at every step of the way in learning about the target agencies.

Each granting agency has its own rules and standards. Many have several committees–or even a profusion of committees–each with its own mandate and standards. Your grant's success will critically depend on a good understanding of the rules and mores of the agency to which you are applying and on the panel that will review your grant.

How can you obtain this knowledge? First, take time to carefully review all the instructions, rules, and guidance from the agency, whether in hard copy or on a Web site. Many grants (even some from senior investigators) have been returned unreviewed as a result of failure to observe formatting rules: specifications about font, character size, margins, and length of the submission.

Your university will have an office responsible for assisting with grant preparation. That office should be able to show you recent successful grants submitted to your target agency, and possibly even your target committee. Review several of these grants carefully. Note their organization, headings, emphasis, and the relative space given to each component. Following formatting, organization, and emphasis directions set by previously successful applicants is likely to serve you well.

You may be uncertain about the eligibility rules, which committee would be best suited to review your grant application, or other administrative or policy issues. There are a number of people to whom you can go to resolve these uncertainties. First, check who sits on the grant review panel of your target committee or committees. Is there someone from your institution? That person may well be able to provide you with the answers to your questions, as well as other insights into how the committee works, and further advice on how to pitch your proposal. (If you fear that this might be "tampering," this person will likely need to declare a conflict of interest when your application is reviewed anyway because they are from your institution.)

Another individual worth talking to is the senior administrative person in charge of the committee to which you are applying. A telephone call in which you explain your situation and your uncertainties is very likely to provide insight. Dealing with such issues is part of the job of the administrative folk at the granting agency, and they are generally very helpful.

Finally, you could call the chairperson of your target review panel. This person will be the one most knowledgeable about the selection process and will be aware of subtleties impossible to glean from written or Web-based information (of which even the agencies' administrative personnel may not be fully cognizant). One such call for a career award resulted in advice to stay very focused; indeed, even if the applicant were engaged in multiple projects, to consider presenting only one. The ultimate result was a submission that was not only successful but also earned the applicant an additional $250,000 of discretionary funds as one of the top five proposals in the country.

Note that the heading of this subsection implies that you will be submitting to more than one agency. If your project is eligible for multiple agencies, apply to them all. Once you have developed one submission, the incremental work for a second application is well worth the incremental gain. If more than one source funds you, you choose the agency that offered the most money or is associated with the most prestige, and politely return the funds to the other agency. There may even be circumstances in which, by dividing the project up, you may get to keep some of the funds from the second agency.

✓ *Ensure optimal collaboration and advice.*

I've already mentioned a number of sources of potential help: the faculty office in charge of facilitating research, previously successful grants, colleagues who sit on grant panels, and granting agency personnel. There are other local sources of help that may be critical to your success.

Almost every research project will benefit from the active help of an established statistician. You should engage a statistician at the earliest stages of protocol development. Both the quality of the proposal and its credibility and feasibility in the eyes of external reviewers will improve as a result.

Your reading of successful grants may raise questions in your mind about the approaches those investigators used and the extent to which they may be applicable to your own proposal. Usually, the principal investigator (PI) will be happy to take some time to discuss the issues with you. Such a conversation may provide substantial insight. If your fields of inquiry are sufficiently similar, that individual may even be willing to review your protocol. Also, some institutions will provide an internal review of *in utero* grant applications for new investigators, organized through the office of the associate dean for research, or the equivalent.

Dave Sackett has written with wisdom and insight about the critical value of a mentor in success in a research career (4). If you have managed to secure the right mentorship, your senior colleague is certain to be helpful in ensuring the success of your protocol. This help will involve working with you to choose an important question, developing the protocol, and tailoring it to the agency or agencies to which you submit your application(s).

Your mentor will also help in putting together the optimal team you need for your project. Because, for almost any study, accruing the ideal sample size is a major challenge, you will often be considering the possibility of a multi-site project. Inter-institutional collaboration is now the norm for clinical research and modern electronic communication has eliminated many of the previous barriers.

Although the ideal mentor will have personal contacts who will help recruit collaborators with expertise, ideas, and established credibility, do not be shy about approaching potential collaborators whom neither you nor your mentor knows personally. Recently, a brilliant, supremely energetic, and ambitious young orthopaedic surgeon, still early in his residency, came to my office to ask for help with his idea for a clinical trial of alternative ways of nailing tibial fractures. Considering the sample size, it quickly became evident that a very large (20 or more institutions) multi-center effort would be required. I suggested to my junior colleague to choose the most prestigious senior investigator in the field and approach that individual about helping to lead the project. When asked, the senior researcher became very enthusiastic and took the role of co-principal investigator. The ultimate result has been a successful, multi-center, randomized trial co-funded by the National Institutes of Health and the Canadian Institutes for Health Research, and international recognition for the young surgeon, while still completing his clinical and research training.

You may be able to recruit expert help for your entire research program despite distance and initial unfamiliarity. A decade ago, a young investigator from an institution more than 800 km from McMaster who was starting to work in quality-of-life measurement approached me about helping with his research. Although I'd never met or heard of him before, he seemed bright and enthusiastic, and I agreed to participate. I made several visits to his institution, and initially put a lot of work into his proposals and papers. Within a few years, he had outgrown the need for my help. In the interval, the collaboration had helped to launch a substantial research program that included seven articles published in peer-reviewed journals.

Finally, if your project involves an important economic component, there is no substitute for engaging a qualified health economist as a co-investigator. The same comments I previously made about involving a statistician also apply here.

✓ *Ensure your proposal is well presented.*

I cannot overemphasize the impact of presentation of a protocol. Your idea may be brilliant and your methodology pristine, but if you do not present it well, you are still unlikely to obtain funding.

Organization, writing, and proofing are the key elements of presentation. Organizational issues arise both in the major headings of the proposal and within sections. In terms of major headings, the organization is likely to differ depending on the nature of your question (are you doing a randomized trial? evaluating a diagnostic test?) and the granting agency to which you are applying. Furthermore, there is no single best way to organize a proposal.

I suggest obtaining several previously successful grants. Ideally, they will be from the granting agency to which you are applying, address the same type of question as your proposal, and (of least importance) are as close to your content area as possible. Note carefully how the applicants have organized their proposal and the logic behind that organization. If the organization is virtually identical in each grant you review, you have the answer about how to organize your proposal. If they differ, you have a number of implicit guides about how to proceed, and can choose an approach that makes most sense to you.

Finding a template for organization within the sections may be more difficult. Focus on creating a logical and appealing flow of ideas. This is particularly critical for the background of your proposal, which is often the most challenging to write.

One broad-stroke approach that works for most background sections is to make the following points:

- We have a problem.
- It's an important problem.
- Here is what has been done to address the problem.
- Here is the key issue that remains unanswered.

In making these points, one tries to create a crescendo leading to the inevitable conclusion that the scientific community must confront the question you are proposing to address.

One strategy that may help you is to lay out the main points of each section in point form. Each point must build on the previous in a logical way. Divide the points in a way that will guide the construction of paragraphs. Each paragraph should have a single idea and clear links to the paragraphs that precede and follow.

In terms of word choice and the structure of sentences and paragraphs, I offer the same comments that you will find in Chapter 16 on preparing reports for publication.

Finally, frequent typos, grammatical *faux pas*, and *non sequiturs* can undermine even the most brilliant application. It can be difficult to stomach proofreading the final version of an application when you have been through so many iterations, but this is an essential task—the more so if you are rushing to meet the application deadline and are bringing everything together at the last minute. If you work in a team and have someone in the team who is a good and willing editor, be sure to assign them this task; otherwise be sure to do it yourself.

✓ *Discuss your prior work.*

Either as a separate heading that is part of the background or in a separate section altogether, discuss your group's prior work in the area of investigation. Any investigation is more likely to be successful if the investigators have conducted similar work in the past and if their current project builds on prior accomplishments. Review panels know this, and will be looking for evidence that you can carry out what you intend.

If you and your group are just entering the field, you have a problem similar to many of the unemployed: They need experience to get a job, but they must first get a job to gain the experience. Here, you need accomplishments to obtain grant funding, but you need grant funding to accomplish anything. Under these circumstances my next suggestion, to first seek funding for a feasibility project, becomes even more compelling.

✓ *Consider a feasibility study.*

If your project is large and complex, without considerable supporting evidence, a grant review panel will be appropriately skeptical about your ability to achieve your goals. You may be able to provide some of that evidence without external funding through minimally expensive pilot work. Many hospitals, universities, and foundations provide small grants to junior investigators to conduct this sort of feasibility study. In addition to, or as an alternative to, a small pilot that requires minimal resources, you may submit an application to a larger agency for a feasibility grant (usually less than $100,000, but sometimes for more). In the last decade, funding agencies have become very receptive to such proposals.

Most feasibility studies include, among their goals, determining the availability of eligible participants. For example, when we were considering our randomized trial of alternative ways of nailing tibial fractures, we began by recruiting 20 centers—7 in Canada and 13 in the United States. We asked each center to conduct a chart review and document, over the period of 1 year, the total number of tibial fractures that they managed and the number of patients who they believed would have met inclusion criteria and agreed to participate in the study. These centers then prospectively, over a period of 2 months, evaluated each patient who presented to their institution with a tibial fracture. They documented the number of such patients and the proportion of those who both met eligibility criteria and were likely to consent to enter the trial. We dropped two centers that were unable to comply with these preliminary steps. We also conducted a reproducibility study of the radiographic interpretation of fracture healing (which we were able to publish).

We concluded, however, that further feasibility work was necessary to convince a granting agency (and ourselves) that we could pull off the study. For our project, and indeed for any feasibility study, specification of objectives and *a priori* criteria for success are critical. For instance, our objectives and success criteria were as follows.

- To estimate recruitment rates in individual centers. We specified that we would consider the pilot successful if we recruited 70 patients during a total of no more than 4 months.
- To determine investigators' ability to adhere to study protocol and data collection procedures. We considered that the feasibility study would be successful if we observed no more than five major protocol deviations in 70 patients.
- To determine our ability to achieve close to 100% follow-up rates. We specified that we would consider the feasibility study successful if we achieved complete follow-up in at least 65 of the 70 patients.

✓ Go early to your Institutional Review Board.

Institutional Review Boards (IRBs) in North America typically meet only once a month and require submissions up to several weeks before the meeting. Furthermore, it is quite common for IRBs to request changes to consent forms, and even to protocols, requiring a second meeting before approval is granted. Applicants often leave IRB approval to just before the grant deadline and are forced to submit with "pro-tem" approval only.

IRBs sometimes can be difficult to convince and appear obstructive, but they can also make insightful comments and suggestions and be quite helpful. Furthermore, even their illogical and obstructive comments may presage some reviewers' reactions, and it is well worth dealing with them before a submission. A submission with full IRB approval is likely stronger not only because the approval is there but also because the investigator has dealt with IRB comments and criticisms.

✓ *Ensure you will get credit for what you do.*

Sadly, as a young investigator, you must always be concerned about issues of credit. Senior investigators taking credit for their juniors' work is a phenomenon as old as scientific investigation. If you have chosen the right mentor, you will at least not have to worry about that individual taking advantage of you. The ideal mentor will not only be personally generous, but will advocate for you aggressively if contentious issues of credit arise.

Issues of credit become particularly salient in preparing grant applications. The reason is that, if you have not come on faculty yet, you may be ineligible to hold a grant. You must, therefore, find a faculty member to front as the PI on your project. Even if you are eligible to hold the grant, you and your team may choose to designate a senior colleague as PI to enhance your grant's competitiveness. Either way, this can be a very risky business.

One of my junior colleague's experiences illustrates the potential problems. My colleague, with whom I was working closely, developed the idea for a project, led our group in bringing together the multi-center team required to conduct the study, conducted the pilot work necessary for the project, and led our group in preparing the grant application. Because my colleague was not yet on faculty, the project's steering committee, of which I was a member, chose from among its membership a senior individual to act as PI. Once the project was funded, my junior colleague did virtually all the work in directing the start-up and running of the trial.

As time passed, the nominal PI reconstructed events, progressively increasing his perceived role in the early phases of the project. The nominal PI, supported by another steering committee member, began to present the project to the world as truly his. My junior colleague, when applying for a personal salary award, found himself with a rejection letter on the basis that his role in the project was unclear. Despite my aggressive support, my colleague had to fight a vigorous and unpleasant battle to ultimately gain the credit he deserved.

Were I going through the process again, I would insist on a written agreement established at the start of the project regarding ultimate credit. This would include public acknowledgement of my colleague's role as the true PI of the project, and transfer of the official PI role as soon as my colleague joined the faculty. In addition, the agreement would ensure first authorship of ultimate publications, including designation as the corresponding author, for my colleague.

Establishing such an agreement may involve appreciable awkwardness because it implies a lack of trust. Unfortunately, this lack of trust is often warranted. Having a mentor to conduct these negotiations on your behalf will substantially decrease the awkwardness.

You and your mentor may bear in mind two useful tips during these negotiations. The first is the manner in which you can make informal discussions formal. Returning to the unpleasant story above, our group implicitly acknowledged my colleague's leadership role when the project started, but that implicit agreement was ultimately forgotten. You or your mentor may follow up a verbal agreement with a letter that reads more or less as follows. "My understanding is that we have agreed on the following ... ," and then lays out how you will distribute credit. The letter concludes with a request for corrections if there have been any errors. When you don't receive any corrections, a second letter lets everyone know that no one has any problems with what the first letter has specified, and so that document reflects your ultimate agreement.

The second tip has to do with dealing with resistance during negotiations. When deciding on authorship of publications, some participants may maintain that since the ultimate distribution of authority, leadership, and work is uncertain, designating authorship at an early stage of the project makes little sense. An effective counter-argument maintains that an early agreement involves a commitment to ensure that you, the junior investigator, will take the lead role in the conduct of the study. In other words, who leads the group in decision making and implementation is very much in the control of the project's leadership. An up-front agreement that the junior person who initiated the project will lead its implementation has an important steering effect on the way leadership and authority plays out in the study's conduct.

REFERENCES

1. Bhandari M, Guyatt GH, Tong D, et al. Reamed versus nonreamed intramedullary nailing of lower extremity long bone fractures: a systematic overview and meta-analysis. *J Orthop Trauma* 2000;14:2–9.

2. Bhandari M, Guyatt GH, Swiontkowksi MF, et al. Treatment of open tibial fractures: a systematic overview and meta-analysis. *J Bone Joint Surg Br* 2001;83:62–68.

3. Bhandari M, Guyatt GH, Swiontkowski MF, et al. Surgeons' preferences for the operative treatment of fractures of the tibial shaft: an international survey. *J Bone Joint Surg Am* 2001;83:1746–1752.

4. Sackett DL. On the determinants of academic success as a clinician-scientist. *Clin Invest Med* 2001;24:94–100.

ONLINE DATA COLLECTION

Dave Sackett

CLINICAL RESEARCH SCENARIO

Sharon Straus, Finlay McAlister, and I wanted to change the way that studies of the accuracy of the clinical examination were carried out. We didn't like asking two or three local experts to examine a few dozen previously diagnosed "cases" and "non-cases" over several months in an academic hot house, publishing their results next year. Instead, we wanted to ask scores of community physicians all over the world to examine hundreds of undiagnosed patients in the hurly-burly of community practice within a month, publishing their results the next week (1). We used electronic mail and the Internet to recruit our scores of clinicians (eventually numbering over 1,000 clinicians from 90 countries). They nominated and designed the studies, posted them on our Web site, and obtained local ethics approvals. For each study, we worked with our Web expert, Douglas Badenoch, to design a simple, self-editing data form and posted it on the Web site. In our first study, participating clinicians worked in pairs. One assigned a local code number to the patient and entered the anonymous results of their clinical examination on-screen. This data entry was done quickly and simply by ticking boxes (smoking history) or by entering numbers as short entries (laryngeal height). This data form is shown in Figure 14–1.

When our overseas collaborator clicked the "submit" button, an instant "robot" editor on our central computer took over. It made sure that all the needed information had been supplied and that no "nonsense" data had been entered; when it detected errors, it refused to accept the record until the errors had been corrected. Once accepted, the clinical collaborator logged off and the robot added the record to the file for immediate analysis. The second clinician, using this same patient code number, logged on later and entered the results of the independent, blind reference standard examination. Our software robot linked the examination and the reference-standard results for each patient, combined the results with those of the other patients, and presented them to our statistician. In our first "CARE" (Clinical Assessment of the

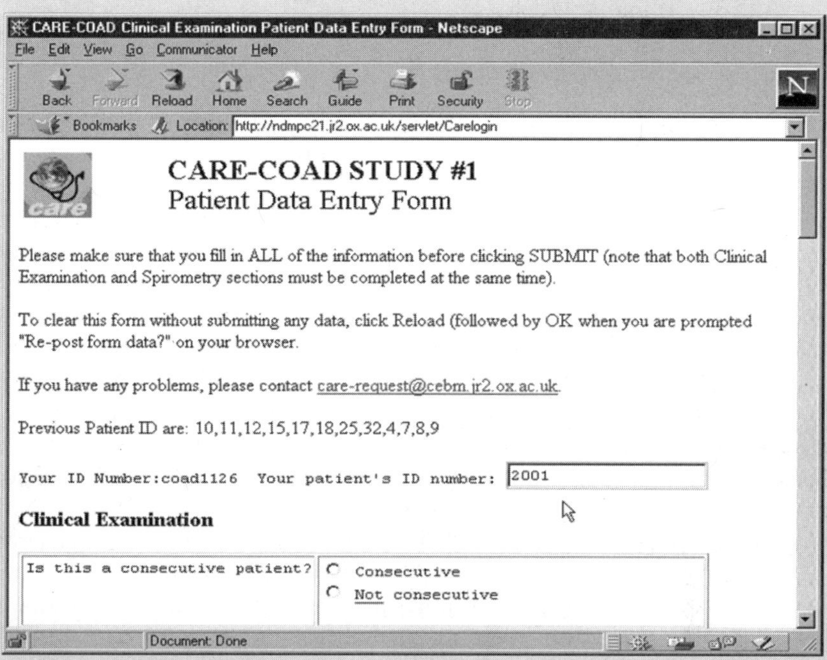

FIGURE 14-1   Online data entry form for the CARE-COAD study.

Reliability of the Examination) study, 25 clinical teams in 14 countries carried out independent, blind clinical examinations, and spirometry on 309 patients in a little over a month (2). Preliminary analyses were available to the participating clinicians the day after the last patient was examined.

Paper forms, completed by hand, have served us well in clinical investigations. However, they have several disadvantages:

- They are bulky.
- They accept, without complaint, doctor's (i.e., indecipherable) handwriting.
- They cost money to mail from the study site to the data center.
- They take time to get to the data center.
- It takes time for the data center to discover that they contain mistakes and missing entries.
- It takes time for the data center to contact the study site to ask for corrections.
- By the time the data center's request for corrections gets back to the study site, the study patient has gone home and her clinical chart has disappeared into the giant maw of medical records.
- It takes time for the study site to track down the study patient's record.

- And so on and so on.
- Finally, it takes time to enter (often in duplicate) and edit data into a record that can be analyzed.

As a result, it can take months between a study patient's visit and the addition of a complete, error-free record to the computer file, if an error-free record can be created at all.

Despite all these disadvantages, paper forms can still serve small, local studies quite well. But as studies get bigger, and as sites become widely scattered and even international, faster and more accurate alternatives to paper data systems become a high priority. As we were writing this book, data collection had already proceeded in two directions.

The first innovation begins with paper but quickly converts it to an electronic format. In Chapter 5, The Tactics of Performing Therapeutic Trials, we described the North American Symptomatic Carotid Endarterectomy Trial (NASCET) of endarterectomy for symptomatic carotid stenosis. Because this trial required multiple examinations, by impatient, computer-illiterate clinicians, of 659 patients in 50 centers, just one of our patients could generate up to 350 pages of data. We therefore faced both the Sisyphusian[1] and Herculean[2] tasks of not only pushing masses of paper but also validating them and generating "clean" data for analysis.

Anticipating this problem, our fearless Principal Statistical Investigator, Wayne Taylor, tried to convert study centers to direct data entry using a distributed computer system. In his own words:

> "When NASCET started we put PCs in all the clinics, trained them to do data entry from the forms (just the important stuff that we printed in red) and called this the NASCET hotline. It was an unqualified disaster. When we compared the data printed on the forms with the data entered over the hotline there were so many mistakes (just keying in the data) that I became discouraged about this method of data collection. It went on anyway but I stopped using hotline data about 2 years into the trial and did not rely on it at all for the stopping rule closure of phase 1 in Feb 1991. By the end of the trial in 1999 only 1 center in 5 was still doing any hotline data entry."

This story preceded the Internet era but does seem to be typical: investigators in the field may not do well with direct data entry into computers, especially if the forms are long and detailed and if the data must be integrated from a number of sources. But what about using paper forms

---

[1]He's the guy who had to endlessly push a boulder (today's mail delivery of data forms) up a mountain, only to have it fall back again each time (tomorrow's mail delivery of data forms).
[2]He's the guy who had to clean up after a thousand cattle in a single day (we leave this analogy to your imagination).

that the computer can "read"? Wayne Taylor next went on to develop an ingenious, automated, "DataFax" system (*http://www.datafax.com/*). Again, in his own words:

> "I started working on DataFax in the fall of 1989 (about the time I gave up on the NASCET hotline). The first DataFax trial, and the resources need to develop it, came from Astra Canada to run a trial comparing Losec and Zantac. The trial contained 1530 patients from 13 sites and went so smoothly and efficiently (with a colleague and me doing all the data management ourselves in hardly any time) that I became hooked on this approach to data management and gave a talk about it at a meeting in May 1991 where I was mobbed by the audience in a crush around the podium that made me feel like a rock star. So I approached the university about this great idea for a business and was essentially told to piss off and go do it myself. So I hired a lawyer and accountants and incorporated in September 1991, with 3 pharmaceutical companies already committed."

DataFax eventually had five vital features:

1. It was very simple at the point where study clinicians saw study patients. Paper forms were completed for baseline visits, treatments, follow-ups, and events of every sort. These "case report forms" were then faxed to the data management center using ordinary fax machines. An example of a case report form appears in Appendix 14.1.
2. The central software read a barcode that identified the study and the type of visit, deciphered both written and tick-box entries, edited them for errors and omissions, and immediately created a "split-screen" that compared the case report form as faxed with the data set that the editor had derived from it.
3. A robot editor checked the data for errors. In addition, data management center staff reviewed the split-screens to pick up any other discrepancies.
4. Any problems found in the robot or human reviews were faxed back to the study sites for fixing, along with reminders about overdue visits and missing forms or pages. Often, these problems could be resolved while study patients or their clinical charts were still readily available.
5. Finally, the system generated census reports, tracked center performance, identified protocol violations, and provided an "audit trail" of who did what to whom, where, why, and when.

This system has had a huge effect on the quality and timeliness of study patient data since its introduction. Moreover, its implementation meant that far fewer research assistants, working in a much smaller space, could edit and manage trial data, and generate "clean" data sets much quicker than before. The DataFax system has been used in several hundred randomized control trials (RCTs) involving tens of thousands of study patients (3). While it might be thought that this paper-to-computer form of data collection would not survive the allure of the Internet, this has not been the case with direct data entry, presumably because paper forms remain more convenient and portable in many forms of patient encounter, at least for computer luddites and during the current era of predominantly prewireless data entry.

The second direction in which data collection has proceeded, illustrated in the scenario at the beginning of this chapter, utilizes the Internet. This strategy permits another exciting approach to clinical-practice research: the ability of the general public to join in. For example, a group of Boston rheumatologists announced a trial of glucosamine for osteoarthritis of the knee on a public-access Web site, and invited interested surfers to apply to become study patients (4). They protected patients' confidentiality with encryption, passwords, and a firewall. Patients' eligibility, utilities, and functional outcomes were determined via the Web, and were augmented by snail mail for consents, clinical records, and distribution of study drugs. They determined that their Internet trial was similar to traditional, "face-to-face" hospital-based osteoarthritis trials in terms of patient characteristics, protocol adherence, and losses to follow-up. However, their per-patient costs (2003 US $914) were about half those of a "face-to-face" trial of similar size and duration (2003 US $1,925).

Alternatives to face-to-face, paper-based data collection are developing rapidly, and by the time this book appears in print, the examples we've given here may be more useful as starting places for literature searches than as the latest word in study implementation.

REFERENCES

1. McAlister FA, Straus SE, Sackett DL, CARE-COAD1 Group. Why we need large, simple studies of the clinical examination: the problem and a proposed solution. *Lancet* 1999;354:1721–1724.
2. Straus SE, McAlister FA, Sackett DL, et al. Accuracy of history, wheezing, and forced expiratory time in the diagnosis of chronic obstructive pulmonary disease. *J Gen Intern Med* 2002;17:684–688.
3. Taylor DW. Ten years with DataFax. *Control Clin Trials* 2000;21(2S):56S–57S.
4. McAlindon T, Formica M, Kabbara K, et al. Conducting clinical trials over the internet: feasibility study. *BMJ* 2003;327:484–487.

APPENDIX 14.1 DATAFAX CASE REPORT FORM

ACE   PATIENT ENTRY FORM (page 1 of 1)   Form 1.0

‖ ‖ ‖ ‖ ‖ ■■■‖ ‖ ‖ ‖ ‖ ‖ ‖ ‖ ■‖ ‖ ‖ ‖ ‖ ‖ ‖ ‖

DataFax #007   Plate 001   Visit 000

Patient No. ☐☐☐ ☐☐☐   **Patient Initials** ☐☐☐   **Entry Date** ☐☐ ☐☐ ☐☐
                                                F M L   month day year

Date of Birth ☐☐ ☐☐ ☐☐   **Sex** ☐ male ☐ female
                 month day year

Race ☐ Caucasian ☐ Black ☐ Asian ☐ Other _____

Recent ASA Consumption
   Has patient taken any ASA in the past 5 days? ☐ No ☐ Yes
   If *Yes*, record total dose (mg) of ASA taken each day. *(enter 0 for none and NA if unknown for each day)*

today	yesterday	2 days ago	3 days ago	4 days ago
☐☐☐☐	☐☐☐☐	☐☐☐☐	☐☐☐☐	☐☐☐☐

Eligibility Criteria

1. Patient is scheduled for carotid endarterectomy by a NASCET surgeon or another surgeon approved by NASCET surgeons at your center.
2. Patient is not already participating in NASCET or another trial.
3. Patient has not received CABG surgery in the past 30 days and is not scheduled for CABG in the next 30 days.
4. Patient will be able to tolerate 1300 mg of ASA/day for 3 months.
5. Patient will not receive ASA from other sources during the trial.
6. Patient will not take other antiplatelet drugs during the trial.
7. If patient has taken ≥ 325 mg of ASA in either of the past 2 days, surgery must be scheduled for 48 hours or more since last dose was taken.
8. If surgery is scheduled within the next 24 hours, patient must be able to take the first days dose of study medication (all 5 pills) at least 8 hours before surgery.
9. Patient has provided informed consent to participate in the trial and to return for follow-up assessments at 30 and 90 days following surgery.

   Does Patient Satisfy All of the Above Criteria for Entry to the Trial? ☐ No ☐ Yes

Surgery is scheduled for ☐☐ ☐☐ ☐☐ at ☐☐ : ☐☐ 24 hr clock
                            month day year

Medication: Patient has been given a 1 week blister pac of study medication and told to start it:

☐ *Immediately if surgery is scheduled within the next 24 hours.*

☐ *7 days before surgery if surgery is more than 1 week away.*

☐ *Today if patient has not been taking ASA and surgery is <7 days away.*

☐ *Tomorrow if patient has been taking ASA and surgery is <7 days away.*

Completed by: _____
                        (Please print)

Please Fax this form today to the ACE Coordinating Center 1-905-574-4755

ANALYZING DATA

Gordon Guyatt, Brian Haynes, and Dave Sackett

This chapter is meant to give comfort to new clinical researchers who are not statisticians. As we've repeatedly pointed out, we are not statisticians and have conducted all our research as part of collaborative teams that included well-trained, experienced, and highly competent statisticians. Our most important advice about analyzing data is that you follow the same approach and ensure that you have high quality statistical collaboration from the planning phases of your research onward.

You, however, will play a key role in planning the analyses of your own studies. To do this well, you must understand the basic concepts of the analytical options that are open to you. By now, we expect that you have participated in one or more introductory courses in statistics and have consulted introductory statistical tests to gain familiarity with the basic approaches. You may have even read one of a substantial number of expositions on statistical approaches that were sometimes written primarily by clinicians (1–3), and always primarily for clinicians (4,5). If you haven't educated yourself in any of these ways yet, please place them high on your "to do" list.

We will not reproduce any of this material here. Rather, we will offer several general observations about the investigator's role in the statistical analysis of clinical studies, some very basic concepts, and then some tips for four specific situations that we have encountered. We must make a number of disclaimers about these examples. The specific examples are obviously not comprehensive and are restricted to non-Bayesian analyses. They are, to an appreciable extent, redundant with material that you will find in the statistical analysis sections of other chapters of this book. Moreover, they are not highly academic, with, for instance, extensive reference to original articles in the statistical literature or statistical texts.

These example situations are, however, common in clinical epidemiological research, and important. They are intended to provide guidance that may be helpful in deciding on optimal approaches to a variety of study questions and designs. Our intent is to give you a sense of the sorts of issues that you will confront when it comes to analyzing your data and the alternative approaches of which you should become aware.

15.1 START SIMPLE

To the fullest extent possible, you should "look at" your data to understand it before you do any statistical analysis. One of the senior statisticians in our department swears that the "eyeball" test is the most important statistical test: Look at your data, arrayed in tables and figures, to see what its message is. The number crunching is just for "blessing" the data.

Ideally, you will have prepared "dummy tables" when you designed the study, and you can now put your data in these tables to provide a "picture" of what you've found, gaining a clear sense of the key messages embedded in your data. Even if you didn't prepare tables during the proposal stage of your project, now is the time to do so, based firmly on your study questions. To these tables you should add measures of central tendency (i.e., means and medians) and dispersion (i.e., ranges, standard deviations, and interquartile ranges), and cross-tabulations. Visual displays (i.e., scatterplots and histograms) are very useful in helping you to gain a good understanding of your data. The better you understand your data from a descriptive point of view, the less likely you are to make serious errors down the road. This is also a good way to review your data for any obvious errors—for data that don't "look right."

15.2 HOW TO BECOME A GOOD PARTNER FOR YOUR STATISTICIAN COLLEAGUES

If you participated in one or more statistical courses, we hope that they were practically oriented. What more do you need to achieve the statistical expertise for your role as a clinical investigator? Some would argue that taking advanced statistics courses and learning to run analyses using the available statistical computer programs will be very helpful (of the most commonly used, SPSS is easier to learn; SAS, the more difficult program, is used more by professionals in the field) and an excellent use of your time. Although this may be the route to go, we don't feel it is necessary, especially if you will be doing research with the advantage of a well-rounded team. Indeed, none of us do our own number crunching. In fact, most of our senior statistician colleagues don't do the analyses themselves. This is usually done by expert research staff who are working under your direction. Your ability to do this comes from a deep understanding of the research you are doing and the methods you've drawn on, a basic understanding of statistical principles, experience you will gain in analyzing the data from your various projects, and the knowledge and advice you will get from your statistician colleagues.

How do you optimize the sort of on-the-job learning of which we are speaking? First, you need to be working with statistician colleagues who are not only highly competent but also ready to help in your education. They will be friendly, good teachers, and willing and able to answer your questions and explain the thinking behind their choice of analytic techniques. You will do your best to respond to their openness by being inquisitive and persistent in learning as much as you can from each analytic challenge you face.

Second, you can add having a "good conceptual understanding of statistical approaches" to the qualities you will seek in your search for an ideal clinical research mentor. Some brilliant statistical teachers will be able to take the clinicians' vantage point, but even good ones will sometimes be bound by their statistical knowledge and experience, which in depth and breadth is far beyond that of most clinical epidemiologists. The advantage of statistical explanation from a clinical mentor is that she will be coming to the problem, having dealt with the same sort of limitations in knowledge and understanding that you are facing. Of course, the mentor must indeed have a good conceptual understanding and must also know her limitations when getting an explanation and further help in understanding is warranted.

15.3 NO ONE KNOWS BEST

New researchers might assume, as we did, that there is a single best approach to any analytic problem. This assumption is proven naïve by the following test. Take any reasonably complex set of findings from a research project, formulate your own approach, and then ask two or three statisticians individually how they would analyze the results. We predict that you will get two or three (if not four or five) seemingly reasonable and valid approaches to analyzing the data. At the end of the process, you will often conclude that the strategy you started with is as reasonable as any of the additional ones that you discover during this exploration.

You can take a number of lessons away from such experiences. First, once you have gained an understanding of the underlying concepts, even if you have never conducted a SAS or SPSS analysis, you should not be shy about offering your opinion and engaging in discussions with your statistician colleagues. Second, there is no single right or best way of conducting an analysis (although there are wrong ways). If you are uncomfortable with what your statistician colleagues suggest, ask around and come back with questions of clarification. Third, it is often informative to run the analysis using more than one strategy. Finding the same results increases your confidence in each of the alternatives. Substantive differences in results should lead to weaker inferences or digging deeper to understand why the results differ. Fourth, you and your statistician colleague must be ready to respond to a statistical reviewer who has her own idea about a superior approach to analysis.

15.4 NOTHING IS STRAIGHTFORWARD

Even after a decade or more of experience, we have been surprised at how often a new study that differs in some (sometimes minor) way from previous projects presents substantial challenges in deciding the optimal approach to analysis. It is useful, indeed crucial, before beginning a study to plan what seems likely to be the best approach to analysis. But having the completed data set available often proves to be a very different experience from the theoretical planning exercise.

Even further down the road in our careers, we are no longer surprised at the extraordinary variety of analytic challenges we face as clinical researchers. The statisticians with whom we have worked have had to develop new methods to deal with a wide variety of issues and have published a number of papers describing and extending these methods.

We find the perpetual new challenges of deciding on optimal analytic approaches and the periodic need to develop new approaches, one of the joys of the clinical research experience. Observing that the minority of analyses are likely to be completely straightforward, we anticipate the need for high-quality statistical collaboration.

15.5 BE SKEPTICAL

We have been blessed with the opportunity of consistently working with a number of excellent statisticians. Typically, after collaboratively planning the analytic strategy for a particular project, an experienced research associate carries out our analyses. Subsequently, we review the analysis as a team, including faculty-level statistical input.

Although our statistician co-workers have all been excellent, mistakes and misunderstandings are not uncommon. Your statistician colleagues may succeed in gaining a sophisticated understanding of the clinical problem that your study has addressed, but your understanding is likely to remain deeper. Furthermore, your statistician colleagues are likely to be working simultaneously on many projects on diverse topics, a situation in which the depth of understanding is more difficult.

Whatever the reason, results will sometimes appear anomalous. Be alert for findings that do not fit together, are inconsistent with what you learned when you examined the data descriptively, or are inconsistent with your clinical understanding of the condition under study. In our experience, when you identify such apparent anomalies, they will very often be due to some analytical error and are quickly corrected. How many such errors end up as part of published papers is unknown, but finding apparent inconsistencies in published data is not uncommon. A constantly critical and questioning attitude will help you to avoid becoming a victim of such problems.

15.6 SPECIFIC ANALYTIC CHALLENGES

We are now entering into a statistical territory proper to review four common and important questions that frequently arise in our work. This section is likely best suited to someone with knowledge of basic statistics, but not much hands-on experience in analysis, or to someone with more advanced statistical skills who wants to know how some clinicians (i.e., we) think about common statistical issues. If you haven't had any statistics, or if you've had a lot of statistics and don't want to get down into the dirt with us, feel free to skip to this section.

Can You Perform Parametric Analysis on Ordinal Data?

Data may be nominal (i.e., categories, not ordered, most commonly two categories), ordinal (i.e., ordered categories, but distance between categories needn't be the same), interval (i.e., ordered categories with distance between the same, but no natural zero) and ratio (i.e., interval with a natural zero). For instance, "A man (*nominal*) walked into my office and told me his joint pain was worse than last month (6 out of 7) (*ordinal*). His temperature was 101°F (*interval*) and his weight was down, at 126 lb (*ratio*)."

One often faces an analysis when an outcome measure has ordinal properties, for example, a seven-point pain scale (as in our patient in the previous paragraph). We deal with such situations most often in surveys, or in clinical trials when the outcome is a quality-of-life measure. In theory, because these ordinal measures do not meet the assumptions of parametric analysis (t-test family), one should use nonparametric methods (chi-square family) to analyze the data. Advances in computer technology have made use of nonparametric approaches, including exact methods, more feasible than in the past.

Nevertheless, parametric methods, if valid, are easier, more flexible, and more familiar. Parametric methods are generally "robust," that is, they are relatively insensitive to violations of their assumptions. Data generally have to be sparse, with gross violations of assumptions, before parametric methods yield importantly misleading results.

Statisticians vary in the extent to which they are willing to use parametric analysis in an ordinal data set. Take a questionnaire with four questions and a seven-point scale response option format for each question. If we use 1 to 7 as the digits for the seven-point scales, patients may score anywhere from 4 to 28 on this questionnaire. Unless the results are very highly skewed, almost all statisticians will be comfortable using parametric methods on such a data set.

Take, on the other hand, a single item with three response options. Many (although not all) statisticians will feel uncomfortable using parametric approaches in this circumstance and will prefer a nonparametric analysis.

What about the in-between situation when you have, say, four to eight ordered categories into which you may categorize respondents on a particular outcome? Here, the first step is to look at the distribution of responses. Let's take a seven-category situation. Assume that 70% of respondents choose an extreme value (e.g., category 1), 28% choose 2, and the remaining 2% are spread over the other five options. Treating these responses as if they represent continuous data would be inappropriate. The distribution of the data suggests that the best approach would be to treat the data as binary (categories being those who choose a value of 1, and those who choose any other value).

What about a distribution in which 70% choose 1, 15% choose 2, and 15% are spread over the 3 to 7 range. Here, treating the data as ordinal with three categories (1, 2, and 3 to 7) is likely to provide the most valid analysis.

If the data are reasonably evenly distributed (reasonably being, of course, in the eye of the statistician-beholder), and respondents use all the seven categories, treating the data as continuous will make your life, and likely that of the clinicians who will have to understand and use your results, easier.

What's the Best Way to Deal with Continuous Data with Repeated Measures?

A common situation we face in our work is a randomized trial, or other longitudinal study, in which patients are exposed to two or more conditions (experimental interventions) and followed serially over time (6). Analytic options for this situation include regression methods and looking at areas under the curve. We have, however, found repeated measures analysis of variance (ANOVA) as the optimal strategy, and a repeated measures ANOVA framework continues to provide a useful conceptual framework.

This framework highlights the factors or variables that may be influencing patients' status on the outcome measure of interest. In one simple design (patients have been randomized to one of two management strategies, baseline values, and two follow-up measurements obtained), the two factors that may systematically influence patients' values on the outcome measure are treatment and time. Furthermore, there may be an interaction between these two factors.

Figures 15–1 to 15–4 illustrate the range of possible results and how these would play out in a repeated measures ANOVA. For instance, time may have no effect, but treatment may have a consistent impact (Figure 15–1). Alternatively, treatment may have no effect, but patient scores may increase

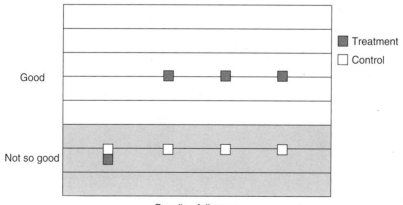

FIGURE 15–1 Treatment effect shown, no effect of time.

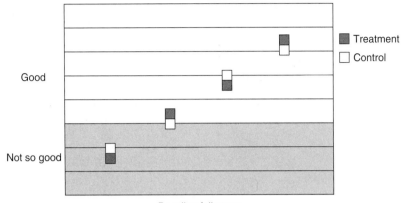

FIGURE 15–2   Time effect shown, no effect of treatment.

with time (Figure 15–2). Third, treatment may have an early effect that disappears on further follow-up (Figure 15–3). Finally, treatment effects may increase over time (Figure 15–4). These latter two results represent interactions between treatment and time (i.e., the treatment effect varies depending on which time point one is considering).

Some investigators using data from this sort of design give the baseline data in this design the same status as the data gathered after individuals in the treatment group began to receive the intervention. If analyzed in this way, a positive effect of treatment is detected as a time by treatment interaction. That is, treatment has no effect at baseline (i.e., before it is administered) but has an effect on subsequent observations.

This way of presenting results will confuse many clinicians to whom the concept of an interaction is foreign. A preferable way of handling the

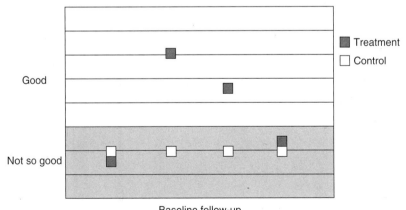

FIGURE 15–3   Treatment shows early effect, but disappears over time.

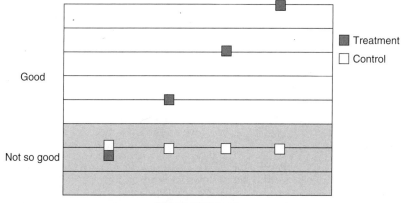

FIGURE 15–4 Treatment effects increase over time.

baseline data is to use it as a covariate in the analysis. This will add power to the analysis as long as the correlation between baseline and follow-up data is at least 0.5 (which it generally is). You can never go wrong with this analysis of covariance approach, and even if correlation between baseline and follow-up is very low, you will never lose power using the baseline data as a covariate.

ANOVA-like models can also be used to deal with missing observations. In the past, statistical program limitations meant that if some of the data were missing, you had challenging decisions to make. If some patients had missing data for some of the observations, the options included eliminating the visit in which the observations were missing, eliminating the patients in whom the observations were missing, or making some sort of estimation for the missing observations. Having decided to estimate, you could choose between a number of estimation strategies.

Nowadays, such data are best analyzed using general linear models. These models are conceptually identical to the repeated measures ANOVA just described. One of their advantages is that they have built-in strategies for dealing with missing data. You can rely on these strategies for accurate inferences if there are not excessive missing data—say, less than 10%—and the missing data is essentially randomly distributed.

When Should You "Degrade" Continuous Data?

A great limitation of continuous data lies in difficulties in clinical interpretation (no doubt an example of the old statistical truism "the mean conceals more than it reveals"). If I lower systolic blood pressure by a mean of 3 mm Hg, is the effect trivial or important? If I improve health-related quality of life by a mean of 0.3 on a scale with extremes of 1 and 7 is the effect trivial or important? If the average compliance with treatment in an intervention group increases by a mean of 5% is the effect trivial or important?

An effective way of making continuous data interpretable is to choose a cut-point and examine distributions of patients in treatment and control groups falling above and below the cut-points. For instance, more than 25 years ago, two of us (Brian Haynes and Dave Sackett) randomized 39 noncompliant hypertensive steelworkers with uncontrolled hypertension to usual care or to an intervention that included home monitoring of blood pressure, monitoring of medication use, tailoring of medication use to daily rituals, and reinforcement of compliant behavior (7).

We reported the results in two ways. We informed readers that compliance increased by 21.3% in the intervention group but fell 1.5% in the control group ($P = 0.025$). We also reported the proportion of patients who had better compliance on follow-up than at baseline (16 out of 20, or 80% in the treated group, and 7 of 18, or 39% in the control group, $P = 0.009$). Note here that, although analysis of continuous data will generally result in greater statistical power than analysis of a dichotomous outcome, in this instance we achieved lower P values in the binary analysis.

In another example, Swedish investigators randomized patients with diabetes to an intensive, multifactor intervention to modify cardiovascular risk factors versus standard management (8). They presented figures that show early and persistent divergence of curves describing the temporal pattern of changes in mean glycosylated hemoglobin level, mean cholesterol level, and mean systolic and diastolic blood pressure in the treatment and control groups. They did not, however, report P values associated with the differences in the curves. They also dichotomized the outcomes to show the percentage of patients who, after a mean follow-up of 7.8 years, achieved the goals of intensive therapy. The percentages were, in the treatment and control groups, respectively, approximately 15% and 3% ($P = 0.06$) for glycosylated hemoglobin levels less than 6.5%; 74% and 21% for cholesterol levels less than 175 mg per dL ($P < 0.001$); 48% and 18% for systolic blood pressure less than 130 mm Hg ($P = 0.001$); and 72% and 60% for diastolic blood pressure of less than 80 mm Hg ($P = 0.21$). Note that two of these four binary comparisons achieve conventional levels of statistical significance. The authors do not say whether the analysis of continuous data yielded significant results.

In both these cases, the authors judge (we suspect rightly) that the percentages of patients achieving particular targets were more meaningful to clinicians than were mean changes in the variables of interest. Although this gain in interpretability is attractive, you must handle this somewhat tricky situation with care. First of all, it is easy to manipulate the data by testing various cut-points and by choosing one that best separates treatment and control groups. For instance, in our hypertension study, we could have presented the proportion of patients achieving a particular target (e.g., 80% compliance) or an increase in compliance of greater than 0 (e.g., 20%). If you plan to dichotomize, you should choose your threshold beforehand, specify the threshold in your protocol, and stick with it. Otherwise, you will be committing the statistical high crime of Data Dredging.

Second, be prepared for the result to reach statistical significance in the analysis of continuous data (with relatively narrow confidence intervals) and, in the binary analysis, to fail to achieve significance (with wide confidence intervals). Personally, we are not terribly troubled by such a discrepancy. Our way of looking at this situation is that the continuous analysis shows that the differences are real (i.e., chance is an unlikely explanation of the findings) and the binary presentation provides a way to understand this true difference. This line of reasoning would argue that presentation of the P values associated with the binary analysis is unnecessary. Indeed, in our randomized controlled trial (RCT) of compliance-enhancement in patients with hypertension, we didn't present the P values associated with the proportion of patients with improved compliance (although those P values were actually lower than those associated with the continuous measures analysis). Others may, however, insist on reporting both sets of P values, and find the loss of significance in the binary analysis, when it happens, troubling. Most awkward, these others may include the reviewers of your manuscript.

Third, be sure that your thresholds really do represent reasonable criteria for importance. In the second example, if you can increase the proportion of patients who achieve the threshold for hypertension or glucose control, have you really made an important change? For the answer to come from within the study itself, long-term follow-up with an adequate number of patients is needed. The Swedish study (8) did so and revealed the convincing evidence of a reduction in the risk for events that matter to patients and their doctors, namely, cardiovascular disease, retinopathy, and nephropathy.

When this type of powerful evidence cannot be generated within a study, then the onus is on the investigator to find other, larger studies that show a direct link between the intermediate variable of interest and an important clinical outcome. Clearly, one can identify strengths and weaknesses in choosing an analysis and presentation restricted to continuous data, restricted to binary outcomes, or both. Currently, we rely heavily on the combined approach in an area where interpretation is particularly challenging: measurement of health-related quality of life (HRQoL). Here, the analysis of the continuous data tells us how likely chance is to explain differences between treatment and control groups, and the proportion who achieve an important benefit with treatment helps us understand what the results mean.

For instance, in a randomized trial of respiratory rehabilitation versus standard care in patients with chronic lung disease (9), the mean differences between rehabilitation and control groups in dyspnea in daily life measured by the Chronic Respiratory Questionnaire was 0.60 on a 1 to 7 scale ($P = 0.006$). Rehabilitation also resulted in gains in emotional function of 0.40 ($P = 0.015$). What is one to make of these differences? Do they represent small or large changes? In other studies, we had established that a change of 0.5 on the seven-point scale represents a small but important difference (10). The mean difference of 0.60, however, does not mean that every patient achieved a small but important difference. Similarly, differences below the threshold of 0.5, such as those seen in the rehabilitation study in emotional function, do not mean that none of the patients experienced considerable improvement. Rather, one would expect a distribution of benefits across patients, some achieving large improvements in HRQoL and others showing trivial or no gains.

Using exactly the same logic as the hypertension compliance and diabetes risk reduction studies, we calculated that 44% of the rehabilitation group met the threshold of a 0.5 improvement in day-to-day shortness of breath, whereas the comparable figure for the control group was 20%. Thus, the net proportion of patients who benefited from rehabilitation was 24% (11). In an approach with which you are now familiar, one can take the inverse of these percentages to determine the number of patients one needs to treat to achieve a small but important improvement in a single patient. One needs to treat 1/0.24, or approximately four patients, to achieve an important reduction in dyspnea for a single patient. The comparable numbers needed to treat (NNTs) for emotional function is 3. These numbers represent an impressive benefit in comparison to many other NNTs and give us a sense of the gains some patients can achieve with rehabilitation.

Regression or Correlation, Anyone?

Establishing associations between variables and trying to establish causal pathways between variables remain key activities in clinical epidemiological inquiry. Whereas other strategies, such as recursive partitioning, have gained some popularity, regression remains the key tool for such analyses.

You probably know some elementary concepts in regression, but they came as such a delightful revelation to us that we cannot resist repeating them. First, correlation and regression are themselves closely related. The difference is that correlation is conceptually used when you are simply interested in the closeness of the relation between two variables rather than trying to establish cause and effect. Regression is designed to try to establish cause and effect.

Given this goal of regression, you have two types of variables: the putative causes and the effect. We refer to the causes as independent variables, and the effects as dependent variables.

We can classify regression into three types, depending on the nature of the dependent variable. If the dependent variable has two categories (binary), we refer to the regression as "logistic" (because the arithmetic relies on logarithms). If the dependent variable is continuous, we refer to the regression as "linear" (because it assumes a linear relation between the dependent and independent variables).

These two categories of dependent variables are by far the most frequently used. In our own work, we have found a third type of regression useful, when the dependant variable is categorical (in our case, not ordered, but it could be ordered). The term for regression in which the dependent variable is categorical is "polytomous" or "polychotomous."

Regression can be "simple" or univariable—only one independent variable—or "multiple" or multivariable, with more than one independent variable. People sometimes use the term "multivariate" synonymously with multivariable. If you wish to be technically accurate, restrict use of the term "multivariate" to situations when you are conducting an analysis with more than one dependent variable—a complexity beyond the scope of the present discussion.

A limitation of simple regression is that it leaves you with no idea of the extent to which the power of apparent predictors is independent. The greater the extent to which the independent variables are related to one another—"co-linearity" is the term that you will sometimes see used to describe the situation when independent variables are correlated with one another—the greater the extent to which simple regressions are liable to mislead.

The usual problem with regression analyses is that there are many independent variables of interest and relatively few participants in your study. A useful rule of thumb is that, in logistic regression, there should be ten events (not ten patients, but ten events) for every independent variable of interest. If you try to conduct an analysis that violates this guide, you are very likely to produce an unreliable and potentially misleading model. When extensive co-linearity is present, or independent variables have multiple categories, the ratio of events to independent variables needs to be even greater to produce a reliable model.

In our experience, an excess of candidate predictors relative to study participants is the rule rather than the exception. The usual approach to this dilemma is to begin by conducting simple regressions with each candidate independent variable. One anticipates that only a relatively small number of independent variables will demonstrate a statistically significant association with the dependent variable. The criterion for significance in this context (as in any other) is somewhat arbitrary, but statisticians often recommend a less strict criterion ($P = 0.10$, or even 0.20) than those (0.05 or 0.01) that we are familiar with seeing in other contexts.

Hopefully, the initial simple regressions leave a smaller number of candidate predictor variables, and therefore you will not be violating the rule of ten. Let us assume that this is the case. The next step is to conduct a multivariable regression, a process appropriately termed "modeling." There are a profusion of strategies. One very commonly used, but probably sub-optimal strategy, is forward "stepwise" regression. Here, the most powerful predictor enters the model first. The predictor that accounts for the greatest portion of the residual unexplained variance enters second. The procedure continues until all available variables have entered the model. One usually sets a cut-off for significance (typically 0.05) and reports all variables that explain a statistically significant additional proportion of the variance.

An alternative approach, favoured by some, is backward "stepwise" regression. Here, you begin by entering all variables into the model. You then eliminate the variable that explains least variance, and rerun the model. You continue until the last variable that you are considering eliminating explains a statistically significant proportion of the variance, and stop there.

Multivariable regression will likely tell you that some of the apparent predictors from univariable modeling fail as independent predictors. For instance, in the study that provided our working example in Chapter 8 on evaluating diagnostic tests, in a univariable regression, sepsis increased the odds of important bleeding by a factor of 7.3 (P <0.001). In the multivariable regression, this apparently powerful predictor of bleeding was no longer significant. The reason is that its apparent power was not due to a causal link between sepsis and ulcers, but rather because patients with sepsis tended to need mechanical ventilation and have a predisposition to coagulopathy, two factors with a stronger link to bleeding.

Whether forward or backward, letting the computer choose the variables for the final predictive model without your input is potentially risky. The risk comes because a true causal variable may be strongly correlated with another, noncausal variable. If this is the case, it is possible that, by chance in a particular data set, the noncausal variable will be more strongly associated with the dependent variable, and will thus be chosen by the model, and the causal variable will be left out.

For instance, could it be that there really is a causal link between sepsis and the risk of bleeding (sepsis compromises the ability of the gastric mucosa to maintain its integrity, perhaps), and that our multivariable model's rejection of sepsis in favor of mechanical ventilation was due to anomaly of this particular data set? The answer, uncomfortably, is yes.

What can you do to avoid this sort of misleading result? You can, before creating your model, specify a hierarchy of predictors on the basis of your understanding of the underlying biology. Then, when you construct the model, limit its flexibility such that predictors higher on the hierarchy enter the model before predictors lower on the hierarchy.

For instance, if we had reason to believe that sepsis is more likely to be causally associated with gastrointestinal bleeding than is mechanical ventilation, we could have specified that in initial construction of the model sepsis entered first (if we were constructing a forward regression model). The model would then test whether, after considering sepsis, mechanical ventilation explained a statistically significant portion of the residual variance.

It remains possible that, if mechanical ventilation explains all the variability explained by sepsis and then some, sepsis would remain absent from the final model. Creating this sort of hierarchy and limiting the model accordingly, however, provides the greatest opportunity for one's *a priori* understanding of the biology to dictate the nature of the final model. Given model-building's susceptibility to serendipity, such constraints are generally welcome.

Let's go back to the point in the process when you have conducted your univariable regressions, hoping to limit the number of your candidate predictors to no more than one tenth of the number of outcome events in your data set. If you still have an excess of independent variables, you have a potentially vexing problem. You can go ahead and run your multivariable regression (there is nothing in the statistical programs to stop you), but the results may be very misleading.

We faced such a situation in a study in which we examined predictors of clinicians' decisions to establish an explicit resuscitation order in critically ill patients and whether that was an order to resuscitate or to not resuscitate (12). When the time came to analyze our data, we found we had 2,916 eligible patients. Sounds like a hefty sample size, right? Of these, 319 had explicit resuscitation orders, the dependent variable, outcome, or "event" in any regression analysis, still a substantial number. Because, however, we were interested in whether the order was to resuscitate or not resuscitate (and thus we conducted a polychotomous regression with three categories: no explicit directive, resuscitate, and do not resuscitate), we had to break down the events further. The orders split almost exactly 50:50; for 160 patients the order was to resuscitate, and for 159 the order was to not resuscitate.

According to the rule of ten, this left us with the potential for simultaneously considering 16 variables. For better or worse, virtually every factor we were considering proved significantly associated with clinicians' resuscitation decisions, and most factors had multiple levels. This situation proved one in which the rule of ten was insufficiently conservative. As a result, our first attempts at model-building provided models that were very unstable (depending on which approach we chose, we obtained quite different results).

To deal with these problems, we grouped our independent variables in four categories. These included demographic factors (i.e., age, APACHE II score, medical or surgical admission); decision-making factors (i.e., ability to participate in decision making within 24 hours of admission, and legal power of attorney for health care); temporal factors [(i.e., time of intensive care unit (ICU) admission (day: 0800 to 1700 hours, versus evening: 1700 to 0800 hours) and day of ICU admission (weekday versus weekend)]; and geographical factors (i.e., center, city, and country). We created four separate polychotomous logistic models, one for each set of factors. Thus, for example, the polychotomous regression analysis involving demographic variables simultaneously considered age, APACHE II score, and admission diagnosis.

The geographic variables offered another statistical wrinkle. Center, city, and country are clearly not independent. If we tell you that we work at the McMaster site within the Hamilton (Ontario) Health Sciences hospitals, you know we work in Hamilton, and you know we work in Canada. Using statistical jargon, city is "nested" within country, and center "nested" within city. The appropriate analysis recognizes this dependency. Thus, we analyzed geographic variables hierarchically; odds ratios for country, city, and center were derived from three unique models.

We're sure you find it evident that we could not have dealt with this data set in a satisfactory manner without high-powered collaboration from statisticians. Once again, the most important message of this section is that, if at all possible, you should obtain highly qualified and experienced statisticians to help with your studies from the planning stages onward.

REFERENCES

1. Jaeschke R, Guyatt G, Barratt A, et al. Measures of association. In: Guyatt G, Rennie D, eds. *Users' guides to the medical literature: A manual for evidence-based clinical practice.* Chicago, IL: AMA Press, 2002.

2. Guyatt G, Jaescke R, Cook D, et al. Hypothesis testing. In: Guyatt G, Rennie D, eds. *Users' guides to the medical literature: A manual for evidence-based clinical practice.* Chicago, IL: AMA Press, 2002.

3. Guyatt G, Walter S, Cook D. Confidence intervals. In: Guyatt G, Rennie D, eds. *Users' guides to the medical literature: A manual for evidence-based clinical practice.* Chicago, IL: AMA Press, 2002.

4. Streiner D, Norman G. *PDQ statistics*, 2nd ed. Hamilton, OH: B.C. Decker, 1997.

5. Altman D. *Practical statistics for medical research.* London. Chapman & Hall, 1991.

6. Frison L, Pocock SJ. Repeated measures in clinical trials: analysis using mean summary statistics and its implications for design. *Stat Med* 1992;11:1685–1704.

7. Haynes RB, Sackett DL, Gibson ES, et al. Improvement of medication compliance in uncontrolled hypertension. *Lancet* 1976;1(7918):1265–1268.

8. Gaede P, Vedel P, Larsen N, et al. Multifactorial intervention and cardiovascular disease in patients with type 2 diabetes. *N Engl J Med* 2003;348:383–393.

9. Goldstein RS, Gort EH, Stubbing D, et al. Randomized controlled trial of respiratory rehabilitation. *Lancet* 1994;344:1394–1397.

10. Jaeschke R, Singer J, Guyatt GH. Measurement of health status: ascertaining the minimal clinically important difference. *Control Clin Trials* 1989;10:407–415.

11. Guyatt GH, Juniper EF, Walter SD, et al. Interpreting treatment effects in randomized trials. *BMJ* 1998;316:690–692.

12. Cook D, Guyatt GH, Rocker G, et al. The Canadian Critical Care Trials Group. Cardiopulmonary resuscitation directives on admission to the intensive care unit. *Lancet* 2001;358:1941–1945.

16

PREPARING REPORTS FOR PUBLICATION AND RESPONDING TO REVIEWERS' COMMENTS

Gordon Guyatt and Brian Haynes

Publishing the findings of your research in highly prestigious, peer-reviewed journals is the *sine qua non* of academic success, short of, say, a Nobel Prize. Although it would be nice to believe that the intrinsic merit of your research is the main determinant of whether your article is published in a given journal, many other factors bear on this, including the target audience of the journal, the number of articles published by the journal compared with the number of manuscripts submitted (the "rejection rate"), whether the journal has recently published something on the same topic, whether the findings are "positive" or "negative," whether the findings are "newsworthy" in the view of the editor, which reviewers assess your article, how well you have written the article, and dumb luck (good or bad). You can do something about most of these factors (see Table 16–1). Sooner or later, you can get virtually any paper accepted by some journal, and this chapter discusses some ways to increase your chances of having your papers accepted sooner rather than later, and by journals that are considered prestigious in your field.

Here is a checklist that will prove useful when preparing reports:

✓ Choose a target journal(s) and write for it.
✓ Choose a clear message.
✓ Achieve high quality in your writing.
✓ Respond to reviewers' comments.
✓ Deal with the editors.

✓ *Choose a target journal(s) and write for it.*

One of the first choices you should make when preparing your manuscript is the category of journal you will target and, on occasion, the target journal itself. Depending on how well matched your project is to the nature

TABLE 16–1 **Determinants of Publication**

Determinant	What You Can Do
Interest to target audience	Choose journal read by those interested in your topic
Rejection rate	Choose lower profile journal
Recent publication on the topic	Choose journal that has recently published on your topic
Whether the findings are "positive" or "negative"	If you have a "negative" study, in your covering letter, you may want to remind the editor of the importance of avoiding publication bias
Whether the findings are newsworthy in the view of the editor	Work hard to vividly highlight the importance of your findings
Who your article is sent to as reviewers	In your covering letter, you may want to suggest reviewers likely to be sympathetic
How well you have written the article	Note the suggestions in this chapter
Dumb luck	Choose a co-author known to have extraordinary and unwarranted good luck

and objectives of the journal you choose, one journal may greet an article with enthusiasm, whereas another will view that same article with disdain. You should consider several issues related to choosing and writing for your target journal.

Tailoring Content to the Target Journal

As a clinical researcher, most of the articles you write will report on the clinical studies you undertake, and your fellow clinicians will constitute the target audience. On occasion, however, you may be writing a paper with a more methodological focus. Such papers explore issues of optimal study design, methods of measurement, or interpretation of findings.

We can think of three categories of journals in which you will publish your research: general medical journals, subspecialty journals, and methodologically-oriented journals. Many articles produced by clinical researchers have the potential for succeeding in more than one category of target journal.

Clinical journals are often interested in papers that focus on methodological issues. By the same token, methodologically-oriented journals often welcome what are fundamentally clinical papers with a methodological slant. Although the *Journal of Clinical Epidemiology* is a common target journal for methodologically-oriented papers, it also deals with a wide range of clinical areas. *Medical Care*, another methodologically-oriented journal, focuses on health services research. You may find methodological journals with a particular focus on your area of exploration. For instance, one of us has conducted many studies in measurement of health-related quality of life (HRQoL), and the journal *Quality of Life Research* is an obvious potential target for these papers. These methodological journals typically have both a smaller and more select readership than even second-tier clinical journals.

You are likely to be submitting an article that might be appropriate to more than one of these three categories of journals. You will write every part of your paper differently depending on the target you ultimately choose.

When writing your introduction, bear in mind that clinical journal audiences will need an explanation of why they should be interested in a methodological topic. For instance, not too long ago we published a paper about a new version of a popular questionnaire for patients with chronic lung disease (1). We targeted a clinical journal that addresses issues of respiratory disease, *Chest*. Our introduction began with the following sentence: "Health-related quality of life (HRQoL) outcomes are gaining importance in clinical trials of patients with chronic airflow limitation (CAL)."

Had we submitted the paper to *Quality of Life Research*, such an opening would elicit groans, because we would be making a statement that readers (and reviewers) would perceive as completely obvious. Clinical journal readers and reviewers, however, must be reminded (or told for the first time) about the importance of HRQoL measurement.

If you are writing for a general medical journal versus a subspecialty medical journal, you may need to provide greater explanation of not only methodological but also clinical issues. For instance, a group of us began the introduction of an article we recently published in the *New England Journal of Medicine* with the following statement: "Mechanical ventilation is the most common form of advanced life support in the intensive care unit (ICU)" (2). Had we been writing for a critical care journal, such an introduction would be self-evident.

Methods sections, including descriptions of statistical analyses, should be much more detailed in a methods journal. Even in a clinical journal, you need to inform reviewers and other researchers (if not clinical readers) of crucial methodological details, and your paper should provide sufficient information that another investigator could reproduce your study. At the same time, clinical journals will want your methods section to be as compact as possible, and you should oblige them. Methods journals will be more indulgent of, and may even demand, detailed descriptions of your methods.

Publishing a methods paper in advance of the results papers for your study is an excellent way to achieve the economy demanded by high-circulation clinical journals. Open access electronic journals such as *BioMed Central* (*http://www.biomedcentral.com*) provide an excellent service for this purpose. If the details of your methods are published there, then your results papers can refer to them for details—and you will gain an additional publication for your resume. If your study is important, many second-tier clinical journals will also accept methods papers, especially if baseline data are included. For example, the North American Symptomatic Carotid Endarterectomy Trial methods paper was published in *Stroke* (3), and the main results paper in the *New England Journal or Medicine* (4). Publishing the methods paper in a timely way can also publicize the trial, provide collaborators with tangible benefits, and stimulate recruitment.

The same issue of level of detail applies to the results. For instance, our HRQoL measure for patients with chronic lung disease has four domains (i.e., dyspnea, fatigue, emotional function, and mastery). One can aggregate the first two domains into a physical function domain and the last two into an emotional function domain. When writing for a methods journal, we always provide information on all four domains. When writing for a clinical journal, however, we may describe only the aggregated two-domain results.

The Discussion section is similar to the Introduction in that, when submitting to a clinical journal, you may need to address issues of the importance of your methodological work. On the other hand, you might have more scope for exploration of methodological issues in a methods journal.

Tailoring Format to Your Target Journal

Virtually every journal has issues of formatting and presentation to which you must attend. Most of these are relatively trivial (such as section headers or reference citation style) and will occupy you when you are polishing the manuscript for submission. Other issues are more substantial, and you should address them early on. For instance, if you are aiming at a very prestigious journal, your total word count is liable to be much more limited than for a lower-profile target. In addition, some journals have special sections that may be particularly suited for your publication, such as "Brief Communications" or "Special Articles."

Choosing a Journal with a Fondness for Your Topic

Some journal editors and editorial boards are fond of particular topics or areas of inquiry. If a journal has previously published a study in an area closely related to your investigation, it qualifies as a likely target for your submission. On the other hand, a dearth of articles in your area or using your methodology provides a message that you should look elsewhere. The *New England Journal of Medicine*, for instance, publishes very few systematic reviews and meta-analyses, whereas other major general medical journals (e.g., *JAMA*, *BMJ*, and *The Lancet*) favor them.

How High to Aim

One question you will confront is how high in the pecking order your paper might climb. Many view five top general medical journals as particularly attractive vehicles for their papers: *New England Journal of Medicine*, *Lancet*, *JAMA*, *BMJ*, and *Annals of Internal Medicine*. Authors often wonder whether it is worth a try at these or other prestigious journals. Even experienced investigators find predicting success (or the lack of it) challenging, and this challenge makes the decision concerning the best target journal more difficult. For instance, knowing that top journals accept few methodology papers (with the exception of papers that are part of a series negotiated with journal editors), one of us strongly discouraged his coauthors from submitting a discussion of the intention-to-treat principle to the *BMJ* (3). They ignored the advice and, lo and behold, the *BMJ* accepted the paper (the price being the need to reduce the word count by 50%, with considerable loss of useful discussion). With electronic publication not burdened by space restraints, clinical journals (including the *BMJ*) are offering a partial solution to this problem by parallel paper (short) and electronic (longer) publication.

Generally, if it is appropriate that you seriously think of submitting to a top journal, it means that your research has been well planned, and well implemented (in other words, you have followed the advice in this book!) and, on top of that, you have gotten lucky. More often, the internal debate (internal to you or to your investigative team) may be whether to make your first submission to a second-tier journal (perhaps, for instance, the top journal in your subspecialty area) or a less prestigious journal more likely to accept your paper. As We've mentioned, reading tea leaves is often as likely to provide as accurate a prediction regarding journal receptiveness as is any other strategy. The resulting uncertainty makes the choice of target journal more difficult.

In advising junior colleagues, we generally ask them about how patient they are feeling regarding the timing of publication. Almost invariably, the timing of publication is not urgent. On rare occasions when you feel you are competing with other investigators whose own submissions may be imminent, you may aim lower to make rapid acceptance more likely, but this may backfire if the lower journal is slower at processing manuscripts, which is often the case. You may, however, be able to negotiate quick review and accelerated publication if you speak directly with the editor.

Top journals typically respond quickly. A local young investigator who asked for expedited review by *The Lancet* and received his rejection 4 hours later probably holds the record for quick rejection. More typically, if rejection is your fate, you can expect to know within 3 months. Other journals take longer. You may want to check with colleagues about your target journal's track record. Unfortunately, rejections after more than 6 months wait are not unusual with some publications.

One benefit of aiming high is that there is a chance that an astute review will help you improve your paper. Our experience is that substantial improvements on the basis of reviewers' comments are unusual, but do happen on occasion. So, if you are feeling patient, and several rejections will not hurt your ego, aim high. If impatience and vulnerability characterize your psychological state, choose a lower status journal more likely to accept your paper on first submission.

✓ *Choose a clear message.*

Your work may be quite complex and a clear conclusion not self-evident. You must keep considering and reconsidering the nature of your results until you have defined a clear message. If your audience is to take away a single point, what is that point to be?

Having decided on your message you need to write your introduction in such a way that readers have no doubt about the importance of your question. The approach should have the same components as a good story. The introduction should raise the reader's curiosity, the results should satisfy that curiosity, and the discussion must show how important the results are.

Recently, we completed an observational study examining the incidence of clinically diagnosed venous thromboembolism (VTE) in critically ill patients (4). We found that only 2.4% of patients had clinically diagnosed VTE. Of patients with diagnosed VTE, approximately half were receiving heparin prophylaxis and half were not. We could have concluded that VTE is infrequent and not a big problem in patients in the ICU. Alternatively, we could have left it to the readers to make their own inferences about the clinical conclusions they should draw. The first approach would have compromised enthusiasm for our ongoing research program in the prevention of VTE. The second would have led to a ho-hum paper that would not likely catch the imagination of reviewers, editors, or readers.

Instead, we chose to focus on the difference between VTE detected in screening studies (approximately 10%) and clinically detected VTE. That choice allowed us to conclude that VTE was clinically underdiagnosed and that clinicians should raise their diagnostic suspicion. The fact that 50% occurred in those not receiving prophylaxis suggested that clinicians should employ strategies to enhance compliance with prophylaxis administration. The fact that 50% occurred in those receiving prophylaxis suggested the need for innovative prophylaxis strategies.

Having made the choice to present the results in this manner, we wrote the Introduction accordingly. The key sentence read as follows: "We hypothesized that the rates of DVT and PE suspected clinically and subsequently confirmed radiologically are lower than those suggested by surveillance testing." The discussion then picks up and echoes the lead-in of the Introduction.

Often, you can structure the first sentence of the Discussion using the PICOT format, but it is framed as an answer rather than a question. For instance, in this case: "In this multi-center cohort study of patients admitted to an ICU during the year 2000, we found that the prevalence and incidence of definite DVT or PE during admission to a medical-surgical ICU or for 8 weeks post-ICU discharge were both approximately 1%." Later, we highlight the concern about underdiagnosis of VTE: "In the ICU, patients are often unable to communicate symptoms, signs of

VTE are non-specific, clinicians are often inattentive to the physical examination of the lower extremities, and there are multiple alternative reasons for changes in hemodynamics and hypoxia in mechanically ventilated patients. All these factors militate against an optimal index of suspicion for VTE in the ICU."

One could argue that any result would have allowed us to emphasize the importance of VTE in the ICU. That is exactly the point. Whether event rates are high or low and whether events occurred in patients with or without prophylaxis, we could have found a clinical problem in urgent need of remedy. Maximizing your chances of acceptance in the journal of your choice requires finding a compelling clinical message and structuring the Introduction and Discussion to highlight that message.

✓ *Achieve high quality in your writing.*

Basic writing skills are necessary for success in publishing your work. All the examples used in this section come from drafts of manuscripts in which we believe we improved on initial wording.

Use the Active Voice

Writing in the passive voice represents a long-standing medical tradition. This tradition persists despite the fact that the passive voice makes writing more awkward and difficult to understand, adds extra words, and robs the work of some of its force. Today's books about the quality of writing from a variety of nonmedical fields, as well as courses on writing conducted by the top medical journals, all recommend use of active voice.

Table 16–2 illustrates the use of passive and active voice.

Moving from passive to active voice creates special challenges in Methods sections. In general, move away from "this was done" and "that was done" to "we did this," and "we did that." The repeated use of "we"

TABLE 16–2 Examples of Passive and Active Voice

Passive Voice	Active Voice
Patients were asked to provide...	*Patients provided...*
Second, longitudinal validity is not influenced by standardization.	*Second, standardization does not influence longitudinal validity.*
Material for this series has been taken from the Users' Guides to the Medical Literature.	*The Users' Guides to the Medical Literature provided much of the material in this series.*
More than 40 candidate HIV vaccines have been tested in Phase I and II clinical trials.	*Phase I and II clinical trials have tested more than 40 candidate HIV vaccines.*

can, however, get repetitive and perhaps egotistical-sounding. We can suggest a number of strategies for dealing with this problem. Consider:

All studies were assessed independently by two appraisers for validity and content.	*Two appraisers independently reviewed all studies for validity and content.*

Here, we have specified the role of the investigators as "appraisers" to avoid use of "we."

Studies using surveys were considered qualitative surveys if questions were asked in an open-ended manner and quantitative surveys if questions were asked in a structured manner.	*Qualitative surveys asked questions in an open-ended manner and quantitative surveys asked questions in a structured manner.*

Here, instead of changing the original construction to "we considered surveys to be qualitative if..." we personify the surveys and they therefore become the subject of the sentence.

Moving away from the passive voice is a challenge for some investigators. We suggest two strategies. First, in every sentence, consider who is the agent; who or what performed the action. Put that agent first in the sentence. Second, conduct one edit of your paper in which your only goal is to change passive to active voice.

Delete Unnecessary Words

Medical writers tend to use unnecessary words. Deleting these words makes your writing easier to read and more forceful. Journal articles are also subject to stringent space limits. In general, use as few adjectives and adverbs as possible. You are often more convincing when you leave it for the reader to decide that your treatment effect is *very* large, your competitor's paper has *serious* flaws, or the imprecision of an estimate leaves an effect *extremely* uncertain. Consider the following examples in Table 16–3 of using unnecessary words.

The last example, aside from pointing out the gratuitous "There are ...," illustrates another common mistake, the misplaced modifying clause.

Avoid Use of the Verb "To Be"

Using the verb "to be" often has the same effect as use of the passive voice. It robs your writing of vigor and energy. Consider Table 16–4.

Here we have changed from "to be" to a more active verb and have also eliminated unnecessary words. Young investigators can experience the goal of decreasing use of the verb "to be" as even more challenging than moving from passive to active voice. Once again, carrying out an edit of

TABLE 16–3   **Deleting Unnecessary Words**

Fat Phrases	Leaner Phrases
The patient tells you that he is a self-employed house-painter ...	*The patient is a self-employed house-painter ...*
The process of evidence-based practice involves acquiring the skills of accessing the highest quality information ...	*Evidence-based practice involves accessing the highest quality information ...*
The 26 eligible studies that matched inclusion criteria utilized several methods of data collection. Five studies used semi-structured qualitative interviews ...	*Of 26 eligible studies, five used semi-structured qualitative interviews ...*
There are many factors that may influence an outcome aside from the intervention being tested.	*Many factors, aside from the intervention being tested, may influence an outcome.*

the paper in which the only goal is to move from "to be" to more active verbs may be helpful.

Keep Your Paragraphs Short

Almost 20 years ago, one of us began to write articles concerning health policy, or health politics, for newspapers. Doing a good job necessitated looking carefully at high-quality newspaper journalism. One revelation was the length of paragraphs used in newspaper writing. If you've never noticed, have a careful look—most paragraphs are one or two sentences long, and a paragraph more than three sentences long is very unusual.

For about three years, one of us wrote a health policy column every 2 weeks. The papers demanded a strict word count of 800 or less, and the articles generally finished with word counts of between 798 and 800. The discipline of writing for a general audience, and newspaper readers at that, is extremely instructive, and can improve medical writing. Newspaper-style writing is extremely revealing in demonstrating just how many unnecessary

Table 16–4   **Banishing the Verb "To Be"**

"To Be"	Not "To Be"
It is challenging for healthcare personnel to be up-to-date.	*Healthcare personnel face challenges in staying up-to-date.*
There are several strengths of this study, including ...	*Strengths of this study include ...*
There is evidence ...	*Evidence suggests ...*

words—extra words that decrease rather than increase the forcefulness of the message—one can delete. In addition, newspaper writing reinforces the need to use the active voice, and highlights the merit of short paragraphs—how keeping to one idea generally enhances clarity.

If you wish to use a rule of thumb, keep your paragraphs to five or less sentences. Clarity is a priority and you can seldom justify paragraphs of greater length.

You must commit to editing and re-editing your own writing. Achieving optimal style and clarity also involves ample use of colleagues, including co-investigators, mentors, and students. For example, at least seven people have reviewed and commented on this chapter. This is a "scratch my back" business, and it follows that you should always try to respond to others when they ask for your help.

✓ *Respond to reviewers' comments.*

Journals will seldom accept your paper exactly as you submit it. Most often, you will have a number of reviewers' criticisms to which you must respond. How you respond is often critical to whether your paper will be published or whether you will have to start the submission process elsewhere from scratch. The following points may help you deal with what some find a particularly onerous task.

- The optimal structure of the response is to state the reviewer's comment, make any introductory statement you need, and then use italics or some other easily seen convention to reproduce the change you have made in your manuscript in response to the reviewers' criticism. It is essential that the editor be able to easily follow how you've responded to each of the reviewers' comments. For instance:

> *Comment:* "We would prefer that you delete from the Interpretation of the Abstract the clause 'in both higher mortality rates.' While true, this interpretation relates to a previous study."
>
> *Response:* We have deleted this clause from the Interpretation of the Abstract and the sentence now reads as follows:
>
> *Private for-profit hospitals* result in higher payments for care than private not-for-profit hospitals.

- It is easiest to do this if you have an electronic copy of the reviewers' comments, so that you can integrate your replies within the comments. An increasing number of journals provide reviews in electronic form to facilitate this. If they don't, you can easily make an electronic version with Adobe Acrobat, and use "cut and paste" to make a word-processed document. You can also help the editor to follow your changes by providing a "redlined" version of the revised

manuscript, using the "track changes" feature in word processing programs, along with a "clean" version.

- Unless the reviewers' suggestion will make the paper substantially
worse, go along with it. It's seldom worth fighting with the reviewer.
We happily make changes that we don't believe improve a paper, as
long as they don't result in a poorer product. Even if the original
is superior, if the suggested change is marginally less attractive, we
are ready to go ahead. Only if the quality drops substantially will
we resist.

- If the reviewer really screws up, say so directly but courteously. For
whatever reason (haste, ignorance, enmity), reviewers can make mistakes or request changes that don't make sense for the study that
you've done or the data you've collected. If so, politely indicate the
mistaken or unreasonable nature of the request.

- You are likely to be outraged on occasion that the reviewer has not
taken the time to read your paper thoroughly. On occasion, they will
manifest this neglect by suggesting a "change" that is already in your
paper. Don't point out the reviewer's negligence. Think whether
what you've written needs to be clearer or better located. If so, make
the change. If, however, you feel that what you've written is fine, simply say that the revised manuscript "emphasizes" the issue the reviewer has raised.

- If you have an excuse to flatter the reviewer, do so. If the reviewer's
point is remotely sensible, let the reviewer know that she has made
an astute observation. Always end off by thanking reviewers for
their helpful comments that have improved the quality of the paper
(well, at least they won't have made it much worse). Facetiousness
aside, you will find that reviewers' comments sometimes help you
strengthen your manuscript substantially.

✓ *Deal with the editors.*

The best way to "deal with" editors is to give them exactly what they want:
well-written, concise papers appropriate for their target audience. But
often the match between your work and the journal's mission is less than
optimal.

On occasion, you may save yourself time, energy, and aggravation
and increase your chance of acceptance if you call the editor before you
submit. "I have a manuscript, and I'm wondering whether you might be
interested," you say, "so I thought I'd run it by you before sending it to
you for review." If the answer is no, you have indeed saved both you
and the editor time and energy. If the answer is yes, you may increase
the chances of thoughtful editorial review, and thereby the chances of
publication.

On occasion, editors exercise poor judgment in rejecting papers. You
may be the victim of such an error. If the reviewers have been positive and
you feel you can deal with the editors' criticisms, don't hesitate to make a

special appeal even if you have received an outright rejection. A colleague secured ultimate acceptance of a rejected manuscript through this artfully worded letter.

Dear Editor:

We have received your letter indicating that your journal was not able to accept our manuscript for publication. We noted the reviewers' comments; we found them to be thoughtful and appropriate, and we feel that attention to their concerns will substantially improve our report. As well, we noted that each of the three reviewers provided positive reviews. Many of the suggested changes involved providing additional details on definitions, which we agree are needed and which we can easily remedy. The more substantial revision suggested was to perform additional statistical analyses. Our data collection was quite detailed, and we would be very willing to recode our data accordingly and conduct the suggested multivariable regression analyses.

We certainly respect the editorial board's decision concerning our manuscript, and we recognize that your journal receives many more submissions that it can accept; however, we also share Reviewer B's view that our manuscript reports on "an important topic for the practicing physician that does not always receive the attention it deserves." We also feel strongly that your journal would provide the best exposure to practicing pediatricians. Once we complete the revisions suggested by the reviewers would it be possible to resubmit our manuscript to your journal for reconsideration?"

If you have carried out meritorious work that you believe is worthy of publication, do not get discouraged by initial rejection. Peer review is often arbitrary, cursory, gratuitously nasty, or just plain dumb. At the same time, reviewers often give insightful assessments and detailed comments and you should carefully consider their advice. In particular, take note if two or more reviewers offer the same criticism—even if they aren't right, other reviewers are likely to share their response.

We have, on occasion, finally gained acceptance by the third or fourth journal to which we submitted. You have worked hard to produce your research. Revise, reformat, and resubmit until you receive a positive response. Nowadays, with a proliferation of electronic journals (most notably *Biomed Central*, *http://www.biomedcentral.com*, and Public Library of Science *http://www.plos.org*) your likelihood of success is greater than ever.

CONCLUSION

Publishing your articles in top journals involves science, good writing, gamesmanship, and human relations. Suggestions in this chapter should promote both your success and your enjoyment of the process.

REFERENCES

1. Schünemann HJ, Griffith L, Jaeschke R, et al. A comparison of the original Chronic Respiratory Questionnaire (CRQ) with a standardised CRQ version. *Chest* 2003;124: 1421–1429.

2. Cook DJ, Rocker G, Marshall J, et al. The Level of Care Investigators and the Canadian Critical Care Trials Group. Withdrawal of mechanical ventilation in anticipation of death in the intensive care unit. *N Engl J Med* 2003;349:1123–1132.

3. North American Symptomatic Carotid Endarterectomy Trial (NASCET) Steering Committee. North American Symptomatic Carotid Endarterectomy Trial: methods, patient characteristics, and progress. *Stroke* 1991;22:711–720.

4. North American Symptomatic Carotid Endarterectomy Trial Collaborators. Beneficial effect of carotid endarterectomy in symptomatic patients with high grade carotid stenosis. *N Engl J Med* 1991;325:445–453.

17

DEALING WITH THE MEDIA

Dave Sackett, Gordon Guyatt, Brian Haynes,
and Peter Tugwell

"The function of good journalism is to take information and add value to it."

—John Chancellor

"Facing the press is more difficult than bathing a leper."

—Mother Teresa

"To a newspaperman, a human being is an item with skin wrapped around it."

—Fred Allen

"Something seems to happen to people when they meet a journalist, and what happens is exactly the opposite of what one would expect. One would think that extreme wariness and caution would be the order of the day, but in fact childish trust and impetuosity are far more common."

—Janet Malcolm

"Fact that is fact every day is not news; it's truth. We report news, not truth."

—Linda Ellerbee

"Journalism—a profession whose business it is to explain to others what it personally does not understand."

—Lord Northcliffe

"It is well to remember that freedom of the press is the thing that comes first. Most of us probably feel we couldn't be free without newspapers, and that is the real reason we want the newspapers to be free."

—Edward R. Murrow

"The press is the enemy."

—Richard Nixon

"Everything you read in newspapers is absolutely true, except for that rare story of which you happen to have first-hand knowledge."

—Erwin Knoll

474

DEALING WITH MEDIA THAT SEEK YOU OUT

Each of us has been "burned" by the media from time to time, and some of these episodes have been seriously troubling. Judging by the quotes above, we're not alone. Indeed, even journalists cast aspersions on themselves (not necessarily with remorse or repentance!). The four of us range in our views about interacting with the media, from highly averse to cautiously optimistic. But we do agree that media disasters can result from us researchers getting ahead of ourselves (talking with the media when we shouldn't or in ways that we shouldn't), as well as from hasty, incompetent, or malicious reporting.

Dave Sackett is the most negative, and he took the lead in preparing this chapter. The most optimistic of us, Gordon Guyatt, declares a "competing interest"—he is a part-time journalist. In this section, we work through some of the cons and pros of responding to media requests and firmly recommend that you take this all "under advisement" for use when your opportunities for interaction with the media arise.

> Returning home from a scientific meeting to which you presented the results of your latest randomized controlled trial (RCT), you discover that a newspaper reporter and a television station want you to return their calls so that they can arrange to interview you. Proud of your work, you are flattered by their interest and are inclined to return their calls. However, you're familiar with reports documenting instances in which research results have been misunderstood (1), misrepresented (2), and sensationalized (3) by the media.

Should you return these reporters' calls? Dave Sackett's blanket advice is "Never!" The rest of us are more inclined to say "Yes," and even Dave would call back under extraordinary circumstances. This section offers seven questions that Dave asks himself in these situations, and we'll identify the spots where the other authors disagree with his answers. The "I" in the subsequent text is Dave unless clearly indicated as one of the rest of us.

Note that none of the following advice applies to investigators who would benefit financially or professionally from having their research results misunderstood, misinterpreted, and sensationalized. These investigators should seek out the most unscrupulous reporters they can find, especially when promised that their conflicts of interest will go unreported (4).

The questions that you might ask yourself are listed in Table 17–1 and will be discussed in turn.

1. *Have your results and conclusions survived external peer review yet?* Although the results and conclusions of our studies have always survived external peer review, this review has always improved their clarity and understandability, and has sometimes prevented their misinterpretation. I think it's a bad idea even to consider being interviewed about a study that hasn't yet survived external peer review.

TABLE 17–1 **Should You Return a Reporter's Call?**

1. Have your results and conclusions survived external peer review yet?
2. Might the top clinical journals reject your manuscript later if you give its details to a reporter sooner?
3. Are you sure that anybody needs to learn about your results by any route other than a peer-reviewed scientific journal?
4. If so, should this notification be left in the hands of a reporter you've never met, who may know very little about the subject, and is extremely unlikely to let you see a draft of his or her article?
5. Who should be the first target audience to learn about and apply your results?
6. What harm might be caused if others learned about the results first?
7. If you decide to return the calls, what strategies can you employ to protect the validity and appropriateness of your message?

2. *Might the top clinical journals reject your manuscript later if you give its details to a reporter sooner?* Most journals are quite specific about limiting the information you give to journalists. They do so for two reasons. First, they share our concern that peer review for validity and clinical application should precede general dissemination. Second, they are in competition with the other media for the "scoop" about your work. Here are the requirements posted on a couple of their Web sites.

The New England Journal of Medicine:
(*http://authors.nejm.org/Misc/Embargo.asp*)

Authors are expected to refrain from discussing their research with reporters prior to the Friday before publication.

The only exception is if an author presents research at a medical meeting. Responding to media inquiries at the meeting, or during the week following the meeting, will not jeopardize publication. We ask that authors follow these guidelines:

- Please do not discuss the fact that the research has been submitted or accepted for publication in the *New England Journal of Medicine.*
- Please do not distribute any copies of the manuscript, tables, or figures. (It is acceptable to use the materials in a presentation, but they should not be distributed.)

Meeting organizers may promote an author's presentation in a press release, plan a press conference, publish the abstract in a meeting proceedings, and/or post the presentation on their Web site. We ask that authors, their institutions, and other organizations sponsoring the research not do any further promotion of the presentation.

The British Medical Journal:
(*http://bmj.bmjjournals.com/advice/media_releases.shtml*)

We do not want material that is published in the BMJ appearing beforehand, in detail, in the mass media. If this happens doctors and patients may be presented with incomplete material that has not been peer reviewed, and this makes it hard for them to make up their own minds on the validity of the message. We accept that reports may appear in the media after presentations at scientific meetings.

   Those authors who wish us to publish their papers can clarify matters for journalists, but should not give the media any further information than was included in their scientific presentations.
Articles may be withdrawn from publication in the BMJ if given media coverage while under consideration or in press at the journal.

You should consider this question in deciding whether to return the reporter's call. And you shouldn't be overconfident that you can withstand their expert strategies for getting you to reveal more than you intended about your study (remember the quote from Janet Malcolm that opened this chapter?).

3. *Are you sure that anybody needs to learn about your results by any route other than a peer-reviewed scientific journal?* Putting this question another way: Would any humanly important purpose be achieved (beyond massaging your vanity) by granting an interview? If your answer is "yes," you should immediately ask the next question:

4. *Should this notification be left in the hands of a reporter you've never met, who may know very little about the subject, and is extremely unlikely to let you see a draft of his or her article?* This question forces you to identify both the target audience for your work and the message you want to give them. The latter issue is discussed in question seven. The former issue is crystallized in the next pair of questions.

5. *Who should be the first target audience to learn about and apply your results?* After the patients and clinicians in the study itself, the targets for most of our research are clinicians elsewhere (and, through them, their patients). However, some of our most important research has been targeted at health policy makers and the general public. For example, during one of the public reviews of the Canadian health care system, PJ Devereaux and his colleagues completed three studies showing that patients were more likely to die in for-profit hospitals (5,6) and dialysis centers (7) than in publicly funded ones. Although these results were published in a peer-reviewed medical journal, the primary target audience was the Canadian public, and those who were recommending changes in the organization and in the financing of health care in Canada. Accordingly, it was not only appropriate but also imperative to reach the public and the policy makers, neither of whom looked to clinical journals as primary sources of information.

As you'll learn in the subsequent text, these investigators had to both select the medium and control the message.

6. *What harm might be caused if others learned about the results first?* When the Women's Health Initiative trial concluded that the risks of postmenopausal estrogen-plus-progestin outweighed its benefits, the first target audience was the women in the trial, who were contacted individually. The next target audience was the thousands of clinicians who needed to understand the results so that they could present and discuss them with the millions of women who were taking these drugs. Plans were made to post the full paper on the journal's Web site so that clinicians could study it as soon as its results were announced by the sponsor; in the meantime, a media embargo was invoked. However, when one newspaper broke the embargo and published the results, other media followed suit (8). Physicians who hadn't yet seen the report were flooded with calls from frightened patients who had read about it in the newspapers or had seen it on the Web. Patients were harmed by having to live with frightening headlines until their physicians could examine the evidence and get back to them. I hope that you'll agree that this answer neither justifies paternalism nor denies patients' rights to know whatever they want to about their health. It simply tries to reduce the harm done to them if they don't have quick access to their own, informed health professionals who can help them appraise the message and decide whether and how to act on it.

This harm is increased when the message is misunderstood, misrepresented, or sensationalized by the media. Examples abound, and here are three. First, Megan MacDonald and Laurie Hoffman-Goetz examined 306 articles about cancer that had appeared in daily newspapers in Ontario, Canada (1). Only 40 of them (13%) even named the sources for their claims. When these 40 were compared with their sources, it was found that more than half of these articles presented erroneous information, omitted important results, and failed to report important qualifications to their results. Half of these articles had misleading titles, and approximately one fifth of them presented speculations as facts. Second, Jeanne Lenzer examined US print and electronic media following a prominent medical journal's publication of an RCT that compared radical prostatectomy with watchful waiting for prostate cancer (2). Although the primary article stated that there was "no significant difference between surgery and watchful waiting in terms of overall survival," she documented several media reports with titles or lead-ins stating, "Prostate removal saves lives." Third, these failures aren't restricted to the lay media. When 127 press releases prepared and distributed by seven major medical journals themselves were critically appraised, it was found that 77% of them exaggerated the results of the studies they were about to publish by failing to report important limitations in their conduct or interpretation (9). Moreover, the source of funding was admitted in only 22% of industry-funded studies.

You can follow the problems with medical reporting on a weekly basis through the UK National Electronic Library for Health's "Hitting the Headlines" feature (*http://www.nelh.nhs.uk/*). This service subjects news reports to a critical appraisal by Bandolier, a prominent UK evidence-based medicine synthesis and translation service.

7. *If you decide to return the calls, are there strategies that you can employ to protect the validity and appropriateness of your message?* The following applies both before and after your report has been published in a scientific journal.

Suppose that, despite all these warnings, you decide to return these calls. Before you do, I suggest that you write down *exactly* the message that you want the readers or listeners to carry away from the interview. You might even want to employ the "reporters' five W's." That is, summarize the application of your results in terms of *Who* should offer *What* to *Whom, When, Where,* and especially *Why.* For example, we summarized the Recent Recurrent Presumed Cerebral Emboli (RRPCE) trial as follows: Neurologists (*who*) should offer aspirin (*what*) to patients referred to them for transient ischemic attacks (*whom*) right away (*when*) in outpatient settings (*where*) because it will reduce their risk of stroke and death (*why*).

However, writing down your message is never enough. You have to protect it from being misunderstood, misrepresented, and sensationalized by the media. Table 17–2 lists some strategies that you can use to protect the validity and appropriateness of the message that gets broadcast.

First, I think it's vital to identify your conflicts of interest (or their absence) to your interviewer before you go on the record and early in the interview. Regardless of how well you protect your study from its sponsors, your message can be lost (along with your reputation) if the interviewer

TABLE 17–2 Strategies for Preserving the Validity and Appropriateness of Your Study Results in the Media

Medium	Strategies
Print	Write (or coauthor) it yourself.
	Work only with reporters with excellent track records.
	Agree only if they commit to sending you a draft for corrections of fact.
Electronic	Only agree to "live" interviews that they cannot edit.
Both	Admit, at the outset, any real or potential conflicts of interest.
	Decide beforehand what message(s) you want to get across.
	Answer every question they pose by ignoring its content and responding with your messages.
	Never agree totally with any proposition or summary statement they offer.

uncovers the fact that your study was funded by big pharma only at the end of the interview.

If you want to maximize the likelihood that readers take home your message, write it yourself and send it to the media as a press release. Alternatively, contact a reporter whose work you admire and offer to co-author the lay report. If you can't do either of these, tell the reporter that you'll consent to interview only if they promise (and you believe them) to send you a draft to confirm that they have their facts straight. When I described how I had successfully done this at a Society for Clinical Trials reporter's workshop, the media stars on the panel became enraged and insisted that no competent, self-respecting reporter would ever let an interviewee see their drafts. Their unwillingness to bother to see whether they had their facts straight solidified my admonition about them: "Never return reporters' calls." Following the session, several other trialists sought me out to say that they had successfully applied this conditional strategy.

When I directed the Center for Evidence-Based Medicine at Oxford, radio and television producers frequently called me requesting interviews. Often, they wanted my reactions to the latest news release claiming that a treatment was a "breakthrough" or a "killer." Wary of being edited, and especially concerned about being reduced to trivial "sound bites," I agreed only if the interviews were to be conducted "live," by the hosts of the relevant programs. This precondition was almost always accepted, and as far as I know, no silly "sound bites" were broadcast.

The key strategy to consider during both print and electronic interviews is to direct your responses to the key elements of the message you want to transmit and not to the questions being thrown at you. If a question matches your message, you can respond directly to it. If it doesn't, I suggest that you ignore it and introduce the next element of your message with phrases such as: "What we'd like your listeners to know about our study is ... " or "The really important thing we found in this study is ... " Surprisingly, perhaps, I've never been interrupted or criticized when I employ this strategy.

I close with an admonition from Charles Barkley, a very outspoken professional basketball player who frequently provided provocative sound bites for the viewers of North American television: "The one thing you have to know about reporters is that they're not your friends." (10)

ADDITIONAL POINTS OF VIEW

Brian Haynes' 2 cents worth

Two "learning experiences" with the media come to mind. Early on in my career, a reporter interviewed me by phone and sent a photographer to get a picture. The photographer took various poses, most of them sensible and dignified as befit my status as a young assistant professor, but one with me aping the camera with the head of my stethoscope above my forehead, taken through a fish lens. I specifically told the reporter not to use that one, which he promised not to do. My good mentor, Dave Sackett, posted the resulting ridiculous picture that accompanied the journal article, over my office door. No doubt, the picture attracted a few curious readers to the piece (which itself was passably written), which I came to understand as the media's prerogative and main goal. In retrospect, it was probably worth the transient humiliation for me. I learned a lesson, consistent with Dave's dictums earlier in this chapter.

The second experience was more aggravating because, by then, I felt that I was doing a reasonable job of getting my message across. I was interviewed live by a well-respected television journalist about the research that I had been involved in, about low patient adherence to medications. The main messages I wished to leave were that it is a serious problem, that there are many reasons for it, and that these reasons did not have anything much to do with the popular notion that patients were themselves the problem, through low intelligence or education or lack of grace or whatever. Exactly as the program was winding up, the interviewer ended with his own pet theory about the reason for low compliance, implying that noncompliers were uneducated or just plain stupid. I had no chance for rebuttal.

To me, talking with the media is like dancing with the devil. We may think we can do it (and are seduced by reporters to think so), but they have and use the last word to their own notion of advantage, which has a lot more to do with titillating their audience and meeting their (admittedly unrelenting) deadlines than it has to do with providing accurate and balanced reporting of our research.

Peter Tugwell

My experiences have been both good and bad. Journalists call more frequently following publication of individual studies than systematic reviews, but the interviews associated with individual study publication have allowed me to emphasize the importance of systematic reviews and of placing the results of the single study in the overall context of the literature on all the studies.

As described in Chapter 10, Assessing Claims of Causation, during my tenure on the US Federal Science Panel on silicone breast implants, the attention of the press was unnerving at times. For example, lawyers for the plaintiffs orchestrated *ad hominem* attacks in the United States national press following the disclosure of our preliminary conclusions that there was no evidence of silicone breast implants causing scleroderma or rheumatoid arthritis. Immediately following these press reports, my wife received calls from three major US morning television shows competing for my appearance. One of them laid out the dire consequences to my reputation if I did not agree to appear on the show to face a panel of women with arthritis and scleroderma post–breast implant. Fortunately, the federal judge ruled that I and my colleagues on the panel were not to appear—and it played out satisfactorily as described in Chapter 10.

We now provide a point–counterpoint e-mail discussion between the most pessimistic (Dave Sackett) and the most optimistic (Gordon Guyatt) authors of our team.

Gordon

My experience with the media, it seems, is far more positive. Personally, I see us having an important educator role with journalists from all media.

Some of what you are saying, Dave, seems to assume that if you don't talk to them, nothing will appear. It seems to me that one needs to distinguish among a number of situations:

1. If you don't talk to them, media folk will ignore your report.
2. If you don't talk to them, media folk will report on your work, and likely do a good job of reporting.
3. If you don't talk to them, media folk will report your work, and at least some are likely to make substantial errors or misrepresentations.

I think the issues differ in these three situations, and it seems difficult to me to approach the problem without distinguishing up front between these.

Dave

The problem is, I think all three happen with every trial report: some reporters ignore it, a small fraction report it accurately, and many report it wrongly. The first two are no trouble (although the second can use press releases that you make yourself or write with them). It's the 3rd group that I refuse to assist by returning their calls.

Gordon

My experience suggests that however wrong they might get it if you talk to them, they get it more wrong if you don't. I believe that we convert a substantial number. Furthermore, there is an education function that goes on.

Another point is that seldom, if ever, do reports come out worse as a result of talking with the journalist. The worst that happens is that one gets nowhere (and suffers the attendant frustration). But for me, that's been unusual.

The third group, those who without talking to the investigator, are destined to write misleading or inaccurate reports, are in fact two subgroups. One are those who are destined to write misleading and inaccurate reports whether they talk to you or not. The second are those who, once they talk to you, will write an accurate report. In advance, one doesn't know which is which (and in the end, it might be difficult to distinguish the second subgroup from those destined to write accurate reports even if they hadn't talked to you). Of course, it's a continuum (they might have been destined to write a very misleading report, but after conversation write only a mildly misleading report) (or they might have been destined to write a good report, but end up with an excellent one—that's unusual, I must admit) but I'm sure you get the idea. I think it's worth trying to move them in the direction of enlightenment, and my sense is substantial proportions do in fact move.

SEEKING OUT THE MEDIA WHEN YOU NEED THEM

We end with an example, based on the experience of Gordon Guyatt and his colleagues, of what to do if the public is a crucial part of your target audience.

PJ Devereaux and I (along with a large team of coworkers) have done a series of systematic reviews that have documented increased death rates in private for-profit hospitals and dialysis centers, and increased charges in hospitals, relative to private not-for-profit hospitals and dialysis centers. We published our results in peer-reviewed medical journals read mainly by physicians, but our primary target audiences included the general public, politicians, health policy analysts, and health policy makers. These audiences (and indeed the physicians who were also part of our target audience as well) were far more likely to hear about and attend to our results if they were prominently reported in newspapers, television, radio, and the Internet.

If you are in our situation, and media coverage is crucial to meeting your goals of research dissemination, how should you proceed? Although by no means absolutely necessary, if you have the money to hire a company that specializes in helping with dissemination, their help will certainly be useful. A charitable foundation funded our reviews, and our budgets included costs associated with dissemination of the order of $5,000 each.

The company can help you with a number of aspects of dissemination. With or without their help, however, you will need to do the following:

1. *Prepare a press release.* Suggestions for constructing such a release are as follows:

    a. Choose a short, strongly declarative title ("Patients more likely to die in private for-profit dialysis centers, major study finds")

b. The first sentence should state the essential message in as dramatic terms as you can manage [If Canada switched to for-profit dialysis centers, approximately 150 additional dialysis patients would die each year, according to a major study to be published in the Journal of the American Medical Association (*JAMA*) tomorrow.]

c. State the most important findings first in a brief one or two sentence paragraphs. Leave background until the end. If you want examples of this general approach, read any well-written newspaper article in a major paper.

d. Early on, provide brief, punchy quotes that you would be happy to have the journalists use directly. ("In both hospital and outpatient settings the profit motive drives up death rates," said PJ Devereaux, lead author of the study.)

e. Provide slightly more expansive explanatory quotes later. ("The reason more patients are dying in for-profit facilities is that administrators must spend 10% to 15% of all expenses satisfying shareholders and paying taxes," said PJ Devereaux. "For-profit providers cut corners to ensure shareholders achieve their expected returns on investment.")

f. Keep it very short; no longer than, say, 350 words.

g. End with another punchy quote. The implications of your research might be a good topic for the finale. ("Our results should raise serious concerns about moves to private for-profit care, whether in hospitals, day surgeries, or other outpatient facilities. It is time to base health care policy on evidence, not ideology.")

2. *Prepare a "backgrounder."* This longer piece can be more expansive, and less constrained in terms of structure and presentation. Here is your chance to educate the journalists, providing them with the information they need to really understand your work. It must still be short (certainly less than 900 words), and you must attend to all the issues we've raised in Chapter 16 on writing well (short sentences and paragraphs; relatively simple language; lots of declarative statements; no unnecessary words; everything in active voice). Show your backgrounder to friends outside the profession who know nothing about your research, and see how they react. Their feedback may help you improve your backgrounder.

3. *Look to the journal to help you.* Most journals love publicity. Make sure the editor knows that you are looking to publicize the piece widely. If you want to keep the journal on your side, also make sure that the media know about the journal embargo. When the *BMJ* chose one of our systematic reviews as its article of the week for the media, the lead author was besieged by a 2-day barrage of media calls (11).

4. *Contact key media people a week or two before the release date.* A phone call to the people whom you would most like to run the story is crucial to successful dissemination. Just a couple of "hits" in key places and you have won the battle. The most relevant reporters in the key newspapers, people responsible for the content of the evening news and commentaries, and the relevant journalists associated with the wire services are all key individuals. Once the story runs on, say, the most respected newspaper in your jurisdiction, or a national wire service, you can be certain of broad coverage. Prior conversation with the key people make this sort of coverage far more likely.

5. *Get help from your hospital or university public relations department.* This is a hit-or-miss exercise. Some PR folk are brilliant, others much less so. The PR department may love your story and push it hard, or may ignore it. It is certainly a mistake to place primary reliance on a local PR department, unless you already know that they are superb and you get the sense that they are deeply committed to your story.

6. *Use media lists for wide dissemination of your press release.* For a few hundred dollars, you can have your press release brought to the attention of a wide range of journalists who, once they know about your story, may well pick it up.

7. *When it comes to the interviews, be well prepared (Dave has already provided you with tips for this stage).* Ideally, your point person(s) for interview will be young, photogenic, articulate, quick on their feet in terms of handling difficult questions, and confident with the media. PJ Devereaux, who led these reviews, conducted brilliant interviews that greatly helped get the message out clearly and succinctly. This likely describes you as well, but if another member of the team fits the description better, that may be the person to front up for the cameras.

The strategies mentioned in the preceding text have served us extremely well. We obtained high-profile national television, radio, newspaper, and international interned coverage for each of our three reviews. Yes, it was a lot of work to achieve this goal, but well worth it.

REFERENCES

1. MacDonald MM, Hoffman-Goetz L. A retrospective study of the accuracy of cancer information in Ontario daily newspapers. *Can J Public Health* 2002;93:142–145.

2. Lenzer J. The operation was a success (but the patients died); how media spin distorted the outcomes of a study comparing radical prostatectomy with watchful waiting. *BMJ* 2002;325:664.

3. Editorial: A health scare in the mass media. *Lancet* 2002;359:1079.

4. Sackett DL, Oxman AD. HARLOT plc: an amalgamation of the world's two oldest professions. *BMJ* 2003;327:1442–1445.

5. Devereaux PJ, Choi PT, Lacchetti C, et al. A systematic review and meta-analysis of studies comparing mortality rates of private for-profit and private not-for-profit hospitals. *CMAJ* 2002;166(11):1399–1406.

6. Devereaux PJ, Heels-Ansdell D, Lacchetti C, et al. Payments for care at private for-profit and private not-for-profit hospitals: a systematic review and meta-analysis. *Can Med Assoc J* 2004;170(12):1817–1824.

7. Devereaux PJ, Schunemann HJ, Ravindran N, et al. Comparison of mortality between private for-profit and private not-for-profit hemodialysis centers: a systematic review and meta-analysis. *JAMA* 2002;288(19):2449–2457.

8. Fontanarosa PB, DeAngelis CD. The importance of journal embargo. *JAMA* 2002;288: 748–750.

9. Woloshin S, Schwartz LM. Press releases: translating research into news. *JAMA* 2002; 287(21):2856–2858.

10. Fish S. Stop the Presses. The Chronicle of Higher Education, 24 May 2002. *http:// chronicle.com/jobs/2002/05/2002052401c.htm.* Accessed of June, 2005.

11. DiCenso A, Guyatt GH, Willan A, et al. Interventions to reduce unintended pregnancies among adolescents: systematic review of randomised controlled trials. *BMJ* 2002;324: 1426–1430.

INDEX